Menopause: Clinical Aspects

Menopause: Clinical Aspects

Editor: Fiona Browning

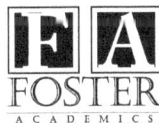

FA
FOSTER
ACADEMICS

www.fosteracademics.com

www.fosteracademics.com

FA FOSTER ACADEMICS

Cataloging-in-Publication Data

Menopause : clinical aspects / edited by Fiona Browning.
  p. cm.
Includes bibliographical references and index.
ISBN 978-1-63242-667-3
1. Menopause. 2. Climacteric. 3. Clinical medicine. I. Browning, Fiona.
RG186 .M46 2019
618.175--dc23

Foster Academics,
118-35 Queens Blvd., Suite 400,
Forest Hills, NY 11375, USA

ISBN 978-1-63242-667-3 (Hardback)

Contents

Preface

The world is advancing at a fast pace like never before. Therefore, the need is to keep up with the latest developments. This book was an idea that came to fruition when the specialists in the area realized the need to coordinate together and document essential themes in the subject. That's when I was requested to be the editor. Editing this book has been an honour as it brings together diverse authors researching on different streams of the field. The book collates essential materials contributed by veterans in the area which can be utilized by students and researchers alike.

Menopause is that period in a woman's life when menstrual periods stop permanently and she becomes incapable of bearing children. It typically occurs between the ages of 49 and 52 years. This period is said to begin when vaginal bleeding stops for more than a year. During this time, there arises a decrease in the hormone production by the ovaries. In the years preceding menopause, women may experience hot flashes, vaginal dryness, emotional changes and sleeping difficulties. It may also occur in women who have undergone chemotherapy or removal of the ovaries. Therapies involving menopausal hormone therapy, selective serotonin reuptake inhibitors and clonidine may be recommended for relieving symptoms. This book is compiled in such a manner, that it will provide in-depth knowledge about the physiological, biological and emotional aspects of menopause. The aim of this book is to present researches that have advanced the understanding of menopause and its implications in a woman's life. The readers would gain knowledge that would broaden their perspective about menopause.

Each chapter is a sole-standing publication that reflects each author´s interpretation. Thus, the book displays a multi-facetted picture of our current understanding of application, resources and aspects of the field. I would like to thank the contributors of this book and my family for their endless support.

Editor

The Passo Fundo Cohort Study: design of a population-based observational study of women in premenopause, menopausal transition, and postmenopause

Karen Oppermann[1,2], Verônica Colpani[3], Sandra C. Fuchs[4] and Poli Mara Spritzer[3,5*]

Abstract

Background: The Passo Fundo Cohort Study (PFS) is a population-based longitudinal observational study of pre-, peri-, and postmenopausal women that has been ongoing since 1995 in Passo Fundo, a city in southern Brazil. This paper describes the rationale and design of the PFS and summarizes objectives and procedures that have been updated during follow-up.

Methods/Design: Women in the PFS have been followed for a variety of diseases that are frequent in menopause. Sampling was conducted in 154 randomly selected census divisions (geographical subdivisions of the city as defined by the Brazilian Institute of Geography and Statistics). One block in each census division was chosen by lot and two women were randomly selected for interview in each block. The first cycle, conducted between 1995 and 1997, included a representative sample of 298 women aged 35 to 55 years. In the second cycle, conducted between 2001 and 2002, additional participants were enrolled based on the same sampling strategy used in 1995, for a final sample of 358 women. In 2010, a third follow-up was initiated, when all 358 participants or their relatives were located. Participants completed a standardized questionnaire on demographic and socioeconomic characteristics. They also answered questions about lifestyle, medical and reproductive characteristics, sexual life, hormone therapy and mental aspects by using validated instruments. Physical activity was assessed and anthropometric measurements, blood sampling and pelvic ultrasound examination were performed. In the third cycle, bone mineral density by dual-energy X-ray absorptiometry and abdominal fat and coronary artery calcium score by computed tomography were also determined.

Discussion: The study findings provide relevant information to evaluate the association between menopausal status, female aging and the risk of cardiovascular diseases, and bone health aspects in a representative sample of women from southern Brazil.

Keywords: Menopause, Cohort studies, Central adiposity, Cardiovascular risk factors, Cardiovascular events, Ovarian volume, Coronary artery calcium, Bone mineral density

* Correspondence: spritzer@ufrgs.br
[3]Gynecological Endocrinology Unit, Division of Endocrinology, Hospital de Clinicas de Porto Alegre, Porto Alegre, RS, Brazil
[5]Department of Physiology, Federal University of Rio Grande do Sul, Porto Alegre, RS, Brazil
Full list of author information is available at the end of the article

Background

Improvements in health care and sanitation have reduced mortality from infectious diseases in developing countries. As a consequence, non-communicable diseases, such as diabetes and cardiovascular disease, are now the leading cause of morbidity and mortality worldwide, with a huge impact on health and society [1, 2]. In Brazil, an upper-middle-income country, only a few observational studies have examined non-communicable diseases, especially regarding women's health [3]. In this respect, the Passo Fundo Cohort Study (PFS) has been conducted for nearly 15 years, investigating pre-, peri-, and postmenopausal women. This paper describes the rationale and design of the PFS and summarizes objectives and procedures that have been updated during follow-up.

The main objective of the first cycle of the PFS was to investigate the prevalence of climacteric symptoms and their association with transvaginal sonographic features and hormone levels in pre- and perimenopausal women. It also investigated lifestyle habits, socioeconomic status, sexual activity, menstrual complaints, and hormone therapy in this population.

In the second cycle, the main goal of the study was to investigate the association of obesity, central adiposity, and ovarian volume with menopausal status, taking into account several confounding factors. In addition, the relationship between physical, psychological, and menopause-related symptoms and minor psychiatric disorders was also studied.

In the third cycle, the objective was to assess cardiovascular risk among pre-, peri-, and postmenopausal women through habitual physical activity, coronary artery calcium, abdominal fat and anthropometric measurements.

Regarding the cohort design, the aim was to assess clinical, hormonal, and metabolic features and bone mass in these women over time in relation to cardiovascular risk and prediction of cardiovascular events.

Methods/design
The design of the Passo Fundo Cohort Study (PFS)

The PFS is a prospective cohort study conducted in Passo Fundo, a city in southern Brazil. The sample consists of women in pre-, peri-, and postmenopause. Figure 1 shows a flow chart of the three cycles of the study.

First cycle

From January 1996 to February 1997, participants were recruited for the study. The sample for the first study was selected from the 16,958 women between 35 and 55 years of age living in Passo Fundo according to the 1991 census. Women with an intact uterus and at least one period in the previous 12 months were invited to participate. Sampling was conducted in two stages. First, 154 geographical subdivisions of the city, defined by the Brazilian Institute of Geography and Statistics [4] as census divisions, were randomly selected. One block in each census division was chosen by lot and two women were randomly selected for interview in each block according to the

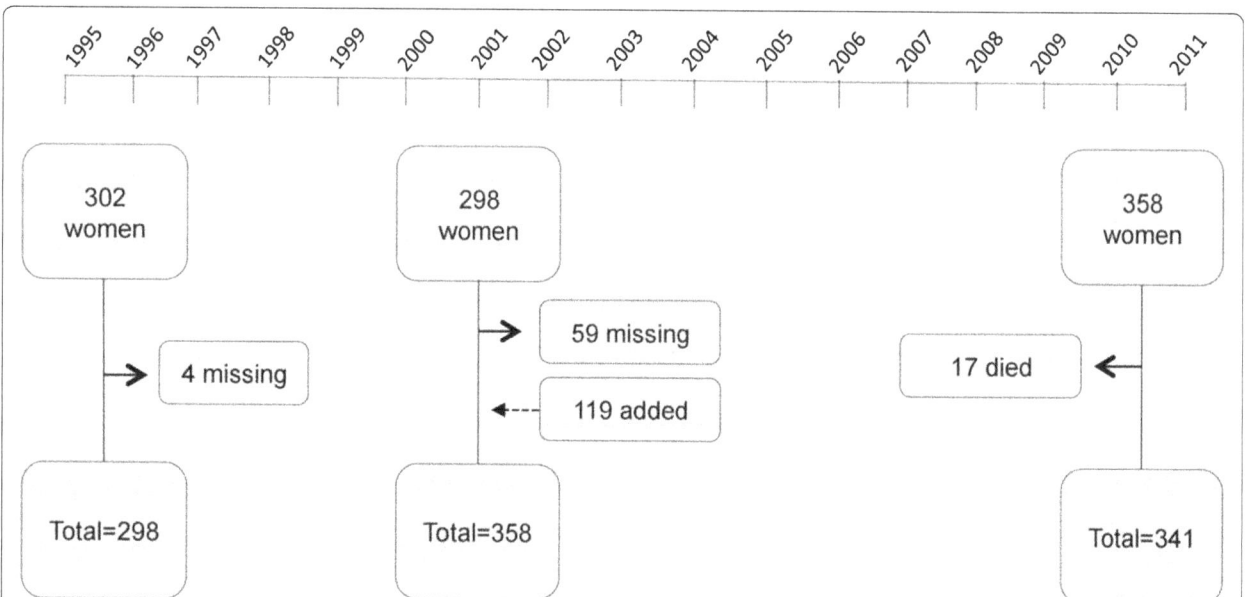

Fig. 1 Cycles of the Passo Fundo Cohort Study (PFS). Year 1995–1996 (first cycle): baseline assessment of the original cohort. Year 2001–2002 (second cycle): baseline reassessment and cohort expansion to include 119 additional women aged 35-62 years. Year 2010–2011 (third cycle): first reassessment of women from the second cycle. Continuous arrows indicate missing or dead/deceased women. Dotted arrow indicates added women. Modified from Colpani et al. 2014 [33]

following procedures: in all blocks, each corner was classified as A, B, C, or D, following the same order from left to right and from bottom to top. To start the interviews, one block was chosen per census division, and one corner per block. Two women were then interviewed in each block. When the drawn corner was A or B, the first woman interviewed was chosen for blood sampling and ultrasound examination; when the drawn corner was C or D, the second woman interviewed was chosen for examination. From the selected corner, the block was investigated in a clockwise direction until an eligible participant was found. Once found, the two nearby houses were excluded, and the third one was screened. If there was more than one eligible woman per household, the one with the most recent birthday was selected for the interview. If the potential participant was not at home, the interviewers returned to the household on another day to interview her. If the selected household was a building, only one interview was performed; the floor and apartment for the interview were also randomly selected. A loss was considered to have occurred when women refused to participate in the study or to undergo ultrasound examination after three attempts by the interviewer. A sample of 302 women aged 35 to 55 years who had had at least one period in the previous 12 months was randomly selected. At the end of the first cycle (1995–1996), a representative sample of 298 women was interviewed (response rate 83.2 %).

Second cycle

A second home visit was conducted between July 2001 and July 2002, when 239 women of the baseline cohort were located and interviewed [5, 6]. The investigators searched for information about first cycle participants with neighbors, in electricity and water company databases, in medical records at Hospital São Vicente de Paulo, and at the Passo Fundo University, the municipal health department, and the Health Information Center (NIS/RS-SES). The retention percent was 80.2 %. Losses were classified as follows: unwilling to participate (19 = 6.37 %), not found (21 = 7 %), moved out of the city (15 = 5 %), and died (4 = 1.3 %).

In view of potential losses to follow-up and considering an increase in population size, 120 additional women aged 35 to 62 years were randomly selected to ensure sufficient statistical power for analysis. Of these, 119 were interviewed (participation percent 99 %, final total sample of 358 participants). The new participants were randomly selected based on the 175 census divisions defined in the 2000 IBGE census. Sixty new census divisions were chosen by lot and one block was chosen per division, following the same randomization procedures used in the first cycle. Eligibility did not include menstrual criteria for this additional sample of women, since some women from the first cycle had already reached postmenopausal status.

Third cycle

In 2010, a third follow-up was initiated in order to assess cardiovascular outcomes [7]. Every effort was made to locate each participant of the previous cycle. For that, contact was made with close relatives, neighbors, and neighboring households; in addition, we reviewed inpatient and outpatient records at Hospital São Vicente and University of Passo Fundo, municipal department of health records in search of women registered to receive medication through the public health system SUS, the city dental registry and the city death records. We also ran an advertisement campaign on two radio stations, Planalto and Uirapuru, reaching 60 municipalities and around 30 thousand listeners per day, and two television stations, RBS TV Passo Fundo and UPF TV, reaching 85 municipalities. All 358 participants or their relatives were located and information on the participant's vital status was obtained for the period ending in November 2011.

Setting

Passo Fundo is a city located in Rio Grande do Sul, the southernmost state of Brazil. The city has a current population of approximately 184 000 inhabitants (data from the 2010 IBGE census) [8]. The economy is based primarily on agriculture and business [8].

Population

The representative sample included in the PFS consists of pre-, peri-, and postmenopausal women living in the urban area of Passo Fundo, although, in the beginning of the study, the sample was composed only of pre- and perimenopausal women. Menopausal status was determined based on the characteristics of menses or time since amenorrhea: premenopause was defined as no change in menstrual frequency or flow, and perimenopause was defined as changes in menstrual frequency or flow in the 12 months before the study; and postmenopause was defined as 12 or more months of amenorrhea occurring naturally or because of surgical intervention, such as bilateral oophorectomy. Questions such as "when was your last period?", "how is your menstrual flow?" and " have you ever been submitted to gynecological surgery (in which organ)?" were asked. A "hysterectomy" category was created for women who had previously undergone hysterectomy without bilateral oophorectomy and whose menopausal status could not be classified.

Eligibility criteria

The PFS was designed as a longitudinal study in order to analyze pre-, peri-, and postmenopausal women. Initially, eligible participants were women aged 35 to 55 years who had at least one menstrual cycle in the past 12 months and who were living in the urban area of Passo Fundo, Brazil.

Exclusion criteria

Women who had undergone bilateral oophorectomy and/or hysterectomy were excluded from the study. An eligible participant was considered a loss if she refused to participate in the study after three attempts of having her accept participation.

Sample size

In the first cycle, the sample size was based on a population of 16,958 women between 35 and 55 years of age. The sample size for prevalence studies was calculated based on the assumption that 20 % of premenopausal and perimenopausal women would have climacteric symptoms, with a 15 % error and 95 % CI. The sample size was increased by an additional 10 % to account for potential missing data, for a targeted sample size of 318 women.

For the second cycle, the sample size was estimated based on population growth for year 2000. The estimated population growth was 2.03 % per year between 1991-1996, and 1.88 % per year between 1996 and 2000. Therefore, the growth in this period was 17.7 %. Based on this information, 54 women were randomly selected. Sixty-six additional women were selected to cover potential follow-up losses. The power of the study was thus maintained.

Ethical considerations

The PFS was approved by the institutional review board of both Passo Fundo University and Hospital de Clínicas de Porto Alegre. Written informed consent was obtained from each participant. During data collection, care was taken to ensure confidentiality of participants' information.

Methods

A standardized questionnaire covering demographic characteristics (age and self-reported skin color), education, medical history, family history, reproductive history, sexual activity (in the last three months), lifestyle/behavioral factors, quality of life, medication/supplement inventory, climacteric symptoms, and hormone therapy was applied. More details regarding which items were included in each cycle are shown in Table 1. In the first and second cycles, participants were interviewed at home and examinations were performed at Hospital São Vicente de Paulo. In the third cycle, all measurements and interviews were conducted at the hospital.

Training

Field training of students and health care professionals was conducted by the PFS coordinators according to the study protocol (interviewer guide). Intra and inter observer reliability was determined. All participants were thoroughly examined at baseline.

A pilot study was conducted in July 1995. The main objective of this pilot study was to test the agreement between ultrasound operators; additional objectives were to probe the participants' understanding of questions and to monitor adherence to hospital visits for collection of blood samples and ultrasound examination. Fifty-six premenopausal women were randomly enrolled from 14 census divisions. Two women were excluded due to total hysterectomy and bilateral oophorectomy. During the pilot study, pelvic ultrasound was performed by two examiners, resulting in 83 % agreement between them. Interviews were tested for reliability and reproducibility. Interobserver reliability for anthropometric and blood pressure measurements was also verified by repeated measurements during the first set of consultations (R values were higher than 0.90, $p < 0.05$).

Study variables
Education

Educational attainment was assessed through the number of years of successful formal education, described as years at school.

Socioeconomic status

Socioeconomic status was assessed using an instrument developed by the Brazilian Association of Market Research Institutes (Associação Brasileira de Institutos de Pesquisa de Mercado, ABIPEME) [9]. It classifies individuals into five socioeconomic groups: A, B, C, D, and E, where A represents the highest socioeconomic level. This classification is based on 10 selected variables: level of education of the household head, number of cars, having a washing machine and videotape recorder, having a vacuum cleaner, having a refrigerator, number of color televisions, number of bathrooms, number of radios, and being able to pay a housekeeper. The participants were classified as working or not working, and by employment status (employer, employee, self-employed, housemaker).

Alcohol intake

From the second cycle onward, alcohol consumption was determined by self-reported alcohol intake (non-drinker or former drinker). In 2001 and 2010, participants were asked what type of alcohol (wine, beer, spirits) they consumed and frequency of consumption.

Smoking

Smoking status was also assessed from the second cycle onward. Participants were considered smokers if they smoked more than five cigarettes per day [10]. Subsequently, in 2010, the amount of smoking and age at smoking onset and cessation were assessed in detail using a self-administered questionnaire. Former smokers were defined as individuals who reported having quit smoking and, in this case, they were also asked how long it had been since they quit smoking. No minimum time

The Passo Fundo Cohort Study: design of a population-based observational study of women in premenopause...

5

Table 1 Questionnaires and clinical information assessed in the PFS

Variable	Method	Cycle (year)
Clinical and demographic characteristics	Self-report	1995/2001/2010
Physical activity		
	Self-report	1995
	Modifiable Activity Questionnaire (MAQ) [19]	2001
	International Physical Activity Questionnaire (IPAQ) [22]	2010
	Pedometer	2010
Quality of life		
	Women's Health Questionnaire (WHQ) [12]	2010
	12-Item Health Survey (SF-12) [14]	2010
Menopausal symptoms		
	Kupperman Menopausal Index [11]	1995/2001/2010
Psychiatric disorders		
	20-Item Self-Reporting Questionnaire (SRQ-20) [17]	2001/2010
Blood samples		
	Hormones	1995/2001/2010
	Cholesterol (mg/dL) (mmol/L)	2001/2010
	Triglycerides (mg/dL) (mmol/L)	2001/2010
	Glucose (mg/dL) (mmol/L)	2001/2010
	Insulin (mU/L)	2001/2010
	DNA samples	2010
Anthropometric measurements		
	Body mass index	1995/2001/2010
	Waist circumference	2001/2010
	Waist-to-hip ratio	2001/2010
Skinfolds	Calipers	2001
Diagnostic imaging		
	Pelvic Ultrasound	1995/2001
	Densitometry	2010
	Computed tomography	2010

since smoking cessation was employed in the definition of former smokers. Because there was no specific question on occasional smoking, occasional smokers were grouped as current or former smokers if they met the aforementioned criteria.

Gynecological data

Women were asked questions about age at menarche, delivery history (vaginal delivery, cesarean delivery, miscarriage), previous gynecological surgery, and sexual activity (in the last three months). Use of oral contraceptive, hormone therapy, estrogen, estrogen plus progestin or tibolone was verified by asking the participants to show the medication box or the physician's prescription and categorized according to duration (in years) of use.

Menopausal symptoms

The Kupperman Menopausal Index was used to evaluate menopausal symptoms [11]. It is a numerical index that ranks menopausal symptoms based on the sum of scores attributed to variables according to the presence and intensity of symptoms. Scores range from 0 to 3, where 0 = absent, 1 = mild, 2 = moderate, and 3 = intense symptoms. Weighted values were assigned to the variables, as follows: hot flashes (4), night sweats (4), vaginal dryness (3), insomnia (2), memory (2), nervousness (2), depression (1), dizziness (1), fatigue (1), and headache (1).

Clinical history
Blood draw

At baseline, blood was collected from a subsample of 140 women. Blood samples were collected on the same day of the ultrasound examination, between 4 and 6 PM. The day of the reproductive cycle was recorded on this occasion; therefore, tests were performed on any day of the menstrual cycle. In the second and third study cycles, blood samples were collected from all participants between 8 and 10 AM after an overnight fast of 10 to 12 h. In the third study cycle (2010), blood was also drawn and stored at –80 °C for future hormone studies, and DNA was extracted from blood samples and stored for future genetic and molecular analysis.

Blood pressure measurements

Standardized blood pressure measurements were performed twice, using the same calibrated mercury manometer. The average of two assessments was used in the analysis. Hypertension was identified by systolic blood pressure greater than or equal to 140 mm Hg or diastolic blood pressure greater than or equal to 90 mm Hg.

Hypertension

At baseline, hypertension was assessed by asking about previous diagnosis of hypertension and measuring blood pressure during the home interview. In the second and third cycles, the question about previous diagnosis was asked again and blood pressure was measured at the clinic. Family history of hypertension (parents and grandparents) was investigated from the second cycle (2001) onward.

Dyslipidemia

In the three cycles, self-reported hypercholesterolemia and use of anti-cholesterol drugs were used to define dyslipidemia. Blood tests were also performed to measure cholesterol and triglycerides levels.

Diabetes

Diabetes was determined by self-report, use of antidiabetic drugs, or a fasting blood glucose level of 126 mg/dL or higher. Metabolic syndrome was defined as the presence of at least three of the following components: waist circumference greater than 88 cm, HDL-c level less than 50 mg/dL, TG level of 150 mg/dL or higher, blood pressure greater than or equal to 130/85 mmHg, and glucose level of 100 mg/dL or higher.

Quality of life

Quality of life was assessed in the third cycle (2010) using the Women's Health Questionnaire (WHQ) [12]. The WHQ consists of 36 items divided into nine domains: depressed mood, somatic symptoms, memory/concentration, anxiety/fears, sexual behavior, vasomotor symptoms, sleep problems, menstrual symptoms, and attractiveness. A score of 0 (zero) indicates good health status, a score of 50 % indicates regular health status, a score between 50 and 100 % indicates low health status, and a score of 100 % indicates poor health status.

The 12-Item Short Form Health Survey (SF-12), a shortened validated version of the 36-Item Short Form Health Survey (SF-36), was also used as a tool to assess quality of life in this population. It is a generic questionnaire, and scores also range from 0 to 100 %. The SF-12 is derived from the functional health and well-being domain of the SF-36 (physical functioning, role limitations due to physical health problems, bodily pain, general health, vitality, social functioning, role limitations due to emotional problems, and mental health) [13, 14].

Psychiatric disorders

From the second cycle onward, the use of medications for insomnia, anxiety, and depression was investigated. In the three cycles, psychiatric disorders were assessed using the 20-Item Self-Reporting Questionnaire (SRQ-20). The SRQ-20 was developed by the World Health Organization to screen for common mental disorders in primary health care settings, and a version of this instrument has been validated for use in Brazil. The questionnaire consists of questions with yes/no answers about symptoms such as sadness, irritability, headache, pleasure in daily activities, crying frequently, decision-making, appetite, sleep disturbance, lack of concentration, sense of usefulness, and fatigue. It is used to screen for minor psychiatric disorders, and a score of 8 or higher indicates a risk of psychiatric disorders [15–17].

Physical activity

From the second cycle onward, physical activity was assessed using structured questionnaires. In the second cycle (2001), physical activity was assessed using a previously tested, standardized questionnaire for each type of physical activity, the Modifiable Activity Questionnaire (MAQ), and metabolic equivalents and total caloric expenditure were calculated [18]. Participants were asked about the type and frequency of the activity performed and time spent standing and sitting. The practice of sports after 18 years of age and in the last year was also evaluated by collecting information on the frequency and duration (in minutes) of each activity. Participants who reached an energy expenditure of at least 1000 kcal/week (approximately 3.5 h per week in activities such as walking, climbing stairs, swimming, playing sports, and yard work) were considered physically active, while all others were classified as physically inactive [19, 20].

In the third cycle (2010), the International Physical Activity Questionnaire (IPAQ) was used. This instrument was developed to facilitate the cross-national assessment of physical activity and inactivity. The short-form questionnaire (IPAQ-SF) was used to evaluate self-reported physical activity at four intensity levels (vigorous-intensity activity, moderate-intensity activity, walking, and sitting) over the last seven days [21, 22].

Pedometer

In the third cycle (2010), habitual physical activity was assessed using a digital pedometer (BP 148; TechLine, São Paulo, SP, Brazil) [7]. The instrument records the number of steps taken per day for seven days. The mean number of steps was calculated by the ratio between the sum of the daily totals and the number of days the pedometer was used [23]. The device was individually configured according to the participant's weight (kg) and average step length (distance between the heels in cm). Each participant was given a pedometer and instructed on how to properly use the device. Participants were also provided with a step-recording diary, where they were asked to record the total daily number of steps and the time they put on (wake-up time) and took off (before going to bed) the pedometer. Participants were also instructed to go about their usual activities and to remove the pedometer while showering or sleeping and at the end of each day.

Anthropometric measurements

At baseline, weight and height measurements were performed on the same day as blood collection and/or ultrasound examination. Measurements were taken without shoes and heavy clothing. Weight was measured using a mechanical scale (Filizola®, Brazil) and height was measured using a stadiometer coupled to the scale.

In the second and third cycles, anthropometric measurements were performed in duplicate and included body weight, height, waist circumference (measured at the midpoint between the lower rib margin and the iliac crest, perpendicular to the long axis of the body, with the participant standing balanced on both feet, approximately 20 cm apart, with arms hanging freely), hip circumference (widest circumference over the buttocks), and waist-to-hip ratio (waist circumference divided by hip circumference). Body mass index was calculated as weight in kilograms divided by the square of height in meters (kg/m^2) and categorized as < 25.0, 25.0–29.9, and ≥ 30.0 kg/m^2 [24]. All measurements were taken without shoes and heavy clothing. Interobserver reliability for anthropometric measurements was verified by repeated measurements during the first round of consultations.

Skinfolds

In the second cycle, skinfold thicknesses (mm) at the triceps, suprailiac, and subscapular were measured using skinfold calipers (Scientific CESCORF, RS, Brazil – similar to the Harpenden model) to the nearest 0.2 mm. Values were the mean of three measurements for each skinfold. The percentage of total body fat was calculated by the Faulkner

formula: percent total body fat = (triceps + subscapular + suprailiac + abdominal skinfolds × 0.153) + 5.783 [25].

Assays

At baseline, blood was assayed for 17-beta-estradiol (E2), luteinizing hormone (LH), follicle-stimulating hormone (FSH), sex hormone-binding globulin (SHBG), and thyrotropin-stimulating hormone (TSH). E2 was measured using a solid-phase radioimmunoassay kit (Coat-A-Coat kit; Diagnostic Products Corporation, Los Angeles, CA, USA), with a sensitivity of 20.0 pg/mL. FSH and LH were measured by a solid-phase immunoradiometric assay (MAIAclone; Biodata Diagnostics, Rome, Italy), with sensitivity of 0.25 mIU/mL. SHBG and TSH were measured by a solid phase chemiluminescent immunometric assay using the DPC Immulite kit (Diagnostic Products Corporation), with sensitivity of 0.2 nmol/L and 0.002 IU/mL, respectively.

Total cholesterol, high-density lipoprotein cholesterol (HDL-c), triglyceride (TG), and glucose levels were determined by a colorimetric enzymatic method (Architect C800 System; Abbott Laboratories, Abbott Park, IL, USA). Low-density lipoprotein cholesterol (LDL-c) was determined indirectly using the following formula: LDL-c = total cholesterol – (HDL-c + TG/5) [26].

Ultrasound

Transvaginal ultrasound was performed with a Toshiba-Tosbee apparatus (Toshiba Corporation, Tokyo, Japan) using a 5.0 MHz transvaginal probe. The maximum transverse (D1), anteroposterior (D2), and longitudinal (D3) diameters of the ovary were measured with electronic calipers. Ovarian volume was calculated using the following formula: volume = D1 × D2 × D3 × 0.523. Ovarian cyst was defined as a lesion with its largest diameter measuring at least 25 mm [27]. The examinations were performed in different phases of the menstrual cycle. Cycle phases were classified as follicular (days 1–10), periovulatory (days 11–17), and luteal (day 18 and later). The association of ovarian volume with menstrual cycle phase was analyzed to minimize any potential bias resulting from the effect of cycle phase on ovarian volume [27–29].

At baseline, all ultrasound examinations were performed by the same examiner. In the second cycle (2001), examinations were also performed by a single examiner and the interobserver correlation coefficient was calculated by comparing results of each case between the first- and second-cycle examiners. Reproducibility of the ovarian volume measurement was evaluated using the intraclass correlation coefficient to calculate the level of agreement with a second observer. Ovarian volume measurement achieved excellent reproducibility, with an intraclass correlation coefficient of 0.957 (95 % CI 0.883–0.94)

Table 2 Main results of the PFS

Author, year	Study design	N participants	Objective	Conclusion
Oppermann et al. 2003 [33]	Cross-sectional	98	To evaluate the relationship between ovarian volume and age, hormone levels, obesity, and menstrual cycle phase in pre- and perimenopausal women.	Ovarian volume was smaller in pre- and perimenopausal women aged 40 years or older compared with younger women.
Bastos et al. 2006 [5]	Cross-sectional	273	To investigate the association of smoking, parity, BMI, oral contraceptive use, and hormone therapy with ovarian volume in pre-, transition, and postmenopausal women.	Obesity was positively related to ovarian volume, menopausal status, and age. Use of contraception was associated with reduced ovarian volume.
Donato et al. 2006 [6]	Cross-sectional	358	To investigate the association between menopausal status and central adiposity measured by two different cutoffs of waist circumference and waist-to-hip ratio.	Postmenopausal women were at greater risk of having central adiposity (waist circumference and waist-to-hip ratio) than premenopausal women.
Oppermann et al. 2012 [15]	Cross-sectional	324	To identify the prevalence of physical, psychological, and menopause-related symptoms and their association with minor psychiatric disorders in pre-, peri-, and postmenopausal women.	Low level of education, memory loss, irritability, and menopausal transition were risk factors for positive findings in screening for minor psychiatric disorders.
Colpani et al. 2012 [7]	Cross-sectional	292	To assess pedometer-determined habitual physical activity in a Brazilian cohort of pre-, peri-, and postmenopausal women and its effect on anthropometric measurements and cardiovascular risk factors.	Walking 6,000 or more steps daily was associated with a decreased risk of CVD and DM in middle-aged women, regardless of menopausal status.
Colpani et al. 2014 [34]	Cross-sectional	292	To compare two methods of assessing physical activity in pre-, peri-, and postmenopausal women.	The agreement (k = 0110; $p = 0.007$) and correlation (rho = 0.136, $p = 0.02$) between the IPAQ-SF and the pedometer were weak.
Colpani et al. 2014 [35]	Longitudinal	358n	To assess mortality rate, causes of death, and associated risk factors in climacteric women.	CVD was an important cause of death in this cohort. DM and/or central adiposity were associated with all-cause mortality.

BMI body mass index, *CVD* cardiovascular disease, *DM* diabetes mellitus, *IPAQ-SF* International Physical Activity Questionnaire-Short Form

for the right ovary and 0.982 (95 % CI 0.940–0.994) for the left ovary.

Densitometry
In the third cycle (2010), bone mineral density was assessed in the lumbar spine (L1-L4), femoral neck, and proximal total femur by dual-energy X-ray absorptiometry (Lunar Prodigy Advance DXA System; GE Medical Systems, Milwaukee, WI, USA) in all participants. The results were expressed in g/cm^2 and estimated z- and t-scores. All measurements were performed in the Division of Radiology at Hospital São Vicente de Paulo.

Computed tomography (CT)
The coronary artery calcium score was assessed by chest CT using a 128-channel multidetector CT scanner (Definition; Siemens Medical Systems, Erlangen, Germany) at Hospital São Vicente de Paulo. The same radiologist read all CT scans at a Siemens Workstation (Leonardo 4.1). The average Agatston score was used in all analyses [30]. Subcutaneous and visceral fat areas were measured on a cross-sectional scan obtained at the umbilicus (L3-L4) as previously described [31].

Mortality data
In the third cycle (2010), medical records were reviewed to collect information on age at death, date and cause of death. The causes of death were coded according to the International Classification of Diseases, 10th revision [32].

Discussion
The study findings provide relevant information on health issues in midlife women and allow us to evaluate the association between menopausal status, aging in women and the risk of metabolic comorbidities and cardiovascular diseases in a representative sample of women from southern Brazil. Key publications to date are summarized in Table 2.

Abbreviations
ABIPEME: Brazilian Association of Market Research Institutes; BMD: Bone mineral density; CAC: Coronary calcium score; CT: Computed tomographic scanning; CV: Cardiovascular; DXA: Dual-energy X-ray absorptiometry; E2: 17-beta-estradiol; FSH: Follicle-stimulating hormone; HDL-c: High-density lipoprotein cholesterol; HT: Hormone therapy; IBGE: Brazilian Institute of Geography and Statistics; IPAQ: International Physical Activity Questionnaire; LDL-c: Low-density lipoprotein cholesterol; LH: Luteinizing hormone; MAQ: Modifiable Activity Questionnaire; NCDs n: Non-communicable diseases; NIS/RS-SES: Center for Health Information; PFS: Passo Fundo Cohort Study; SF-12: 12 Item Health Survey; SF-36: Short Form Health Survey -36; SHBG: Sex hormones binding globulin; SRQ-20: Self-Reporting Questionnaire;

TG: Triglyceride; TSH: Thyrotrophin stimulating hormone; WC: Waist circumference; WHQ: Women's Health Questionnaire; WHR: Waist-to-hip ratio.

Competing interests
The authors declare that they have no competing interests.

Authors' contributions
KO and PMS conceived of this protocol study and participated in its design and drafted the manuscript.
VC drafted the manuscript.
SCF helped to draft the manuscript and revised it critically.
All authors read and approved the final manuscript.

Acknowledgements
The study was supported by grants from Conselho Nacional de Desenvolvimento Científico e Tecnológico (CNPq INCT 573747/2008-3), Brazil.

Author details
[1]School of Medicine, Passo Fundo University, Passo Fundo, RS, Brazil. [2]Hospital São Vicente de Paulo, Passo Fundo, RS, Brazil. [3]Gynecological Endocrinology Unit, Division of Endocrinology, Hospital de Clinicas de Porto Alegre, Porto Alegre, RS, Brazil. [4]Department of Social Medicine, School of Medicine, Federal University of Rio Grande do Sul, Porto Alegre, RS, Brazil. [5]Department of Physiology, Federal University of Rio Grande do Sul, Porto Alegre, RS, Brazil.

References
1. Jaspers L, Colpani V, Chaker L, Van der Lee SJ, Muka T, Imo D, et al. The global impact of non-communicable diseases on households and impoverishment: a systematic review. Eur J Epidemiol. 2015;30(3):163–88.
2. (WHO) WHO. Gender and Health: Gender, Health, & Aging. 2003.
3. Aquino EM, Barreto SM, Bensenor IM, Carvalho MS, Chor D, Duncan BB, et al. Brazilian Longitudinal Study of Adult Health (ELSA-Brasil): objectives and design. Am J Epidemiol. 2012;175(4):315–24.
4. Oppermann-Lisboa KFS, Spritzer PM. Premenopause cross sectional study: sexual hormones profile, age and body mass index. A population based study. Gynecol Endocrinol. 1999;13 Suppl 2:171. Abstract 166.
5. Bastos CA, Oppermann K, Fuchs SC, Donato GB, Spritzer PM. Determinants of ovarian volume in pre-, menopausal transition, and post-menopausal women: a population-based study. Maturitas. 2006;53(4):405–12.
6. Donato GB, Fuchs SC, Oppermann K, Bastos C, Spritzer PM. Association between menopause status and central adiposity measured at different cutoffs of waist circumference and waist-to-hip ratio. Menopause. 2006;13(2):280–5.
7. Colpani V, Oppermann K, Spritzer P. Association between habitual physical activity and lower cardiovascular risk in pre-, peri- and postmenopausal women: a population-based study. Menopause. 2013;20:525–31.
8. IBGE IBdGeE. Cidades@. 2010; http://cidades.ibge.gov.br/xtras/perfil.php?lang=&codmun=431410&search=%7C%7Cinfogr%E1ficos:-informa%E7%F5es-completas. Accessed May 6, 2015.
9. [ABIPEME] ABdldPdM. Proposição para um novo critério de classificação socioeconômica. São Paulo, Brazil: LPM/Burke; 1991.
10. Hijjar M, Silva V. Smoking epidemiology in Brazil. J Bras Med. 1991; 60:50–54.
11. Kupperman HS, Blatt MH, Wiesbader H, Filler W. Comparative clinical evaluation of estrogenic preparations by the menopausal and amenorrheal indices. J Clin Endocrinol Metab. 1953;13(6):688–703.
12. Silva Filho EA, Costa AM. Evaluation of quality of life of climacteric women assisted at a school hospital of Recife, Pernambuco, Brazil. Rev Bras Ginecol Obstet. 2008;30(3):113–20.
13. Camelier A. Avaliação da qualidade de vida relacionada à saúde em pacientes com DPOC: estudo de base populacional com o SF-12 na cidade de São Paulo-SP. São Paulo: Universidade Federal de São Paulo; 2004.
14. Ware JE, Kosinski M, Keller SD. SF-12: how to score the SF-12 physical and mental health summary scales, 3rd edn. Lincoln: QualityMetric Incorporated, 1998.
15. Oppermann K, Fuchs SC, Donato G, Bastos CA, Spritzer PM. Physical, psychological, and menopause-related symptoms and minor psychiatric disorders in a community-based sample of Brazilian premenopausal, perimenopausal, and postmenopausal women. Menopause. 2012;19(3):355–60.
16. Beusenberg M, Orally J. A User's Guide to Self-Reporting Questionnaire (SRQ). Geneva, Switzerland: World Health Organization; 1994.
17. Mari JJ, Williams P. A validity study of a psychiatric screening questionnaire (SRQ-20) in primary care in the city of Sao Paulo. Br J Psychiatry. 1986;148:23–6.
18. Vuillemin A, Oppert JM, Guillemin F, Essermeant L, Fontvieille AM, Galan P, et al. Self-administered questionnaire compared with interview to assess past-year physical activity. Med Sci Sports Exerc. 2000;32(6):1119–24.
19. Kriska AM, Pereira MA, Fitzgerald SJ, Gregg EW. Modifiable activity questionnaire. In: A collection of physical activity questionnaires for health-related research. Med Sci Sports Exerc. 1997;29:S73–8.
20. Paffenbarger Jr RS, Hyde RT, Wing AL, Hsieh CC. Physical activity, all-cause mortality, and longevity of college alumni. N Engl J Med. 1986;314(10):605–13.
21. Papathanasiou G, Georgoudis G, Georgakopoulos D, Katsouras C, Kalfakakou V, Evangelou A. Criterion-related validity of the short International Physical Activity Questionnaire against exercise capacity in young adults. Eur J Cardiovasc Prev Rehabil. 2010;17(4):380–6.
22. Craig CL, Marshall AL, Sjostrom M, et al. International physical activity questionnaire: 12-country reliability and validity. Med Sci Sports Exerc. 2003; 35(8):1381–95.
23. Graff SK, Alves BC, Toscani MK, Spritzer PM. Benefits of pedometer-measured habitual physical activity in healthy women. Appl Physiol Nutr Metab. 2012; 37(1):149–56.
24. WHO WHO. Obesity: Prevention and Management of the Global Epidemic. Report of the WHO Consultation. Geneva: WHO; 1998.
25. Faulkner JA. Physiology of swimming and diving. In: Falls H, editor. Exercise physiology. Baltimore: Academic; 1968. p. 415–45.
26. Friedewald WT, Levy RI, Fredrickson DS. Estimation of the concentration of low-density lipoprotein cholesterol in plasma, without use of the preparative ultracentrifuge. Clin Chem. 1972;18(6):499–502.
27. Borgfeldt C, Andolf E. Transvaginal sonographic ovarian findings in a random sample of women 25-40 years old. Ultrasound Obstet Gynecol. 1999;13(5):345–50.
28. Filly R. Ovarian masses…What to look for…What to do. In: Callen P, editor. Ultrasonography in obstetrics and gynecology. Philadelphia: WB Saunders; 1994. p. 625–40.
29. Spritzer PM, Lisboa KO, Mattiello S, Lhullier F. Spironolactone as a single agent for long-term therapy of hirsute patients. Clin Endocrinol (Oxf). 2000; 52(5):587–94.
30. Agatston AS, Janowitz WR, Hildner FJ, Zusmer NR, Viamonte Jr M, Detrano R. Quantification of coronary artery calcium using ultrafast computed tomography. J Am Coll Cardiol. 1990;15(4):827–32.
31. Yoshizumi T, Nakamura T, Yamane M, Islam AH, Menju M, Yamasaki K, et al. Abdominal fat: standardized technique for measurement at CT. Radiology. 1999;211(1):283–6.
32. CID-10 CEldDePRàS. Classificação estatística internacional de doenças e problemas relacionados à saúde: 10a rev. http://www.datasus.gov.br/cid10/V2008/cid10.htm. Accessed May 5, 2015.
33. Oppermann K, Fuchs SC, Spritzer PM. Ovarian volume in pre- and perimenopausal women: a population-based study. Menopause. 2003; 10(3):209–13.
34. Colpani V, Spritzer PM, Lodi AP, Dorigo GG, Miranda IA, Hahn LB, et al. Physical activity in climacteric women: comparison between self-reporting and pedometer. Rev Saude Publica. 2014;48(2):258–65.
35. Colpani V, Oppermann K, Spritzer PM. Causes of death and associated risk factors among climacteric women from Southern Brazil: a population based-study. BMC Public Health. 2014;14:194

2

Bone mineral density in midlife long-term users of hormonal contraception in South Africa: relationship with obesity and menopausal status

Mags E. Beksinska[1][*] [iD], Immo Kleinschmidt[2] and Jenni A. Smit[1]

Abstract

Background: In South Africa, hormonal contraception is widely used in women over the age of 40 years. One of these methods and the most commonly used is depot-medroxyprogesterone acetate (DMPA) which has been found to have a negative effect on bone mass. Limited information is available on the effect of norethisterone enanthate (NET-EN) on bone mass, and combined oral contraceptives (COCs) have not been found to be associated with loss of bone mass. The aim of this study was to investigate bone mineral density (BMD) in pre and perimenopausal women (40–49 years) in relation to use of DMPA, NET-EN and COCs for at least 12 months preceding recruitment into the study and review associations with body mass index (BMI) and menopausal status.

Methods: One hundred and twenty seven users of DMPA, 102 NET-EN users and 106 COC users were compared to 161 nonuser controls. Menopausal status was assessed, BMI and forearm BMD was measured at the distal radius using dual X-ray absorptiometry. Comparison analysis was conducted at baseline and 2.5 years.

Results: There was no significant difference in BMD between the four contraceptive user groups ($p = 0.26$) with and without adjustment for age at baseline or at 2.5 years ($p = 0.52$). The BMD was found to be significantly associated with BMI ($p = < 0.0001$) with an increase of one unit of BMI translating to an increase of 0.0044 g/cm^2 in radius BMD. Follicle stimulating hormone (FSH) level ≥ 25.8 mIU/mL was associated with a decrease of 0.017 g/cm^2 in radius BMD relative to women with FSH < 25.8 mIU/mL. Significant interaction between FSH and BMI in their effect on BMD was observed ($p = .006$).

Conclusion: This study found no evidence that long-term use of DMPA, NET-EN and COCs affects forearm BMD in this population at baseline or after 2.5 years of follow-up. This study also reports the complex relationship and significant interaction between FSH and BMI in their effect on BMD. BMD research in older women needs to ensure that women are assessed for menopausal status and BMI.

Keywords: Depot-medroxyprogesterone acetate, Norethisterone enanthate, Combined oral contraceptives, Bone mineral density, Menopause, Follicle stimulating hormone, Body mass index

* Correspondence: mbeksinska@matchresearch.co.za
[1]MatCH Research Unit [Maternal, Adolescent and Child Health Research Unit], Department of Obstetrics and Gynaecology, Faculty of Health Sciences, University of the Witwatersrand, 40 Dr AB Xuma Street,11th floor, Suite 1108-9,Commercial City, Durban 4001, South Africa
Full list of author information is available at the end of the article

Background

In South Africa hormonal contraceptive use is high as reported in the last South African Demographic and Health Survey [1]. Of the two available hormonal injections, older women (> 40 years) almost exclusively use depot medroxyprogesterone acetate (DMPA) (81%) compared to norethisterone enanthate (NET-EN) (19%) [1]. These highly effective methods of contraception may be the method of choice for many women over 40 who have completed childbearing and are concerned about avoiding pregnancy. Hormonal injectables are not generally recommended in perimenopausal women where use of these methods is viewed as "contraceptive overkill" [2]. Most studies have found that current users of DMPA have lower BMD compared to nonusers [3–7]. However, a recent Cochrane review concludes that existing information cannot confirm whether steroidal contraceptives influence future fracture risk [8].

Specifically there is limited information on the effect of hormonal contraception on BMD in women in their midlife (> 40 years of age) [9–12]. As few studies have included women in this age group. Results of these studies have been mixed with some finding no differences in BMD between older DMPA users and nonusers or normal population means [9–11], while one study found a negative effect of DMPA on BMD compared to nonusers [12].

Studies investigating combined oral contraceptive (COC) use in perimenopausal users have not found a negative impact on BMD compared to nonusers of COCs [3]. Two cross-sectional studies have looked at BMD in NET-EN users. In one of these studies [13], current NET-EN users aged 40–44 had lower ultrasound measures in the calcaneus compared to nonusers, while the second study found no difference in forearm BMD between current users and controls [10].

Other potential factors that may play a role in BMD in midlife include menopausal status [14] and obesity [15]. However, evidence suggesting that being overweight / obese may be protective of BMD, is conflicting [16]. This study aimed to investigate BMD in pre and perimenopausal users (40 to 49 years) of DMPA, NET-EN, COC and nonusers of contraception in a 4–5 year follow-up study and review associations with BMI and menopausal status.

Methods

A cohort of women aged 40 to 49 years old using DMPA, NET-EN, or COCs, and nonusers of hormonal contraception were recruited from a large family planning clinic in Durban, South Africa. For inclusion as a hormonal contraceptive user, women had to have used either DMPA, NET-EN or COCs for at least 1 year. For inclusion in the nonuser control group women should not have used any form of hormonal contraception in the past year. Women who were postmenopausal were

excluded from the study at screening using menstrual history (no bleeding for 2 years or more) and follicle-stimulating hormone (FSH) levels from blood samples. An FSH level of ≥25.8 m International Units per milliliter (mIU/mL) was considered to be in the menopausal range (King Edward VIII Hospital Durban; Chemical Pathology Laboratory criteria using Roche Elecsys FSH expected values). Women with an FSH ≥25.8 m (mIU/mL) who reported irregular bleeding within the last 2 years were classified as perimenopausal and were eligible for this study.

On recruitment, a questionnaire was administered to elicit information on lifetime contraceptive history, fertility history, menopausal symptoms and regularity of the menstrual cycle. The examination included height, weight, blood pressure and waist and hip measurement. Forearm BMD was measured by dual energy x-ray absorptionmetry (DXA model DTX-200). Osteometer MediTech A/S Co, Rodovre, Denmark). BMD was measured in grams/centimetre^2 (g/cm^2) in the distal forearm (radius). The DXA equipment was standardized daily using a phantom as prescribed by the manufacturers instructions. Accuracy to the standard during the recruitment period was 0.53%. and in vivo precision was 0.94%. Study participants were followed-up at six-monthly intervals for a total of four to 5 years depending on time of recruitment. BMD was measured at each 6-monthly follow-up visit. Final comparison analysis was conducted at 2.5 years as the majority of women (87%) had stopped using a method of contraception by end of study. The study was conducted between 2000 and 2008.

The characteristics of women in the study were quantified as means ± standard deviations (SD), medians, or percentages. FSH levels were divided into two categories according to laboratory cut-off levels for premenopausal (< 25.8 mIU/mL) and perimenopausal/menopausal (≥25.8 mIU/mL). Differences in BMD between contraceptive groups, and the associations between BMD and selected characteristics of the study participants by contraceptive group were assessed using one-way analysis of variance and multiple variable linear regression.

The study aimed to be able to detect a half standard deviation difference in BMD between users and non-users of injectable contraceptives. This would be of biological significance as this difference would translate into a large difference in the risk of fracture in the older woman. Information on the mean and standard deviation of cross sectional measurements of forearm bone mass made in white, European, premenopausal, women as was reported by Nordin [17], was used to estimate sample size. The sample size required for each category assuming a two-tailed statistical test with a probability value (alpha) of 0.05 and with a power (beta) of 0.80 was 63 subjects. Loss to follow up was estimated at 8–10% per year. Sample size was adjusted to 100 per user group to ensure that a statistically significant difference could be detected. Data were analysed using the statistical package STATA (V.12 College station, TX, USA).

Ethical approval was granted by the University of the Witwatersrand, Human Subjects Research Committee (ref M981001), and by the Scientific and Ethical Review Group of the World Health Organization.

Results

In total, 496 women were recruited. Baseline demographic and reproductive characteristics are summarised in Table 1. The mean age was approximately 43 years in the three hormonal contraceptive user groups with the nonusers on average 2 years older. Almost all women were African except for the COC group which included a higher proportion of Indian and Coloured women. Most women took no regular exercise and the mean BMI of the women in each user group fell into the upper end of obese class 1 (30–34.99 kg/m^2) group [18]. Women in the contraceptive groups had used their method for approximately four of the previous 5 years prior to recruitment, with all having used the method without a break for the last 12 consecutive months. Only 19.7% of women in the DMPA group and 33.0% of the

NET-EN group reported a regular menstrual cycle (between 21 and 35 days), compared with 90.0% of the COC group and 93% of the non-users.

In total, 48.5% of women in the non-user group were classified as perimenopausal (reported at least one vasomotor symptom in the last 3 months and had an FSH in the perimenopausal/menopausal range). This was a higher proportion than in the other 3 groups (40.2% DMPA, 31.4% NET-EN, 30.1% COCs); however, after adjusting for age, there was no evidence of a difference between the 4 groups in terms of menopausal status (DMPA $p = 0.48$; NET-EN $p = 0.93$; COC $p = 0.29$).

There was no significant difference in BMD at baseline between the four contraceptive user groups at the radius ($p = .26$), with and without adjustment for age (Table 2). Although a small decrease in BMD was noted per year over the age range – 0.0017 g/cm^2 (95% CI -0.0041-0.0008) this was not statistically significant ($p = .18$). Length of use of method in the last 5 years and total lifetime use was not associated with difference in BMD.

Body mass index, FSH level (equal to and above 25.8 mIU/mL versus below 25.8 mIU/mL) and interaction of BMD with FSH level were all significantly associated with BMD in a multiple regression model ($r^2 = 0.2$). According to this model, for women of median BMI of

Table 1 Baseline characteristics of subjects in the 40–49 year age range by contraceptive method use

Characteristics	DMPA (n = 127)	NET-EN (n = 102)	COC (n = 106)	Non-user Controls (n = 161)	P-value
Mean age, years (SD)	43.6 (2.7)	43.0 (2.2)	43.7 (2.5)	45.4 (2.5)	< 0.001
Ethnicity %					
African	98.4	95.2	67.0	94.4	0.007
Coloured	1.6	1.0	7.5	2.5	
Indian	0	3.8	25.5	3.1	
Exercise					
No regular exercise (%)	96.9	96.0	94.3	93	0.48
Dieted in last 6 months (%)	0	0	4.7	< 1	0.003
Current smoker (%)	4.7	5.6	5.7	9.9	0.23
Parity (median)	4	3	3	3	0.04
Ever lactated %	88.2	91.3	87.7	83.2	0.34
Mean age at menarche, years(SD)	15.2± 1.7	15.5 ± 1.7	14.8 ± 1.7	14.8 ± 1.6	0.014
Lactation (yrs) median	3.5	3.2	3.0	3.2	0.06
FSH					
< 25.8 mIU/mL, %	72	94	90	68	< 0.0001
≥ 25.8 mIU/mL, %	28	6	10	32	
Use of group method*					
Median use last 5 yrs. (months)	53	45	52	NA	
Median lifetime use (months)	84	49	89	NA	
Median age at first use	36	37	36	NA	
Radius BMD g/cm^2	0.514	0.514	0.500	0.518	0.26

*Only group method shown i.e. group to which women using that method at the time of recruitment were allocated

Table 2 Factors potentially associated with Radius BMD (unadjusted) at baseline

Factors	Radius BMD g/cm² 95% CI	P value
Contraceptive group		0.26
DMPA	0.514 (0.501–0.527)	
NET-EN	0.514 (0.499–0.528)	
COC	0.500 (0.486–0.514)	
Nonuser	0.518 (0.506–0.529)	
Ethinicity		
African	0.516 (0.509–0.523)	
Indian	0.491 (0.451–0.531)	0.007
Coloured	0.479 (0.456–0.503)	
Age, per year	−0.0017 (−0.0041–0.0008)	0.188
BMI, change per kg/m²	0.0044 (0.0036–0.0052)	< 0.001
FSH		0.029
< 25.8 mIU/mL, %	0.516 (0.508)-0.524)	
≥ 25.8 mIU/mL, %	0.498 (0.483–0.512)	

33.9 units, mean radius BMD varied from 0.514 g/cm² [95% CI 0.507–0.521] with FSH < 25.8 mIU/mL, to 0.501 g/cm² [95% CI 0.488–0.513] for women with FSH ≥ 25.8 mIU/mL, ($p = 0.066$). The effect of FSH on BMD was significantly modified by BMI, and vice-versa ($p = .006$). For women with FSH < 25.8 mIU/mL, BMD increased by 0.0038 [95%CI 0.0028–0.0047] (g/cm²) per unit increase in BMI, whereas for women with FSH ≥ 25.8 mIU/mL, BMD increased by 0.0067 g/cm² [95% CI 0.0048–0.0086] for each unit increase in BMI (Table 3).

Follicle-stimulating hormone level was found to be significantly different between user groups ($p = < 0.0001$). However, after adjusting for age, the difference between the 4 groups was no longer significant ($p = 0.13$). An increase of 1 year in age increased FSH level by 3 mIU/mL ($p < 0.001$).

Although differences were noted between the contraceptive groups, most were not associated with BMD except for BMI, ethnic group and FSH level. A statistically significant difference in BMD was found between the Indian and African women ($p = .014$); however after adjusting for BMI the difference in BMD was no longer significant.

During follow-up all nonusers of hormonal contraception remained as nonusers, however many women in the user groups continued participation in the study but ceased using a contraceptive method. At baseline 32% of women recruited were nonusers of contraception, this increased to 71% after 3 years of follow-up and by end of the follow-up period the majority of women (87%) had ceased using a method of contraception. Due to small numbers of hormonal contraceptive users from 3 years of follow-up, comparison of user groups was conducted at the 2.5 year visit. At this follow up visit 278 women continued with the same method they were using at baseline. Women were excluded from the analysis if they stopped or changed their method. No difference was found in BMD between the groups at the 2.5 year visit (Table 4).

Discussion

This longitudinal study found no difference in forearm BMD between pre and perimenopausal users and nonusers of hormonal contraception at baseline or after 2.5 years of follow-up. This is in agreement with other studies of COC users in the perimenopause, where no change in BMD occurred [3]. The populations investigated in previous studies looking at the effect of DMPA and NET-EN on BMD have included women using the method in their 40s but there is limited information in this age group specifically. The age ranges of women in some studies have included users up to the age of 52, however the numbers have been small. In one cross-sectional study older DMPA users were disaggregated in the data [11] and no differences were found in BMD in women aged between 40 and 49 and a slightly older group of 50–52 compared to a normal population mean in the lumber spine and femoral neck. Tang et al., conducted a 3-year prospective study of perimenopusal women (mean age 43 years) who had used DMPA for 5 years or more [12]. At baseline significantly lower BMD in the spine, femoral neck, trochanter and ward's triangle were reported compared to never users. At the three-year follow up, women had a mean age of 46 years

Table 3 Results of multiple regression model with BMI and FSH level

Factors	Radius BMD units 95% CI	P value
Effect of [a]FSH (for women of median BMI = 33.9 kg/m²)		
< 25.8 mIU/mL	0.514 (0.507–0.521)	< 0.066
≥ 25.8 mIU/mL	0.501 (0.488–0.513)	
Effect of BMI, unit BMD per unit change in BMI For		< 0.001
FSH < 25.8 mIU/mL For	0.0038 (0.0028–0.0047)	
FSH ≥ 25.8 mIU/mL	0.0067 (0.0048–0.0086)	

[a]Significant interaction between FSH level and BMI ($p = 0.006$)

Table 4 Mean Radius BMD at 2.5 years by contraceptive group[a]

	N	Radius BMD g/cm² (SD)	P value
Contraceptive group			0.522
DMPA	63	0.511 (.071)	
NET-EN	38	0.501 (.081)	
COC	48	0.500 (.082)	
Nonuser	129	0.504 (.075)	

[a]Only women continuing with the same method from baseline were included in this analysis

with a mean length of DMPA use of 10.1 years. At this follow up it was projected that the loss from baseline would be linear, however only small losses were noted of less than 1% in all sites aside from the trochanter where a small increase was noted [12]. The authors of the Tang study concluded that rate of BMD loss may be faster in the first 5 years of DMPA use with a levelling off thereafter. Our DMPA user sample was of similar age and reported length of DMPA use to the Tang study. It may be that users in our study had reached a steady state and further bone loss had not occurred. A further longitudinal study [9] followed up women who had been long-term users of either DMPA or the IUD until menopause. This study found no difference in BMD between these two groups at each of the three forearm sites at one-year follow-up post-menopause.

The absence of differences between the groups in BMD at baseline and follow up in our study is in agreement with some studies of BMD in hormonal contraceptive users in the midlife [3]. Although most studies adjust for BMI as it is a known to be associated with BMD [15], it may also be important to review the overall weight of the sample population to assess the proportion that may be obese. The majority of women in our study were classified in the upper range of obese class 1 which may have conferred some protective effect on their BMD. In 2013, South Africa had an obesity rate of 42% for women and 13.5% for men, the highest overweight and obesity rate in sub-Saharan Africa [19].

Another possible reason for the lack of difference in BMD between the groups may be related to the sensitivity of the measurement using forearm BMD. Forearm DXA has been shown to give good precision [20] and accuracy [21] with the added advantages of equipment that is portable and considerably less cost to purchase and maintain compared to DXA equipment measuring central sites. In a large European osteoporosis cohort, a logistic regression analysis for identification of group (HRT or control), the prediction was best for whole body (82.6%) and spine (80.9%), followed by total hip (78.5%) and lastly, forearm (74.7%). The authors concluded that for clinical diagnosis axial DXA is recommended [22].

The study recruited from a public sector urban family planning clinic in a South African city. There was no locally available public health facility with DXA equipment to measure central body sites due to the high cost of the equipment, maintenance and staff to undertake scans. The Forearm DXA scanner was purchased through the study funding which was only able to cover the cost of a forearm DXA scanner.

Many women may continue to use hormonal injectables into their late forties and beyond menopause as menopausal symptoms such as amenorrhea may be masked by use of progestogen-only hormonal contraceptives which also cause amenorrhea [2]. DMPA has been shown to relieve vasomotor symptoms in perimenopausal women [23, 24]. and DMPA and NET-EN are known to suppress the midcycle surge of follicle-stimulating hormone (FSH) and luteinising hormone (LH), thereby reducing raised FSH levels, although the tonic release of these gonadotrophins continues at luteal phase levels [25]. Data from South Africa presents some evidence that a raised FSH level, although initially supressed, will return to its raised level within the three monthly DMPA and two-monthly NET-EN cycles of use and could be potentially used to assist as a menopausal indicator without interrupting method use in this group of contraceptive users [26]. Detection of menopause or perimenopause does therefore present some challenges in this group of injectable contraceptive users, whose BMD may be compromised by any risk associated with hormonal contraception use.

Conclusions
This study adds to evidence on the effect of hormonal contraception on BMD in the midlife. This study also reports the complex relationship and significant interaction between FSH and BMI in their effect on BMD. BMD research in older women needs to ensure that women are assessed for menopausal status and BMI.

Acknowledgements
Not applicable.

Funding
Funding for the study was provided by the World Health Organization. The funding body had some input into the design of the study and final approval of the protocol and had some minimal input into the interpretation.

Authors' contributions
MB developed the protocol and data collection instruments, assisted in the analysis of the data under the supervision of IK and interpreted the results and led the manuscript writing. IK analysed and interpreted the data. JS interpreted the data and was a major contributor in writing the manuscript. All authors read and approved the final manuscript.

Competing interests
The authors declare that they have no competing interests (MB IK JS).

Author details
[1]MatCH Research Unit [Maternal, Adolescent and Child Health Research Unit], Department of Obstetrics and Gynaecology, Faculty of Health Sciences, University of the Witwatersrand, 40 Dr AB Xuma Street,11th floor, Suite 1108-9,Commercial City, Durban 4001, South Africa. [2]London School of Hygiene and Tropical Medicine, Keppel Street, London WC1E, England.

References
1. Department of Health South Africa, Medical Research Council and Measure DHS. South African demographic and health survey 1998, full report. Pretoria (South Africa) Department of Health; 2002.
2. Guillebaud, J. 2001. Contraception: your questions answered. Edinburgh : Churchill Livingstone: 1993. 280
3. Curtis KM, Martins SL. Progestogen-only contraception and bone mineral density: a systematic review. Contraception. 2006;73:470–87.
4. Wanichsetakul P, Kamudhamas A, Watanaruagkovit P, Siripakam Y, Visutakul P. Bone mineral density at various anatomic bone sites in women receiving combined oral contraceptives and depot-medroxyprogesterone acetate for contraception. Contraception. 2002;65:407–10.
5. Petitti DB, Piaggio G, Mehta S, Cravioto MC, Meirik O. Steroid hormone contraception and bone mineral density: a cross-sectional study in an international population. Obstet Gynecol. 2000;95:736–43.
6. Scholes D, Lacroix AZ, Ott SM, Ichikawa LE, Barlow WE. Bone mineral density in women using depot medroxyprogesterone acetate for contraception. Obstet Gynecol. 1999;93:233–8.
7. Cundy T, Farquhar CM, Cornish J, Reid IR. Short-term effects of high dose oral Medroxyprogesterone acetate on bone density in premenopausal women. J Clin Endocrinol Meta. 1996;81:1014–7.
8. Lopez LM, Grimes DA, Schulz KF, Curtis KM, Chen M. Steroidal contraceptives: effect on bone fractures in women. Cochrane Database Syst Rev. 2014;6:CD006033. https://doi.org/10.1002/14651858.CD006033.pub5.
9. Sanches L, Marchi NM, Castro S, et al. Forearm bone mineral density in postmenopausal former users of depot medroxyprogesterone acetate. Contraception. 2008;78:365–9.
10. Beksinska M, Smit J, Kleinschmidt I, Farley T, Mbatha F. Bone mineral density in women aged 40-49 years using depot-medroxyprogesterone acetate, norethisterone enanthate or combined oral contraceptives for contraception. Contraception. 2005;71:170–5.
11. Globade B, Ellis S, Murphy B, Randall S, Kirkman R. Bone density amongst long term users of medroxyprogesterone acetate. Br J Obstet Gynaecol. 1998;105:790–4.
12. Tang OS, Tang G, Yip PSF, Li B. Further evaluation of long-term depot-medroxyprogesterone acetate use and bone mineral density; a longitudinal cohort study. Contraception. 2000;62(4):161.
13. Rosenberg L, Zhang Y, Constant D, Cooper D, Kalla AA, Micklesfield L, et al. Bone status after cessation of use of injectable progestin contraceptives. Contraception. 2007;76:425–31.
14. Salamat MR, Salamat AH, Janghorbani M. Association between obesity and bone mineral density by gender and menopausal status. Endincrinol Metab. 2016;31(4):547–58. https://doi.org/10.3803/EnM.2016.31.4.547.
15. Cummings SR, Black DM, Nevitt MC, Browner W, Cauley J, Ensrud K, et al. Bone mineral density at various sites for prediction of hip fractures. The study of osteoporotic fractures research group. Lancet. 1993;31:72–5.
16. Migliaccio S, Greco EA, Fornari R, Donini DM, Lenzi A. Is obesity in women protective of osteoporosis? Diab Metab Syndrome Obes Targets Ther. 2011;4:273–82.
17. Nordin BE. The definition and diagnosis of osteoporosis. Calcif Tissue Int. 1987;40:57–8.
18. World Health Organisation Global data on body mass. BMI Classification. http://apps.who.int/bmi/index.jsp. Accessed 11 Mar 2018.
19. Ng M, Fleming T, Robinson M, Thomson B, Graetz N, Margono C, Mullany EC, Biryukov S, et al. Global, regional, and national prevalence of overweight and obesity in children and adults during 1980–2013: a systematic analysis for the Global Burden of Disease Study 2013. Lancet. 2014;384(9945):766–81.
20. Davis JW, Ross PD, Wasnich RD, MacLean CJ, Vogel JM. Long-term precision of bone loss rate measurements among postmenopausal women. Calcif Tissue Int. 1991;48:311–8.
21. Stock JL, Coderre JA, Mallette LE. Effects of a short course of estrogen on mineral metabolism in postmenopausal women. J Clin Endocrinol Metab. 1985;61:595–600.
22. Abrahamsen BL, Stilgren LS, Hermann AP, Tofteng CL, Barenholdt O, Vestergaard P, et al. Discordance between changes in bone mineral density measured at different skeletal sites in perimenopausal women—implications for assessment of bone loss and response to therapy: the Danish osteoporosis prevention study. J Bone Miner Res. 2001;16:1212–9.
23. Bullock JL, Massey FM, Gambrell RD Jr. Use of medroxyprogesterone acetate to prevent menopausal symptoms. Obstet Gynecol. 1975;46:165–8.
24. Morrison JC, Martin DC, Blair RA, Anderson GD, Kincheloe BW, Bates GW, et al. The use of medroxyprogesterone acetate for the relief of climacteric symptoms. Am J Obstet Gynecol. 1980;138:99–104.
25. Franchimont P, Cession G, Ayalon D, Musters A, Legros JJ. Suppressive action of norethisterone enanthate and depo medroxyprogesterone acetate on gonadotropin levels. Obstet Gynecol. 1970;36:93–100.
26. Beksinska ME, Smit JA, Kleinschmidt I, Rees HV, Farley TM, Guidozzi F. Detection of raised FSH levels among older women using depo medroxyprogesterone acetate and norethisterone enanthate. Contraception. 2003;68:339–43.

3

The Midlife Women's Health Study – a study protocol of a longitudinal prospective study on predictors of menopausal hot flashes

Ayelet Ziv-Gal[1], Rebecca L. Smith[2], Lisa Gallicchio[3], Susan R. Miller[4], Howard A. Zacur[4] and Jodi A. Flaws[5*]

Abstract

Background: The Midlife Women's Health Study (MWHS) was developed to address some of the gaps in knowledge regarding risk factors for hot flashes among generally healthy midlife women during their menopausal transition. This manuscript describes the methods from the study and the main findings that were published to date, with a focus on predictors of hot flashes. This study was initially funded to test the hypothesis that obesity is associated with an increased risk of hot flashes through mechanisms that involve ovarian failure, altered sex steroid hormone levels, and selected genetic polymorphisms.

Methods/Design: The MWHS was conducted between 2006 and 2015 as a prospective longitudinal population-based study of generally healthy midlife women (ages 45 to 54 years) during their natural menopausal transition. Women were eligible if they had intact uteri and both ovaries and reported having at least 3 menstrual periods in the last 12 months. Exclusion criteria included pregnancy, cancer, and use of hormonal/hormone-like supplements. Overall, 780 women were recruited into the study. The majority of study participants were followed for 4 to 7 years. At annual visits, women donated blood and urine samples, completed questionnaires, had a vaginal ultrasound, and had their anthropometric measurements taken.

Discussion: Several risk factors for menopausal hot flashes were identified or confirmed, including older age, perimenopausal status, current and former cigarette smoking, lower estradiol levels, lower progesterone levels, black race, and depressive symptoms. Factors that were associated with decreased odds of hot flashes included moderate alcohol consumption and more than 5 years of cessation of cigarette smoking. Body mass index was not associated with hot flashes. The MWHS has provided important information regarding hot flashes. The study methods are rigorous and can be easily adopted by research groups investigating naturally occurring menopausal hot flashes.

Keywords: Hot flash, Menopausal transition, BMI, Cigarette smoking, Race, Study protocol

Background

Hot flashes are the most common symptom reported by women during their menopausal transition [1, 2]. They are described as sudden transient periods of intense heat in the upper parts of the body, arms, and face. Hot flashes are often followed by flushing of the skin, profuse sweating, chills, palpitations, and anxiety [1]. In the United States, it is estimated that the health care expenditures due to hot flashes can be as high as 339 million dollars per year [3]. Additionally, symptomatic women can suffer from difficulties in overall daily functioning [4]. Despite the high prevalence of menopausal hot flashes and the overall public burden, the etiology and longitudinal changes/dynamics of natural occurring and untreated hot flashes are still unknown.

Few risk factors have been consistently reported to be associated with the occurrence of midlife hot flashes [5, 6]. Cigarette smoking, later menopausal stage, and low

* Correspondence: jflaws@illinois.edu
[5]Department of Comparative Biosciences, University of Illinois, 2001 S. Lincoln Avenue, Urbana, Illinois 61802, USA
Full list of author information is available at the end of the article

estrogen levels have been associated with an increased risk of hot flashes [5, 6]. Additionally, moderate alcohol consumption has been found to be associated with a reduced risk of hot flashes, whereas body mass index (BMI) and body fat composition have been shown to be associated with both increased and decreased risk of hot flashes [5, 6]. However, previous studies were mostly cross-sectional, investigated hot flashes with a limited number of questions, encompassed limited time periods, or focused on treatment efficacy rather than on untreated hot flashes. A recent study by Avis et al. examined hot flashes dynamics, but it focused only on frequent hot flashes instead of examining other aspects of hot flashes (e.g., severity, less frequent hot flashes) [7]. Thus, overall, there was a need for a study such as the Midlife Women's Health Study (MWHS) to examine the dynamics of natural occurring and untreated hot flashes over time. This information was needed to fill some of the gaps in our knowledge about hot flashes, including events that predispose women to develop hot flashes, the estimated duration of hot flashes, and changes in hot flashes severity over time.

The MWHS was conducted between 2006 and 2015 as a prospective longitudinal population-based study of generally healthy midlife women recruited during their menopausal transition. The overall goal of the study was to expand findings from a previous cross-sectional study that was conducted by the same team [8–23], while focusing on the mechanisms by which obesity is associated with an increased risk of hot flashes. Specifically, the MWHS was developed to test the hypothesis that obesity is associated with an increased risk of hot flashes through mechanisms that involve ovarian failure, altered sex steroid hormone levels, and selected genetic polymorphisms. The study working model is shown in Fig. 1.

Specific analyses that have been completed to date in the MWHS include: 1) identification of risk factors associated with longer duration of hot flashes and the time of peak hot flashes severity [24]; 2) examination of the

associations between demographic characteristics, health behaviors, hormone concentrations, and the experience of any, current, more severe, and more frequent midlife hot flashes [25]; 3) examination of the association between quitting smoking and midlife hot flashes [26]; 4) examination of the associations between BMI, BMI change, and weight change and midlife hot flashes [27]; 5) examination of whether higher urinary levels of phthalate metabolites are associated with an increased risk of midlife hot flashes [28]; 6) examination of the associations between BMI, cigarette smoking, alcohol intake, and hormone concentrations with ovarian volume among midlife women [29]; and 7) identification of factors associated with sexual activity during the menopausal transition [30].

In the next sections we describe in detail the main methods that were used during the MWHS for recruitment of the study participants, handling of biological samples, data collection, and analyses. Additionally, we describe the main findings that have been published to date along with a concise discussion of the results.

Methods
Study design
The Midlife Women's Health Study (MWHS) was a prospective longitudinal population-based study. It was innovative as it included generally healthy midlife women who were either late premenopausal or perimenopausal women. The inclusion criteria allowed the research team to examine, prospectively, the associations between specific variables (e.g., demographic, health habit, and clinical factors) and the occurrence, frequency, severity, and duration of hot flashes over time. Additionally, the detailed questionnaires completed by the study participants allowed for the examination of other commonly reported symptoms/issues during the menopausal transition, including sexual function, mood, and medical conditions (e.g., hypertension, allergies, diabetes).

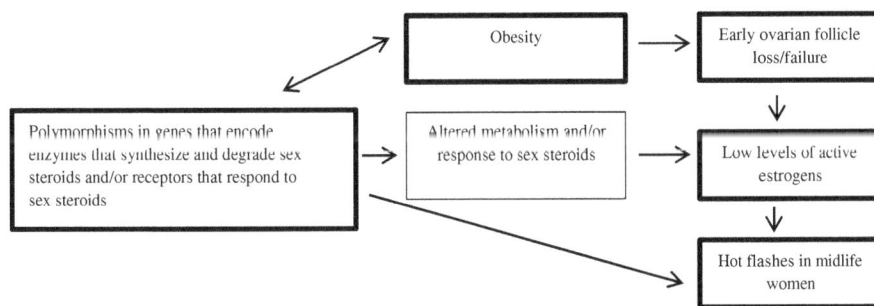

Fig. 1 The MWHS study was designed to test the hypothesis that obesity is associated with hot flashes through: a) early ovarian follicle loss/failure, b) selected genetic polymorphisms in the genes that encode enzymes that synthesize and degrade sex steroids and/or the receptors that allow tissues to respond to sex steroids, or c) mechanisms involving early follicle loss/failure, altered sex steroid hormone levels, and genetic polymorphisms in genes that encode enzymes that synthesize and degrade sex steroids and/or receptors that respond to sex steroids (this part of the study is yet to be conducted)

Sample selection and recruitment

The MWHS team used predetermined eligibility and exclusion criteria to ensure that during the initial recruitment period, women were not postmenopausal and were undergoing a natural process of reproductive aging. Specifically, women in the age range of 45 to 54 years were included as these women are typically perimenopausal and this is when women are most likely to have hot flashes [2]. Eligibility criteria also included having intact uteri and both ovaries; hence, only those women who were naturally undergoing the menopausal transition were eligible, whereas women who had surgical menopause were excluded from participation. Lastly, women who reported having at least 3 menstrual periods in the last 12 months were included, whereas women who did not have a menstrual period for ≥12 months were excluded because they are clinically considered postmenopausal [31].

Additional exclusion criteria were used to avoid known factors that may interfere with the natural menopausal transition and the natural occurrence of hot flashes. Specifically, currently pregnant women were excluded because the study focused on women who were transitioning from a reproductive to non-reproductive stage of their lives. Additionally, women currently using hormone therapies or oral contraceptives were excluded because the study focused on women's natural experiences of hot flashes, and hormone therapies and oral contraceptives are often used to prevent/reduce hot flashes. Lastly, women with any history of cancer were excluded because chemotherapeutic agents used to treat cancer can deplete ovarian follicles and increase risk of hot flashes [32]. Figure 2 summarizes the eligibility strategy for initial recruitment of participants.

Mailing addresses of women aged 45 to 54 years residing in the Baltimore, Maryland metropolitan area (USA) and its surrounding counties were purchased from AccuData America (Fort Myers, FL, USA). Recruitment letters were then sent to addresses located nearest to the clinical site at Johns Hopkins, Greenspring Station and then in concentric circles out from the site until reaching the target number of enrollees. To avoid potential reporting bias, the study was presented as a general "Midlife Women's Health Study." Women who were interested in enrolling in the study were asked to call the clinic to obtain more information.

Once a woman called the clinic, a clinic staff member determined if the woman met the eligibility criteria. Based on a woman's interest and eligibility, a baseline clinic visit was scheduled. At this baseline clinic visit, the woman was informed again of the general purpose of the study, and her questions were answered. All participants provided written informed consent according to procedures approved by the University of Illinois and

Johns Hopkins University Institutional Review Boards and each woman received a copy of the consent form.

During the baseline clinic visit, each participant was asked to complete a detailed baseline study questionnaire, donate urine and blood samples for hormone measurements, and have her weight, height, waist and hip circumferences and blood pressure measured. In addition, each participant underwent a transvaginal 2D ultrasound to measure ovarian volume and follicle numbers. Generally, baseline clinic visits were scheduled in the mornings (8:30–10:00 AM) to minimize daily fluctuations in hormone levels between the participants. Women were also instructed to fast overnight to avoid any potential dietary effects on hormone levels.

Each participant was then asked to visit the clinic once a week on each of the 3 weeks following the baseline visit to provide additional blood and urine samples. At the fourth clinic visit (the last of the three weekly visits following the baseline visit), each woman also completed another shorter questionnaire. Further details about the questionnaires are provided below.

During the clinic visits, a staff member reviewed each questionnaire for completeness and recorded any medications that the participant was taking on a regular basis. Hot flash status was assigned using the participant's answer to the question "Have you ever had hot flashes?" ("yes" = ever experienced hot flashes, "no" = never experienced hot flashes). After each visit, the participant was given $10 US to cover the expense of time and travel to the clinic, and was provided with a voucher for a snack after the fasting blood work.

These four consecutive weekly clinic visits were then repeated on a yearly basis throughout the woman's participation in the study, with visits proceeding similarly to the first year as described above. During these visits, the clinic staff examined any change that potentially affected a woman's eligibility for further participation in the study. Specifically, the study team discontinued follow-up of women who reported the current use of hormone therapy, ever had an oophorectomy and/or hysterectomy, or ever were diagnosed with cancer. Generally, women were followed over a total of 4 years because they became postmenopausal at the end of the 4 year follow up. However, some participants were followed for more than 4 years because they were not postmenopausal at the end of the 4th year follow up.

A total of 126,000 recruitment letters were mailed, 2507 women called the clinic for more information and were screened for eligibility. Of these women, a total of 780 women were recruited and were active participants during the first year of the MWHS. About 5.5% of 780 women withdrew after year 1 and approximately 3% dropped out after each subsequent year. Some of the reasons for withdrawal included lack of time, a medical issue, or the participant moving out of town. The study

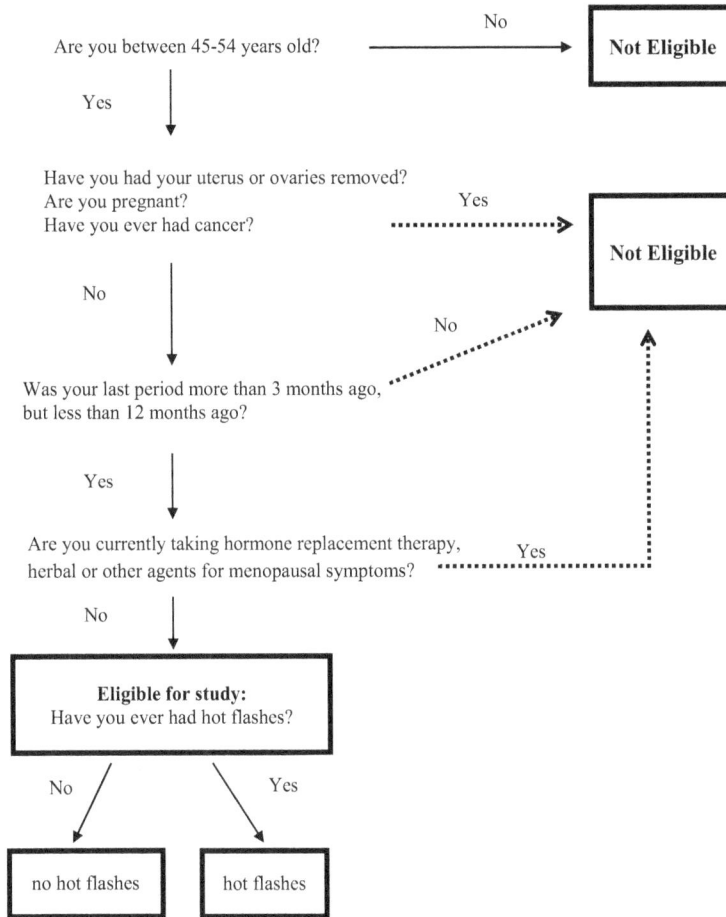

Fig. 2 Potential participants in the MWHS were screened for eligibility based on the described selection algorithm. Specifically, women between the ages of 45 and 54 years, with an intact uteri and both ovaries, not pregnant, who have not had cancer, who have had their last menstrual period within the last 12 month period, but not within the last 3 month period, and who have not used hormone replacement therapy, herbal or plant substances for treatment of hot flashes were eligible for the MWHS

team discontinued follow-up of women who reported the use of hormone therapy (*n* = 30), had an oophorectomy and/or hysterectomy (*n* = 25), or were diagnosed with cancer (*n* = 12) [29]. Figure 3 provides a flow chart of women enrolled in the study.

If a woman missed a single visit or a year of visits, she was still asked to remain in the study and data from those skipped visits were considered missing. Lastly, to protect the participants' privacy, each participant received a unique identification code. All records and data were stored in a locked file cabinet in a designated office and only personnel directly involved in the study had access to the files.

Questionnaires
During the first visit and the last visit of each year of participation, women were asked to complete a self-administered questionnaire while seated in a private comfortable room. During the first visit, participants completed a 20-page, single-sided survey that took about

an hour to complete. This detailed questionnaire contained questions regarding demographic information, reproductive history and menstrual cycle characteristics, hormonal and other supplement consumption, menopausal symptoms, medical and family history, and health behaviors such as smoking and alcohol use.

During the last yearly visit, the participant completed a condensed version of the questionnaire (9 pages, single-sided) that took about 30 min to complete. This survey assessed only factors that may have changed during the course of a 2 to 4-week time period (the time between the 'same year' visits). For example, the survey included questions on medical history, hot flashes history, smoking history, whereas factors such as birth date and race were excluded from the condensed version of the questionnaire.

Anthropometric measurements
On the day of each visit, women were weighed without shoes in street clothing to the nearest 0.05 kg, rounding

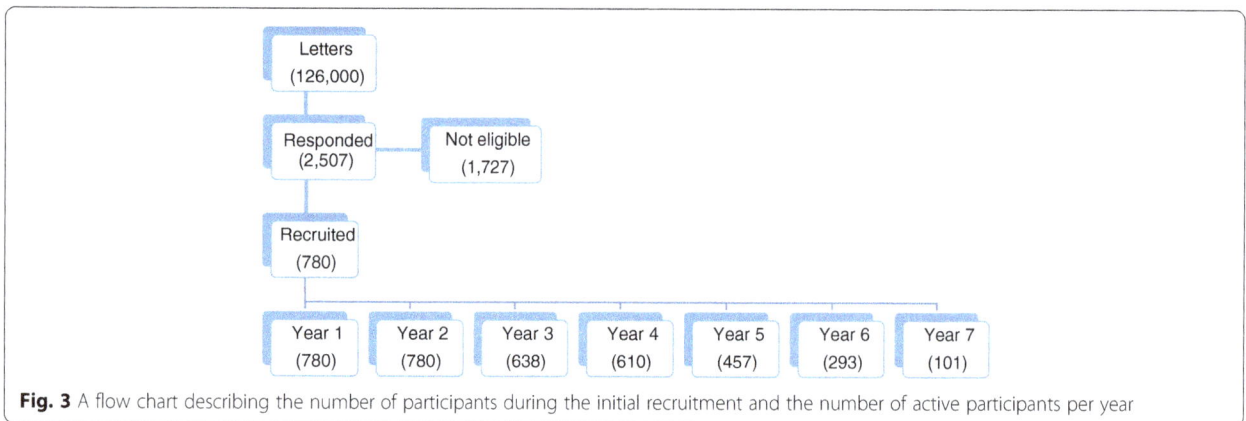

Fig. 3 A flow chart describing the number of participants during the initial recruitment and the number of active participants per year

down, on a calibrated scale. Height was measured without shoes to the nearest 0.5 cm, rounding down, with a standard stadiometer. Body mass index (BMI) was calculated using the National Institutes of Health on-line BMI calculator [33]. Normal, overweight, or obese status was categorized as BMI less than 25 kg/m^2, 25–29 kg/m^2, and 30 kg/m^2 or greater, respectively. Waist circumference was measured at the narrowest part of the waist. Hip circumference was measured at the fullest part of the hips.

Measurement of ovarian volume and antral follicle numbers
Transvaginal ultrasounds were performed on each study participant on a yearly basis by a licensed, highly trained physician in the Department of Gynecology and Obstetrics at Johns Hopkins University. All transvaginal ultrasounds were performed using the 7.5 MHz transvaginal probe on a GE Logig 200 Alpha/Pro Model. All measurements were conducted without knowledge of the woman's age, menopausal status, or hot flash status. Examination of the ovary was established by scanning from the outer to the inner margin. All follicles 2–10 mm in size were measured and counted in each ovary. Follicle size was calculated from 2 to 3 perpendicular measurements. The volumes of each follicle and ovary were calculated by applying formulas of an ellipsoid (LxWxDxpi/6). Total ovarian volume was obtained by summing the volumes of both ovaries.

Blood collection and measurement of hormone levels
Blood was collected via venipuncture conducted by a trained phlebotomist. Aliquots of whole blood samples were either stored in –20 °C for future genetic analyses or were further processed for serum extraction. For serum extraction, samples were centrifuged at 2000 g for 20 min in a cooled centrifuge. After centrifugation, the serum was aspirated and stored at –70 °C until hormone analysis.

Because the participants were going through the menopausal transition, they had irregular cycles during the study. To minimize variability between measurements,

samples were collected from fasting women, at the same time of day, but not on the same day of the cycle. Additionally, four different blood samples (one per week within a month) per each year of the study were collected. The values from these samples were averaged per year in the statistical analyses.

Serum concentrations of estradiol, testosterone, progesterone, and sex hormone-binding globulin (SHBG) were measured by enzyme-linked immunosorbent assays (ELISAs; DRG, NJ USA). All assays were performed without knowledge of participant characteristics by the same laboratory (Dr. Flaws, University of Illinois, Urbana, IL, USA). Each sample was quantified in duplicate within the same assay. Some samples were run in multiple assays to ensure that the assay values did not dramatically shift over time. Overall, the averaged inter-assay variability was less than 5%. A mean value, per participant, was used in all statistical analyses. When a participant's hormone levels were below the limit of detection, a value between zero and the detectable limit (based on uniform distribution) was randomly assigned to ensure a more accurate estimate of the variance.

Determination of menopausal status
Menopausal status was determined based on woman's answers to several questions on the study questionnaire on menstrual cycle history (e.g., age at menarche, regularity of menstrual cycles, and number of menstrual cycles in the past year). Specifically, premenopausal women were those who experienced their last menstrual period within the past 3 months and reported 11 or more periods within the past year. Perimenopausal women were either those who experienced their last menstrual period within the past year, but not within the past 3 months or had their last menstrual period within the past 3 months and overall 10 or fewer periods within the past year. Postmenopausal women were those who had no menstrual periods within the past year. During

the study, the follow-up of women who became post-menopausal ($n = 120$) was discontinued.

Hot flashes variables

A detailed hot flash history was obtained through a series of questions in the study questionnaires. These specific questions have been used to collect data on hot flashes in the previous studies conducted by the MWHS team for more than 12 years [10, 11, 13, 15, 22, 27, 29, 34]. Women were asked: if they ever had hot flashes; whether they had experienced hot flashes within the last 30 days; the number of hot flashes experienced within the last 30 days; the age when hot flashes first occurred; the severity and frequency of the hot flashes; and the length of time a woman had been experiencing hot flashes.

Hot flashes severity was classified as moderate or severe if a woman had hot flashes that were described as a sensation of heat accompanied by sweating that may interrupt usual activity. A woman was classified as having mild hot flashes if she had hot flashes that were described as a warm sensation without sweating or disruption of usual activity. Hot flashes frequency was determined based on detailed questions on the occurrence of hot flashes. Specifically, the participants were asked if they experienced hot flashes every hour, every 2–5 h, every 6–11 h, every 12–23 h, 1–2 days per week, 5–6 days per week, 2–3 days per month, 1 day per month, less than 1 day per month, or never.

Time to peak severity was calculated as the difference between the age at which hot flashes were most severe and the age at which hot flashes were first experienced. By default, peak severity was the age at which hot flashes were reported to be most severe during the baseline visit. If, during the study, a woman reported a higher severity on a survey than reported on the baseline visit survey, the time of the later survey was considered to be the participant's peak severity.

Additionally, women were asked whether any other female relatives (e.g., mother, sister, aunt) experienced hot flashes. Lastly, several questions inquired about quality of sleep and hot flashes experienced during the night (i.e., night sweats). Specifically, women were asked about the occurrence, number of events during the night (frequency), and severity (need to change clothes/sheets at night and frequency in a typical week) of night sweats.

Sexual activity

Sexual activity was determined by several questions that inquired whether the participant was sexually active, her level of satisfaction in the case of being sexually active, and the reasons for not being sexually active (partner related or individual reasons). A subset of outcomes was generated based on items included in the Short Personal Experiences Questionnaire [35] such as frequency of sex, enjoyment of sex, arousal during sex, orgasm during sex, passion for partner, satisfaction with partner, pain during sex, lubrication during sex, and sexual fantasies. A variable for a group of the outcomes was created, and participant scores were calculated using Likert scale values ("1" = Not at all; "5" = A great deal).

Lifestyle habits

Previous studies, including our preliminary cross-sectional study, indicated that cigarette smoking is associated with increased risk of hot flashes [11, 17, 36]. In the MWHS, cigarette smoking status was assessed using the questions: "Have you ever smoked cigarettes?" and "Do you still smoke cigarettes?" Cigarette smoking status was then categorized as current, former, and never. For smokers, information was also collected on the frequency, amount, and type of smoking.

Similarly, data on alcohol consumption were collected using the following questions: "During your entire life, have you had at least 12 drinks of any kind of alcoholic beverage?" and "In the last 12 months, have you had at least 12 drinks of any kind of alcoholic beverage?" Further queries for those responding affirmatively on having at least 12 drinks in the last 12 months were made to assess the average number of days per month that the woman drank and the number of drinks on those days.

Physical activity was assessed by the participant's response to questions regarding their levels of activity at work and at leisure time. These included questions such as "At work, I sit/stand/walk/lift heavy loads/tired/sweat" [choices: never, seldom, sometimes, often, and always], "In comparison with others my own age, I think my work is physically" [choices: much heavier, heavier, as heavy, lighter, and much lighter], "In comparison with others my own age, I think my physical activity leisure time is" [choices: much more, more, as much, less, and much less], and "During leisure time, I play sport/watch television/walk/cycle" [choices: always, often, sometimes, seldom, and never].

Mood/Emotional status

The experience of depressive symptoms was assessed using the Centers for Epidemiologic Studies – Depression Scale (CES-D) [37]. The study questionnaire included multiple questions in which women were asked to describe themselves during the visit at the clinic and during the past week. These questions included statements that best described what a woman felt (e.g., 'I was happy', 'I thought my life had been a failure', 'I had crying spells', 'I had trouble keeping my mind on what I was doing'). The participant was asked to check the best fit on a given scale [choices: rarely, some of the time, moderately, most of the time].

Other health related outcomes

The women were asked about their medical history using a series of several questions. The first question provided a list of selected illnesses/medical conditions of which the participant was asked to mark "Yes/No" and to indicate the age first diagnosed. The list included illnesses/conditions such as uterine fibroids, diabetes, epilepsy, and asthma. Other questions presented other symptoms that may be experienced by women in this age group such as incontinence, vaginal discharge, and headaches. The participant was asked to mark how frequently she had experienced each symptom during the past year [choices: never, rarely, sometimes, frequently, and regularly]. Lastly, a staff member queried the participants on medication use and that information was documented separately.

The questionnaire also included questions on hormone replacement therapy and herbal supplements. This allowed confirmation that participants were not taking hormonal or herbal agents. The questionnaire also included questions on the participant's reproductive history (e.g., number of pregnancies, use of oral contraceptives).

General information

Employment status was categorized as employed (either full-time or part-time) and not employed. Data on occupation and total family annual income, marital status, race/ethnic background, and education level were also collected on the detailed questionnaire administered at the first visit each year.

Phthalate metabolite levels

Phthalates can be readily found in personal care products and are considered endocrine disrupting chemicals [38–40]. Because women are likely to use these phthalate-containing products, a subset of samples from 195 participants (96 with hot flashes and 99 without hot flashes) was evaluated for urine phthalate metabolites levels. To minimize potential confounding, this subset of samples included only nonsmokers and white women with similar BMIs. Urine samples were analyzed by isotope dilution high-performance liquid chromatography negative-ion electrospray ionization-tandem mass spectrometry (HPLC-MS/MS) at the Environmental Health Laboratory & Trace Organics Analysis Center, School of Public Health at the University of Washington. Detailed methods are described by Ziv-Gal et al. [28].

Statistical analyses

In MHWS publications, data have been analyzed using various statistical approaches. The approaches included, but are not limited to, univariate and bivariate analyses [24, 25], logistic regression and generalized estimated equation models [24–29], survival analysis [24], and Bayesian network analysis [24, 30]. For each analysis, potential effect modifiers and confounders were examined as described in detail in the published manuscripts.

Published results to date

Sample characteristics and hot flashes

At baseline, 45.4% of the study participants reported experiencing hot flashes [27]. The majority of these women reported experiencing hot flashes in the previous 30 days (72.3%) [27]. Approximately 55.7% of women reported hot flashes that were moderate in severity, and about a quarter of those women with hot flashes reported experiencing them daily (23.2%) or weekly (26.2%) [27]. The majority of women had experienced hot flashes for more than 1 year (63%) [25]. In the longitudinal analysis, women experienced hot flashes over 2.5 years on average when including only those who reported an end to their hot flashes within the first 4 years of the study [24]. When including all women during all years of study, hot flashes duration was 6 years on average [24].

At baseline, older age, higher education level, having depressive symptoms, and use of anti-hypertensive medications were significantly associated with increased odds of hot flashes [27]. In contrast, marital status and physical activity were not significantly associated with hot flashes outcomes [27]. In the longitudinal analysis, shorter mean duration of hot flashes (i.e., the difference between the age first experiencing hot flashes and the age first reported not having hot flashes) was significantly associated with higher education level during the study period [24]. Additionally, longer mean duration was associated with delayed time to peak severity [24].

Menopausal status, hormone levels, and hot flashes

At baseline, women experiencing hot flashes were more likely to be of perimenopausal status (56%) [27] and to have significantly lower estradiol and progesterone levels compared to women without hot flashes [25]. Additionally, mean ovarian volume was significantly lower in women experiencing hot flashes compared to women without hot flashes [25]. Testosterone levels were similar between women with and without hot flashes [25]. In the longitudinal analysis, shorter mean duration (in years) of hot flashes was significantly associated with higher estradiol and progesterone levels among women with hot flashes during the study period [24]. Higher progesterone levels were associated with decreased time to peak severity [24]. Lastly, similar to baseline results, testosterone levels were not statistically associated with hot flashes [24].

Weight, BMI, and hot flashes

The main objective of the funded MWHS study was to evaluate the association between body weight and menopausal hot flashes. Baseline data of MWHS indicated that BMI was not associated with any of the hot flashes outcomes [27]. Similarly, longitudinal analysis indicated no association between BMI, BMI change, or weight change and any of the hot flashes outcomes [27].

Race and hot flashes

At baseline, race was not associated with menopausal hot flashes [24, 25, 27]. However, race was significantly associated with experiencing hot flashes over time [24]. Specifically, black women were more likely to have hot flashes over a longer duration (in years) when compared to white women; however, white women had a significantly earlier peak of hot flashes severity compared to black women [24].

Cigarette smoking and hot flashes

At baseline, both current and former cigarette smoking were significantly associated with increased odds of hot flashes outcomes, independent of estradiol levels [27]. Similarly, in the longitudinal analysis, cigarette smoking was significantly associated with a longer mean duration (in years) of hot flashes during the study period [24].

The association between quitting cigarette smoking over time and hot flashes was further examined in the MWHS [26]. Findings from the MWHS were suggestive for a differential effect of cigarette smoking on hot flashes outcomes. Specifically, women who quit smoking for more than 5 years were less likely to suffer from hot flashes (any, severe, or frequent) compared to women who continued smoking; however, they remained at higher risk for having any, severe, and frequent hot flashes compared to women who never smoked cigarettes [26].

Alcohol consumption and hot flashes

At baseline, higher alcohol consumption was associated with decreased odds of menopausal hot flashes [25]. In the longitudinal analysis, women who consumed at least 12 drinks in the previous year had significantly shorter hot flash duration and shorter mean time to peak severity (in years) compared to women who consumed less than 12 drinks in the previous year [24].

Sexual activity and hot flashes

When comparing the frequency of hot flashes and sexual activity, women with less frequent hot flashes (weekly) were more likely to be sexually active than those with more frequent hot flashes (daily). These results were independent from having a partner [30].

Phthalate metabolite levels and hot flashes

The association between levels of urinary phthalates and the risk of menopausal hot flashes was statistically analyzed using baseline data from a subset of participants as described above [28]. The results indicated that levels of phthalate metabolites commonly found in personal care products were positively associated with an increased risk of ever experiencing hot flashes, hot flashes in the past 30 days, and more frequent hot flashes [28].

Findings independent of hot flashes

Given the detailed nature of the MWHS questionnaire, investigators were able to examine a variety of outcomes other than hot flashes. The key findings from some of these analyses are described below.

Ovarian volume

These analyses were based on data collected at baseline and the fourth year of the MWHS. Results indicated that a significant reduction in ovarian volume was associated with older age and later stage of the menopausal transition [29]. Additionally, ovarian volume was found to be significantly and positively associated with estradiol levels in the entire cohort and when stratified by race [29]. In contrast, progesterone levels were significantly and positively associated with ovarian volume only among white women [29]. Lastly, BMI, alcohol intake, and cigarette smoking were not associated with ovarian volume at baseline or at the fourth year of the study. These results were observed for the entire cohort and when stratified by baseline menopausal status [29].

Age at menarche and midlife obesity

An analysis of baseline MWHS data showed that age at menarche was significantly associated with midlife obesity, independent of testosterone and estradiol concentrations in adulthood [41]. Other variables significantly associated with higher BMI and obesity were black race, perimenopausal status, lower education level, higher weight at the age of 18, and never smoking [41].

Sexual activity

Several factors were found to be positively associated with sexual activity during the menopausal transition. Such factors included higher estradiol levels, higher income, heavy physical work, and better mental condition (i.e., less depressed, less fatigue, and less irritable) [30]. In contrast, some variables such as alcohol consumption, race, testosterone levels, and the amount of smoking cigarettes were not significantly associated with any of the sexual activity outcomes [30].

Discussion

The MWHS followed midlife women over time to examine their experience of hot flashes in a detailed manner. The study design allowed for the longitudinal examination of various factors (e.g., race, BMI, hormone levels) that were shown to be associated with hot flashes in cross-sectional studies. It also allowed for the examination of factors that could not be assessed in cross-sectional studies (e.g., hot flashes peak severity, quitting cigarette smoking). Overall, the results from the MWHS, as well as others, strongly suggest that menopausal symptoms are likely multi-factorial [42, 43].

Some of the longitudinal results of the MWHS are consistent with those reported in other longitudinal studies. Specifically, the MWHS study showed that menopausal hot flashes were significantly associated with age, menopausal stage, education level, race, some hormonal changes, and cigarette smoking [24]. Similarly, the Study of Women's health Across the Nation (SWAN) showed that education level, age, race, smoking cigarettes, and hormone levels were associated with menopausal hot flashes [6, 45]. The Penn Ovarian Aging Study showed that race, menopausal stage, hormone levels, education level, and smoking cigarettes were associated with menopausal hot flashes [44, 46]. The Australian Longitudinal Study on Women's Health showed that education levels and menopausal stage were associated with menopausal hot flashes [47]. Lastly, the Norwegian Hordaland Women's Cohort Study showed that education levels and smoking status were associated with hot flashes [48]. A unique contribution of the MWHS is the observation that some personal interventions such as quitting smoking may be beneficial in reducing the odds of hot flashes [26].

In contrast, some results from the MWHS are not in agreement with findings from other longitudinal studies and hence necessitate further investigation. For example, findings from the MWHS indicated that neither BMI change nor change in weight during the menopausal transition were associated with the risk of hot flashes [27], whereas findings from SWAN indicated that body fat gain measured by bioelectrical bio-impedance was associated with increased odds of hot flashes [49]. Differences in study design (e.g., cohorts, evaluation, collection methods) can explain some of these differences in results. For example, the cohort compositions were different with respect to their geographical location and ethnic representation. The MWHS recruited mostly white and black women from the Baltimore area [25, 45, 50], whereas SWAN [45] recruited participants from multiple locations around the United States and included a greater representation of Hispanic women compared to the MWHS. In addition, various cohort studies differ in the duration of the study. For example, the Penn Ovarian Aging Study was conducted over 16 years

(n = 255), whereas the MWHS was conducted over 7 years (n = 780). Further, some of the outcomes under study were calculated differently. In the MWHS, timing of hot flashes peak severity was calculated relative to the time that hot flashes were first experienced [24], whereas in the Penn Ovarian Aging Study, timing of peak severity was calculated relative to the timing of the final menstrual period [44].

The data from the MWHS showing that BMI was not associated with hot flashes outcomes were surprising because our previous cross-sectional study, which formed the basis for the development of the MWHS, showed that obesity was associated with increased odds of hot flashes [9, 15, 27]. The reasons for the discrepant findings between the MWHS and our previous cross-sectional study are unclear. It is possible that the perimenopausal women in the MWHS were later in perimenopause than women in our previous cross-sectional study. Although the MWHS obtained information on the participants' menopausal stage, it was not possible to know from our data how early the participants were in each stage and how this compares to other studies. Thus, we can only speculate that reported differences in the association between BMI and hot flashes among studies may be due to differences in where participants were in each stage of the menopausal transition or due to other unknown factors that were not evaluated.

The MWHS had several limitations. The results of the MWHS are generalizable to women during their natural menopausal transition, only to some degree. Recruitment was based on similarities in demographic factors between the study population and the target regions. Yet, the target area was comprised of a limited number of women of race/ethnicities other than black and white. Consequently, in the MWHS, a total of 780 women were enrolled with a dominant representation of black (32%) and white (67%) women. Hence, the MWHS has identified specific factors that may be useful in informing the hot flash experience for these two racial/ethnic groups.

Additionally, many participants were going through their menopausal transition, a period that is characterized by irregular menstrual cycles. Therefore, biological samples were not collected on a specific day or phase of the menstrual cycle. To minimize biases that occur with the collection of biological samples at random time points, the participants were asked on a yearly basis to donate samples each week during four consecutive weeks. Hormone levels of these samples were averaged for each participant over these 4 weeks for each year of participation. Lastly, during the study duration, women who reported having at least one of the initial exclusion criteria (e.g., pregnancy, taking hormone replacement therapy) were discontinued from the study. Their data were not used from the time of reporting having one of these criteria and onward. This approach was taken because the MWHS was originally designed to identify risk factors (including hormone levels) related to natural occurring hot flashes. These participants were discontinued regardless if they reported having hot flashes or not, and only a relatively small number of participants were discontinued.

The MWHS also has several notable strengths. First, the MWHS included a relatively large sample size with a fairly high retention rate over the study years. It is also one of the few studies to have collected detailed data regarding the dynamics of past and present experience of hot flashes. Although hot flashes history was self-reported, this approach is similar to what was used in other population-based studies and is a valid indicator of hot flashes that is accepted by the National Institute of Health [11, 51, 52]. Further, during the MWHS, multiple biological samples, general measurements (e.g., weight, blood pressure), and other data from the participants were collected. This allowed the examination of specific changes over the study period (e.g., change in weight, lifestyle habits) and their association with menopausal hot flashes.

Conclusion

The MWHS followed hundreds of women over several years during their menopausal transition by collecting multiple biological samples and measurements and self-reported questionnaire data. The study was designed and conducted by an experienced research team using well-established research tools. The MWHS results contribute a substantial amount of information relevant to women during their menopausal transition and clinicians who take care of these women. Some of the findings include the need to raise public awareness of changes in lifestyle habits that may alleviate menopausal hot flashes. The MWHS recently ended recruitment and data are still being analyzed. Therefore, more findings will be reported in the future.

Acknowledgements
We are grateful for all the MWHS participants that contributed their time, information, and biological samples. In addition, we thank all the staff members at the Johns Hopkins Greenspring Station clinic site and at the University of Illinois at Urbana Champaign who helped with this study.

Funding
The MWHS was supported by the National Institute on Aging (R01 AG18400) and the National Institute of Environmental Health Sciences (R01 ES026956-01A1).

Authors' contributions
All authors contributed to writing, read the manuscript, and approved the final version.

Authors' information
JAF: Study design and Principal Investigator of the MWHS study. RLS: Co-investigator, data analysis and interpretation. LG: Co-investigator, study design, data analysis. SRM: Co-investigator, collection of questionnaires and biological samples. HAZ: Co-investigator, oversight of the clinical site. AZG: Co-investigator, data analysis and interpretation, manuscript preparation.

Competing interests
The authors declare that they have no competing interests.

Author details
[1]School of Health Sciences, Massey University, Palmerston North, New Zealand. [2]Department of Pathobiology, University of Illinois, Urbana, Illinois, USA. [3]Epidemiology and Genomics Research Program, Division of Cancer Control and Population Sciences, National Cancer Institute, Bethesda, Maryland, USA. [4]Johns Hopkins University School of Medicine, Baltimore, Maryland, USA. [5]Department of Comparative Biosciences, University of Illinois, 2001 S. Lincoln Avenue, Urbana, Illinois 61802, USA.

References
1. Kronenberg F. Hot flashes: epidemiology and physiology. Ann N Y Acad Sci. 1990;592:52–86. discussion 123-133
2. Kronenberg F. Menopausal hot flashes: a review of physiology and biosociocultural perspective on methods of assessment. J Nutr. 2010; 140(7):1380S–5S.
3. Sarrel P, Portman D, Lefebvre P, Lafeuille MH, Grittner AM, Fortier J, Gravel J, Duh MS, Aupperle PM. Incremental direct and indirect costs of untreated vasomotor symptoms. Menopause. 2015;22(3):260–6.
4. Thurston RC, Blumenthal JA, Babyak MA, Sherwood A. Emotional antecedents of hot flashes during daily life. Psychosom Med. 2005;67(1):137–46.
5. Ziv-Gal A, Flaws JA. Factors that may influence the experience of hot flushes by healthy middle-aged women. J Women's Health (Larchmt). 2010;19(10): 1905–14.
6. Thurston RC, Joffe H. Vasomotor symptoms and menopause: findings from the Study of Women's Health across the Nation. Obstet Gynecol Clin N Am. 2011;38(3):489–501.
7. Avis NE, Crawford SL, Greendale G, Bromberger JT, Everson-Rose SA, Gold EB, Hess R, Joffe H, Kravitz HM, Tepper PG, Thurston RC, Study of Women's Health Across the N. Duration of menopausal vasomotor symptoms over the menopause transition. JAMA Intern Med. 2015;175(4):531–9.
8. Visvanathan K, Gallicchio L, Schilling C, Babus JK, Lewis LM, Miller SR, Zacur H, Flaws JA. Cytochrome gene polymorphisms, serum estrogens, and hot flushes in midlife women. Obstet Gynecol. 2005;106(6):1372–81.
9. Gallicchio L, Visvanathan K, Miller SR, Babus J, Lewis LM, Zacur H, Flaws JA. Body mass, estrogen levels, and hot flashes in midlife women. Am J Obstet Gynecol. 2005;193(4):1353–60.
10. Schilling C, Gallicchio L, Miller SR, Babus JK, Lewis LM, Zacur H, Flaws JA. Current alcohol use is associated with a reduced risk of hot flashes in midlife women. Alcohol Alcohol. 2005;40(6):563–8.
11. Gallicchio L, Miller SR, Visvanathan K, Lewis LM, Babus J, Zacur H, Flaws JA. Cigarette smoking, estrogen levels, and hot flashes in midlife women. Maturitas. 2006;53(2):133–43.
12. Miller SR, Gallicchio LM, Lewis LM, Babus JK, Langenberg P, Zacur HA, Flaws JA. Association between race and hot flashes in midlife women. Maturitas. 2006;54(3):260–9.
13. Schilling C, Gallicchio L, Miller SR, Langenberg P, Zacur H, Flaws JA. Genetic polymorphisms, hormone levels, and hot flashes in midlife women. Maturitas. 2007;57(2):120–31.
14. Schilling C, Gallicchio L, Miller SR, Langenberg P, Zacur H, Flaws JA. Current alcohol use, hormone levels, and hot flashes in midlife women. Fertil Steril. 2007;87(6):1483–6.
15. Schilling C, Gallicchio L, Miller SR, Langenberg P, Zacur H, Flaws JA. Relation of body mass and sex steroid hormone levels to hot flushes in a sample of mid-life women. Climacteric. 2007;10(1):27–37.

16. Romani WA, Gallicchio L, Flaws JA. The association between physical activity and hot flash severity, frequency, and duration in mid-life women. Am J Hum Biol. 2009;21(1):127–9.

17. Cochran CJ, Gallicchio L, Miller SR, Zacur H, Flaws JA. Cigarette smoking, androgen levels, and hot flushes in midlife women. Obstet Gynecol. 2008; 112(5):1037–44.

18. Brown JP, Gallicchio L, Flaws JA, Tracy JK. Relations among menopausal symptoms, sleep disturbance and depressive symptoms in midlife. Maturitas. 2009;62(2):184–9.

19. Alexander C, Cochran CJ, Gallicchio L, Miller SR, Flaws JA, Zacur H. Serum leptin levels, hormone levels, and hot flashes in midlife women. Fertil Steril. 2010;94(3):1037–43.

20. Gallicchio L, Miller SR, Zacur H, Flaws JA. Hot flashes and blood pressure in midlife women. Maturitas. 2010;65(1):69–74.

21. Nakano K, Pinnow E, Flaws JA, Sorkin JD, Gallicchio L. Reproductive history and hot flashes in perimenopausal women. J Women's Health (Larchmt). 2012;21(4):433–9.

22. Ziv-Gal A, Gallicchio L, Miller SR, Zacur HA, Flaws JA. Genetic polymorphisms in the aryl hydrocarbon receptor signaling pathway as potential risk factors of menopausal hot flashes. Am J Obstet Gynecol. 2012;207(3):202 e209–18.

23. Montasser ME, Ziv-Gal A, Brown JP, Flaws JA, Merchenthaler I. A potentially functional variant in the serotonin transporter gene is associated with premenopausal and perimenopausal hot flashes. Menopause. 2015;22(1): 108–13.

24. Smith RL, Gallicchio L, Miller SR, Zacur HA, Flaws JA. Risk factors for extended duration and timing of peak severity of hot flashes. PLoS One. 2016;11(5):e0155079.

25. Gallicchio L, Miller SR, Kiefer J, Greene T, Zacur HA, Flaws JA. Risk factors for hot flashes among women undergoing the menopausal transition: baseline results from the Midlife Women's Health Study. Menopause. 2015;22(10):1098–107.

26. Smith RL, Flaws JA, Gallicchio L. Does quitting smoking decrease the risk of midlife hot flashes? A longitudinal analysis. Maturitas. 2015;82(1):123–7.

27. Gallicchio L, Miller SR, Kiefer J, Greene T, Zacur HA, Flaws JA. Change in body mass index, weight, and hot flashes: a longitudinal analysis from the Midlife Women's Health Study. J Women's Health (Larchmt). 2014;23(3):231–7.

28. Ziv-Gal A, Gallicchio L, Chiang C, Ther SN, Miller SR, Zacur HA, Dills RL, Flaws JA. Phthalate metabolite levels and menopausal hot flashes in midlife women. Reprod Toxicol. 2016;60:76–81.

29. Gallicchio L, Miller SR, Kiefer J, Greene T, Zacur HA, Flaws JA. The associations between body mass index, smoking, and alcohol intake with ovarian volume in midlife women. J Women's Health (Larchmt). 2016;25(4):409–15.

30. Smith RL, Gallicchio L, Flaws JA. Factors affecting sexual activity in midlife women: results from the midlife health study. J Women's Health (Larchmt). 2017;26(2):103–8.

31. Hall JE. Endocrinology of the menopause. Endocrinol Metab Clin N Am. 2015;44(3):485–96.

32. Leon-Ferre RA, Majithia N, Loprinzi CL. Management of hot flashes in women with breast cancer receiving ovarian function suppression. Cancer Treat Rev. 2017;52:82–90.

33. Shen Y, Xu Q, Ren M, Feng X, Cai Y, Gao Y. Measurement of phenolic environmental estrogens in women with uterine leiomyoma. PLoS One. 2013;8(11):e79838.

34. Gallicchio L, Miller S, Zacur H, Flaws JA. Race and health-related quality of life in midlife women in Baltimore, Maryland. Maturitas. 2009;63(1):67–72.

35. Dennerstein L, Randolph J, Taffe J, Dudley E, Burger H. Hormones, mood, sexuality, and the menopausal transition. Fertil Steril. 2002;77(Suppl 4):S42–8.

36. Whiteman MK, Staropoli CA, Langenberg PW, McCarter RJ, Kjerulff KH, Flaws JA. Smoking, body mass, and hot flashes in midlife women. Obstet Gynecol. 2003;101(2):264–72.

37. Radloff LS. The CES-D scale: a self-report depression scale for research in the general population. Appl Psychol Meas. 1977;1(3):385–401.

38. Hauser R, Skakkebaek NE, Hass U, Toppari J, Juul A, Andersson AM, Kortenkamp A, Heindel JJ, Trasande L. Male reproductive disorders, diseases, and costs of exposure to endocrine-disrupting chemicals in the European Union. J Clin Endocrinol Metab. 2015;100(4):1267–77.

39. Marsee K, Woodruff TJ, Axelrad DA, Calafat AM, Swan SH. Estimated daily phthalate exposures in a population of mothers of male infants exhibiting reduced anogenital distance. Environ Health Perspect. 2006;114(6):805–9.

40. Hannon PR, Brannick KE, Wang W, Flaws JA. Mono(2-ethylhexyl) phthalate accelerates early folliculogenesis and inhibits steroidogenesis in cultured mouse whole ovaries and antral follicles. Biol Reprod. 2015;92(5):120.

41. Gallicchio L, Flaws JA, Smith RL. Age at menarche, androgen concentrations, and midlife obesity: findings from the Midlife Women's Health Study. Menopause. 2016;23(11):1182–8.

42. Baber RJ. East is east and West is west: perspectives on the menopause in Asia and The West. Climacteric. 2014;17(1):23–8.

43. Avis NE, Stellato R, Crawford S, Bromberger J, Ganz P, Cain V, Kagawa-Singer M. Is there a menopausal syndrome? Menopausal status and symptoms across racial/ethnic groups. Soc Sci Med. 2001;52(3):345–56.

44. Freeman EW, Sammel MD, Sanders RJ. Risk of long-term hot flashes after natural menopause: evidence from the Penn Ovarian Aging Study cohort. Menopause. 2014;21(9):924–32.

45. Gold EB, Colvin A, Avis N, Bromberger J, Greendale GA, Powell L, Sternfeld B, Matthews K. Longitudinal analysis of the association between vasomotor symptoms and race/ethnicity across the menopausal transition: study of women's health across the nation. Am J Public Health. 2006;96(7):1226–35.

46. Freeman EW, Sammel MD, Lin H, Gracia CR, Pien GW, Nelson DB, Sheng L. Symptoms associated with menopausal transition and reproductive hormones in midlife women. Obstet Gynecol. 2007;110(2 Pt 1):230–40.

47. Herber-Gast GC, Mishra GD, van der Schouw YT, Brown WJ, Dobson AJ. Risk factors for night sweats and hot flushes in midlife: results from a prospective cohort study. Menopause. 2013;20(9):953–9.

48. Gjelsvik B, Rosvold EO, Straand J, Dalen I, Hunskaar S. Symptom prevalence during menopause and factors associated with symptoms and menopausal age. Results from the Norwegian Hordaland Women's Cohort study. Maturitas. 2011;70(4):383–90.

49. Thurston RC, Sowers MR, Sternfeld B, Gold EB, Bromberger J, Chang Y, Joffe H, Crandall CJ, Waetjen LE, Matthews KA. Gains in body fat and vasomotor symptom reporting over the menopausal transition: the study of women's health across the nation. Am J Epidemiol. 2009;170(6):766–74.

50. Green R, Santoro N. Menopausal symptoms and ethnicity: the Study of Women's Health Across the Nation. Womens Health (Lond). 2009;5(2):127–33.

51. Freeman EW, Sammel MD, Lin H, Liu Z, Gracia CR. Duration of menopausal hot flushes and associated risk factors. Obstet Gynecol. 2011;117(5):1095–104.

52. Miller HG, Li RM. Measuring hot flashes: summary of a National Institutes of Health Workshop. Mayo Clin Proc. 2004;79(6):777–81.

4

Depressed mood during the menopausal transition: is it reproductive aging or is it life?

Ellen Sullivan Mitchell[1] and Nancy Fugate Woods[2*]

Abstract

Background: Although there has been noteworthy attention to both depressed mood symptoms and majordepressive disorder during the menopausal transition (MT), recently investigators have questioned whether there is an over-pathologizing of the MT by emphasizing hormonal effects on depression and deflecting attention from the everyday conditions of women's lives as they relate to depressed mood. In addition, fluctuation of mood over short periods of time may not be captured by measures of depressed mood symptoms such as the CESD, especially when administered using a reference period such as a week or more. The purpose of this study was to examine the association of menopausal transition factors, health-related factors, stress factors, social factors and symptoms with repeated measures of depressed mood reported for a 24 h period.

Methods: Seattle Midlife Women's Health Study participants ($n = 291$, 6977 observations) provided data from 1990 to 2013 including annual questionnaires, symptom diaries and urine specimens assayed for hormones several times per year. Multilevel modeling was used to test bivariate and multivariable models accounting for depressed mood severity.

Results: In individual models with age as the measure of time, being in early postmenopause, exercising more, and being partnered were associated with less severe depressed mood; greater perceived stress, having a history of sexual abuse, difficulty getting to sleep, early awakening, and awakening at night were each associated with higher depressed mood severity. In a multivariable model ($n = 234$, 6766 observations), being older, being in the early postmenopause, exercising more, being partnered, were associated with less severe depressed mood; reporting greater perceived stress, history of sexual abuse, difficulty getting to sleep and early awakening were associated with more severe depressed mood.

Conclusions: Clinicians need to consider the context in which midlife women experience the menopausal transition and mood symptoms as well as hormonal transitions during this part of the lifespan.

Keywords: Depressed mood, Menopausal transition stages, Early postmenopause, Urinary estrone, Health-related factors, Stress factors, Social factors, Abuse history, Sleep disruption symptoms

Background

Gender differences in reports of depressed mood, as well as episodes of major depressive disorder, have prompted investigators to examine periods of biological variability in women's lives, such as phases of the menstrual cycle, pregnancy and postpartum, and the menopausal transition (MT), as windows of vulnerability [1, 2]. Progress in understanding stages of reproductive aging has provided a framework for understanding biological variability during the menopausal transition and early postmenopause as related to depression and depressed mood [3–7]

Longitudinal studies of community-based cohorts experiencing transitions of reproductive aging, including the Melbourne Midlife Women's Health Project (MMWHP) [8], the Study of Women's Health Across the Nation SWAN) [9], the Penn Ovarian Aging Study (POAS) [10], and the Seattle Midlife Women's Health Study (SMWHS) [11] included data on a variety of measures of depressed

* Correspondence: nfwoods@uw.edu
[2]Biobehavioral Nursing and Health Informatics, University of Washington, Seattle, USA
Full list of author information is available at the end of the article

mood symptoms from multi-ethnic community-based cohorts of women studied annually (some more frequently) for 20 years or longer. These studies have revealed a pattern of increasing depressed mood symptoms during the menopausal transition. Massachusetts Women's Health Study investigators had documented an increase in depressive symptoms, measured by the Center for Epidemiologic Studies Depression Scale (CES-D), especially among women who experienced a lengthy MT [12]. SWAN investigators found that dysphoric mood symptoms, measured by 4 mood symptoms, increased during early MT [13]. The Harvard Study of Moods and Cycles investigators found an elevated odds ratio (2.5) of experiencing depressive symptoms (CES-D) during the MT vs premenopause (late reproductive stage) [14] and POAS investigators reported elevated odds ratios of 1.5 to 5.4, depending on women's past history of depression [15, 16]. In addition, evidence supports a decrease in negative mood as women transition to early postmenopause. MMWHP investigators found an improvement in negative mood, measured by 10 negative adjectives, during the late MT stage and a decrease in negative mood as women progressed to PM [17]. POAS investigators found that reaching the final menstrual period (FMP) played a pivotal role in reduced prevalence of depressive symptoms (CES-D) [18].

Patterns of increasing incidence of major depressive disorder mirror those of depressed mood symptoms. SWAN investigators studying major depressive disorder found an increase in prevalence of new depression during the MT and early PM [19, 20].

Given the relationship seen between reproductive aging stages and depressed mood, it is tempting to attribute this association to hormonal changes. Investigations of the relationship of estrogen, testosterone, DHEAS, inhibin B, LH and FSH levels and variability to depressed mood have yielded a lack of definitive conclusions, likely attributable to variability in the endocrine measures, their timing and frequency, variability in the depressed mood measure and various analytic strategies used to assess hormone effects [21]. Nonetheless, there is some evidence implicating some hormones: POAS investigators found evidence for effects of increased levels of estradiol, FSH, decreased levels of inhibin B and LH, and greater estradiol, LH, and FSH variability on depressive symptoms (CES-D) [16, 17]. SWAN investigators found effects of both testosterone levels and their increase during the MT on depressive symptoms, but no associations between FSH or estradiol levels and their changing levels with depressive symptoms or with major depressive disorder [22, 23]. MMWHP investigators found declining estradiol levels were associated with depressive symptoms in a sample of women studied primarily during the PM [24].

The SMWHS team analyzed factors influencing depressive symptoms measured annually with the CES-D, finding no significant relationships with urinary estrone,

FSH, testosterone, or cortisol [25, 26]. Instead, depressive symptoms were a function of age (being younger) and being in late MT stage when the severity of depressive symptoms increased. Hot flashes, life stress, family history of depression, history of postpartum blues, sexual abuse history, BMI, and use of antidepressants were also related to depressive symptoms. Age at entry into and duration of late MT stage were unrelated to depressive symptoms. These findings suggest that factors accounting for depressive symptoms earlier in the life span, as well as contemporary stressors, influenced depressive mood symptoms during the MT.

Although there has been noteworthy attention to both depressed mood symptoms and major depressive disorder during the MT, recently investigators have questioned whether there is an over-pathologizing of the MT by emphasizing hormonal effects on depression and deflecting attention from the everyday conditions of women's lives as they relate to depressed mood [27]. In addition, fluctuation of mood over short periods of time may not be captured by measures of depressed mood symptoms such as the CESD, especially when administered using a reference period such as a week or more. Indeed, investigators have recently used ecological momentary assessment, a data capture technique involving repeated sampling made close in time to the experience in naturalistic environments [28]. Moore and colleagues found that among adults 65 years of age and older, sensitivity to change of the same symptoms of depressed mood, anxiety, and mindfulness varied across two different assessment methods: ecological momentary assessment (EMA) and traditional paper and pencil measures. Indeed, results indicated greater sensitivity of the ecological momentary assessment measures of depression, anxiety, and mindfulness in response to a mindfulness-based stress response intervention than a control intervention when the same symptoms were reported using the same items administered by EMA and by paper and pencil measures with a one week reference period.

The SMWHS team had obtained a single symptom measure of depressed mood, defined as an emotional state experienced over the past 24 h (reference period was today), on multiple occasions throughout multiple years of the study. Overnight urine samples were provided on the same day as the depressed mood rating and assayed for a variety of endocrine measures (e.g. urinary estrone-3-glucuronide (E1G)) [25]. The purpose of the analyses reported here was to test a longitudinal model of the effects of MT factors (menopausal transition stages, estrone, FSH), health-related factors (alcohol use, BMI, amount of exercise), stress factors (perceived stress, history of sexual abuse), social factors (partner status, number of live births), and symptoms (hot flashes and sleep symptoms) on depressed mood severity reported for a 24 h period. (See Fig. 1). We hypothesized that depressed mood would be positively related to perceived stress, history of sexual abuse, hot flashes, sleep symptoms, BMI, alcohol use, and FSH levels, and negatively related to age, being in the early postmenopausal stage, estrone levels, amount of exercise, being partnered, and number of live births.

Methods
Design
The data for these analyses are from a longitudinal study of the MT, the Seattle Midlife Women's Health Study (SMWHS), described in greater detail elsewhere [29]. Women entered the cohort between 1990 and early 1992 when most were not yet in the MT or were in the early stages of the transition to menopause. Eligibility for the parent study included ages 35–55, at least one ovary, a period within the previous 12 months, not pregnant or lactating and able to speak and read English. Screening all households within selected multi-ethnic neighborhoods in Seattle (11,222 households) yielded 820 women eligible for the study and 508 were able to participate in an interview during the recruitment window. After completing an initial in-person interview (n = 508) administered by a trained Registered Nurse interviewer, participants (n = 390) began providing data annually by questionnaire, menstrual calendar, and health diary. The health diary included a symptom checklist that included depressed mood and other symptoms, as well as indicators of health behaviors and stress. Diary data were obtained on days 5, 6 and 7 of the menstrual cycle and a first morning voided urine specimens was collected on day 6. The women provided urine specimens 8 to 12 times per year for endocrine assays (from late 1996 through 2000), and then quarterly for 2001–2005. These data were in addition to an annual health questionnaire and menstrual calendars.

Sample
Eligible participants for this study (N = 291) were those who contributed ratings of depressed mood severity from the health diaries beginning in 1990 and were in either the late reproductive, early or late MT stages, or within 5 years from FMP at data collection during the course of the study. Women not eligible for this study either did not keep a daily diary or were not able to be classified into one of the eligible stages due to hormone use, inadequate calendar data, hysterectomy, chemotherapy or radiation therapy.

Women eligible for inclusion had a mean age of 41.5 (SD = 4.3) years at the beginning of the study, 15.9 years of education (SD = 2.8), and a median family income of $38,200 (SD = $15,000). Most (87%) were currently employed, 71% married or partnered, 22% divorced or separated or widowed, and 7% never married or partnered. They described their racial/ethnic identity as African American (7%), Asian American (9%), and White (82%). Women included in these analyses were similar with respect to employment status, marital status, and age to those who were ineligible. The only significant differences between those who were included and those who were not were higher incomes, greater likelihood to be White, and more years of education than those in the study. (See Table 1). Data obtained on any occasion when the woman was using hormones were excluded.

Measures
Measures used in these analyses include: age; MT-related factors (MT stages, urinary estrone and urinary FSH); health-related factors (BMI, alcohol use and amount of exercise); stress factors (perceived stress and history of sexual abuse), social factors (number of live births and partner status), symptoms (hot flash severity and sleep symptoms) and depressed mood severity.

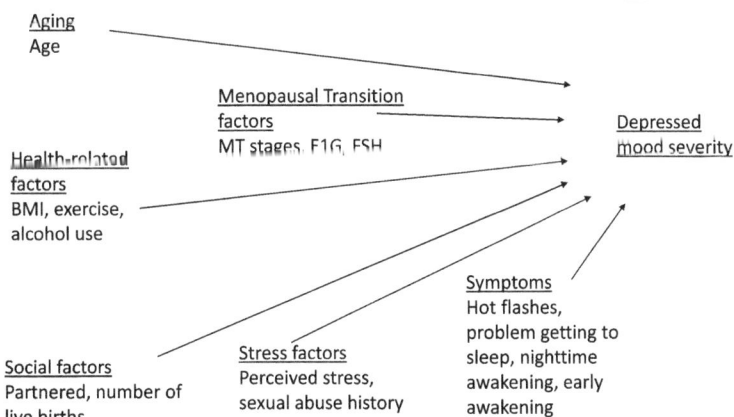

Fig. 1 Factors influencing depressed mood severity during the menopausal transition and early postmenopause

Table 1 Sample characteristics at start of study (1990–1991) of the eligible and ineligible women in the mixed effects modeling analyses of depressed mood severity

Characteristic	Eligible Women (n = 291) Mean (SD)	Ineligible Women (n = 217) Mean (SD)	p value*
Age (years)	41.5 (4.3)	42.0 (5.0)	0.18
Years of education	15.9 (2.8)	15.3 (3.0)	0.03
Family income ($)	38,200 (15,000)	35,200 (17,600)	0.04
BMI wt kg/ht. m^2)	25.3 (5.4)	27.1 (7.2)	0.002
Exercise (min/week)	187.8 (286.9)	179.0 (368.5)	0.76
Characteristic	N (Percent)	N (Percent)	p value**
Currently employed			0.42
Yes	254 (87.3)	184 (84.8)	
No	37 (12.7)	33 (15.2)	
Race/ethnicity			0.001
African American	20 (6.9)	38 (17.5)	
Asian /Pacific Islander	27 (9.3)	16 (7.4)	
White	238 (81.8)	153 (70.5)	
Other (Hispanic, Mixed)	6 (2.1)	10 (4.6)	
Marital Status			0.20
Married/partnered	278 (71.1)	141 (65.0)	
Divorced/widowed/not partnered	63 (21.7)	62 (28.6)	
Never married/ partnered	21 (7.2)	14 (6.5)	
Alcohol Use			0.001
Yes	264	174	
No	26	42	

*Independent t-test
**Chi-square test

Depressed mood severity

Depressed mood severity was assessed in the health diary using one item that asked women to rate the severity of their feeling "depressed/sad or blue" on a scale where 1 indicated not present, 2 mild, 3 moderate and 4 extreme. The reference period was for "today". This single item has been validated in the PROMIS measures [30–32].

Menopausal transition-related factors

Menopausal transition-related factors included MT stages as well as urinary estrone glucuronide and FSH. Using menstrual calendar data, women not taking any type of estrogen or progestin were classified according to stages of reproductive aging: late reproductive, early MT, late MT, or early PM, based on staging criteria developed by Mitchell, Woods and Mariella [11] and validated by the Re-STAGE collaboration [3–5]. The names of stages match

those recommended at the Stages of Reproductive Aging Workshop (STRAW) [6]. The time before the onset of persistent menstrual irregularity during midlife was labeled the late reproductive stage when cycles were regular. Early stage was defined as persistent irregularity of 7 or more days absolute difference between any two consecutive menstrual cycles during the calendar year, with no skipped periods. Late stage was defined as persistent skipping of one or more menstrual periods. A skipped period was defined as 60 or more consecutive days of amenorrhea during the calendar year [3–5]. Persistence means the event, an irregular cycle or skipped period, reoccurred one or more times in the subsequent 12 months. Onset of early MT stage was the date of Day 1 for the bleeding segment when the irregularity criterion was first met. Onset of late stage was the date of Day 1 of the first bleeding segment with skipping. Final menstrual period was identified retrospectively after one year of amenorrhea without any known explanation. The first day of the FMP is synonymous with the term menopause and was used to determine age of onset of FMP. Early PM refers to the years within five years of the FMP.

Urinary assays

Urinary assays were performed in our laboratories using a first-voided morning urine specimen provided on day 6 of the menstrual cycle, if menstrual periods were identifiable. For women with no bleeding or spotting or extremely erratic flow, a consistent date each month was used. Women abstained from smoking, caffeine use, and exercise before the urine collection. All assays were adjusted for urinary creatinine which was assayed in urine specimens using the method of Jaffe [33]. More assay details are reported elsewhere [34].

Urinary estrone glucuronide (E$_1$G)

Urinary estrone glucuronide (E$_1$G) was selected to assess estrogens because it is stable, can be reliably measured without special preparation, and is highly correlated with serum estradiol levels [35–40]. Urinary E$_1$G was measured by a competitive enzyme immunoassay (EIA) that cross-reacts 83% with estradiol glucuronide and less than 10% with free estrone, estrone sulfate, estriol glucuronide, estradiol and estriol [35]. The assay is described in detail elsewhere [41].

Urinary FSH

Urinary FSH was assayed using Diagnostic Products Corporation (DPC) Double Antibody FSH Kit, using a radioimmunoassay (RIA) was designed for the quantitative measurement of FSH in serum and urine [42]. The procedure is described in detail elsewhere [41].

Health-related factors

Health-related factors included women's use of alcohol, amount of exercise and BMI. Women were asked to indicate in the daily health diary whether or not they drank alcohol on that day (coded as 0 for no and 1 for yes). They estimated their exercise in response to the question: how many total minutes of non-work related exercise did you do today? (walking, running, biking, swimming, aerobics, sports, work out, gardening, yard work). In addition, height and weight were reported annually from which the BMI was calculated (wtkg/htm^2).

Stress factors

Stress factors included perceived stress and history of sexual abuse. Perceived stress was assessed in the diary with a question "how stressful was your day?" that women rated from 1 (not at all) to 6 (extremely, a lot). Brantley, Waggoner, Jones, & Rappaport found that a global stress rating and the sum of stress ratings across multiple dimensions correlated significantly ($r = .35$, $p < .01$) [43] Sexual abuse history was assessed by asking "Have you ever been sexually assaulted, abused, or molested?" These data were obtained in 1999–2002. Also, beginning in 1996 and through the end of the study, women were asked "during the past year did you experience any sexual abuse or sexual assault?" A cumulative variable was created to represent any history of sexual abuse or assault and coded as 1 for yes and 0 for no at each data point.

Social factors

Number of live births and partner status were assessed yearly from two items in the annual health questionnaire as were income and employment status. Race/ethnicity was established by self-report at beginning of the study.

Symptoms

Hot flashes severity and sleep symptoms were assessed in the diary with single items that women rated from 0, not present to 4, extreme. Sleep symptoms included difficulty getting to sleep, awakening during the night, and early morning awakening.

Analyses

To determine which covariates in the conceptual model (Fig. 1) had a significant effect when examined individually, bivariable mixed effects modeling was used. Finally, to test the multivariable model to determine which predictors had a significant effect on depressed mood severity over time, those individual variables from the bivariate analyses with a significance of $p \leq 0.1$ were entered together in a multivariable mixed effects model [42–47].

Before testing the conceptual model, an initial series of statistical models tested age alone as a predictor of depressed mood severity to learn whether a random intercept, fixed slope model or a random intercept, random slope model was the best fit. It was first postulated that overall levels of depressed mood severity would differ from woman to woman (random intercept), but the scores would change with age in a common manner (fixed slope). The second statistical model extended the first to postulate that each woman had a different mean level of depressed mood severity and rate of change (random intercept, random slope). The best fitting model (fixed slope or random slope) was determined by using the maximum likelihood estimation with Akaike Information Criterion (AIC) [48].

Using the best fitting model, individual covariates were added iteratively to test the effect on depressed mood severity over time. Because these analyses were for exploration and to stimulate further mechanistic studies, a p value of ≤ 0.10 was used as the criterion of significance for the univariate model and ≤ 0.05 for the final model. Different numbers of women and observations occurred with each covariate tested because the analysis required pairing observations of the outcome and predictor variables at each time point. In all analyses, age was centered at the group mean to enable the interpretation of the effect of age on depressed mood severity.

Results

Participants whose data were included in these analyses reported moderate levels of symptoms, with awakening during the night and problems getting to sleep, depressed mood, early awakening, and hot flashes in decreasing order of average severity. There were large standard deviations. Also 34% of these participants reported a history of sexual abuse. (See Table 2).

With age as a measure of time, a random intercept, random slope model was used to test separately each covariate in the model for effect on depressed mood. Being in the early PM was significantly and negatively associated with depressed mood as was reporting a higher amount of exercise. In addition, perception of stress, history of sexual abuse, and each of the three sleep symptoms were associated with an increase in depressed mood. Being partnered was negatively associated with depressed mood. Age, estrone and FSH levels, BMI, alcohol intake, number of live births, and hot flash severity were not associated significantly with depressed mood. (See Table 3).

When the significant factors ($p \leq 0.1$) from the univariate analysis listed above were included in a multivariate model, perceived stress, history of sexual abuse, problem getting to sleep, and early awakening significantly predicted an increase in depressed mood while increased age, being in the early postmenopause, greater amount of exercise and being partnered were associated with a decrease in depressed mood. (See Table 4).

Discussion

In a multivariable model, depressed mood severity reported for a 24 h period was not associated with age, MT markers (reproductive aging stages, levels of estrone or FSH), or symptoms of hot flashes or awakening at night. Instead, factors reflecting the context of women's lives, including perceived stress, history of sexual abuse, being partnered, amount of exercise, and sleep symptoms (early awakening, problem getting to sleep), were associated with severity of depressed mood.

In the analyses presented here, depressed mood severity reported for a 24 h period was not related to any of the MT markers. Although prior research has provided limited evidence linking endocrine changes and the MT stages to depressive symptoms and also to episodes of major depressive disorder among women with no prior history of depression, Freeman's recent review concluded that the contribution of the changing endocrine milieu to the development of depressive symptoms was small [21]. She reminded us that only a minority of women experience debilitating depressive symptoms during this part of the lifespan and that hormonal change is not the only factor to consider in disentangling the complex pathways to depression.

There was not a significant relationship between hot flashes and depressed mood over the past 24 h in the diary-based data reported here. In contrast, Freeman's review [21] indicated that although the association between hot flashes and depressive symptoms predominantly measured with the CES-D was confirmed, the direction of the relationship was unclear and evidence for a relationship between hot flashes and major

Table 2 Sample characteristics at start of study (1990–1991) of the eligible women in the mixed effects modeling analyses of depressed mood severity

Characteristic	Eligible Women
	Mean (SD)
Depressed mood severity (0–4)	0.41 (0.63)
Hot flashes (0–4)	0.11 (0.41)
Problem getting to sleep (0–4)	0.32 (0.67)
Awakening during the night (0–4)	0.57 (0.87)
Early morning awakening (0–4)	0.34 (0.66)
Perceived stress (1–6)	2.77 (1.09)
Characteristic	N (Percent)
History of sexual abuse (N = 233)	
Yes	80 (34%)
No	153 (66%)

depressive disorder was much less clear. Although hot flashes predicted negative mood on the next day in SWAN daily diary data, negative mood did not predict hot flashes on the subsequent day [49]. On the other hand, studies evaluating the risk of women with high levels of depressive symptoms (CES-D) indicated that depressive symptoms were likely to precede hot flashes among women who had not experienced either type of symptoms earlier in life [50, 51]. Women with consistently high levels of depressive symptoms in the SMWHS (CES-D) were more likely to experience hot flashes than those without more severe depressive symptoms [50]. Among POAS participants, 24% without high depressive symptoms (CES-D) or hot flashes at baseline reported depressive symptoms before reporting hot flashes over a 10 year follow up period, but only 8% reported hot flashes before reporting depressive symptoms [51].

Sleep symptoms and depressed mood co-occur frequently among midlife women. Indeed, use of poor sleep as one indicator of clinical depression makes it difficult to determine whether there is a causal relationship between the two symptoms. Awakening during the night was the only sleep symptom significantly related to MT stages in the SMWHS [52], but in the analyses reported here, both trouble getting to sleep and early awakening were associated with depressed mood over the past 24 h, while awakening during the night was not. Self-reported difficulty sleeping was associated with next-day negative mood in SWAN participants [49]. Burleson and colleagues tracked midlife women over 36 weeks during which they experienced the highest weekly frequency of vasomotor symptoms. They found that sleep problems occurring on one day predicted next-day negative mood (mean of 8 negative adjectives) more robustly than did vasomotor symptoms [53].

In a review of studies of sleep and the MT, Shaver [54] concluded that although the MT is associated with poor sleep beyond that anticipated with aging, perceptions of sleep are likely to be influenced by an emotional overlay on symptom reporting. Depressed mood and poor sleep are likely to be related in bidirectional ways [55]. Thus attention to mood as a factor contributing to sleep problems as well as sleep problems contributing to mood experiences is warranted. Induced poor sleep has been associated with more negative mood, but effects of improved sleep on mood during the MT remain to be examined. Induced poor sleep has been associated with more negative mood, but effects of improved sleep on mood during the MT remain to be examined. To date, a single clinical trial of cognitive behavioral therapy for insomnia delivered by telephone to women who were experiencing the menopausal transition or early postmenopause revealed that the treatment effect, when compared to a menopause education control, had the

Table 3 Random effects models for depressed mood severity with age as predictor (β_2) and with individual covariates (β_3)

Predictor	Mean Values (p values)			Standard Deviations			Number	
	β_1^a	β_2^a	β_3^a	σ_1^b	σ_2^b	σ_ϵ^b	Women	Observations
Age (47.7)	0.51	<0.001 (0.84)	–	0.49	0.03	0.60	291	6977
Menopausal Transition Factors								
MT-stage	0.52 (<.001)	0.005 (0.25)		0.49	0.03	0.60	291	6977
Early			0.02 (0.56)					
Late			−0.006 (0.88)					
Early PM			−0.10 (0.05)					
Estrone (1.3)	0.62 (<.001)	−0.01 (0.04)	−0.03 (0.32)	0.50	0.04	0.60	131	4908
FSH (1.1)	0.58 (<.001)	−0.01 (0.04)	−0.02 (0.23)	0.50	0.04	.060	131	4996
Health-related factors								
BMI (26.0)	0.37 (<.001)	<0.001 (0.97)	0.005 (0.20)	0.49	0.03	0.60	291	6977
If drinks alcohol	0.51 (<.001)	<0.001 (0.84)	−0.001 (0.97)	0.49	0.03	0.60	291	6977
Amount of exercise	0.54 (<.001)	0.001 (0.69)	−0.001 (<.001)	0.49	0.03	0.60	291	6977
Social factors								
If partnered	0.58 (<.001)	<0.001 (0.87)	−0.11 (0.002)	0.49	0.03	0.60	291	6977
Number of live births	0.51 (<.001)	<0.001 (0.83)	−0.002 (0.93)	0.49	0.03	0.60	291	6977
Stress								
Perceived Stress	0.06 (0.10)	0.008 (0.02)	0.18 (<.001)	0.47	0.03	0.58	291	6977
History of sexual abuse	0.42 (<.001)	<0.001 (0.82)	0.25 (<.001)	0.47	0.03	0.60	234	6766
Symptoms								
Hot flashes	0.50 (<.001)	<0.001 (0.88)	0.003 (0.78)	0.49	0.03	0.60	291	6977
Problem getting to sleep	0.42 (<.001)	−0.0003 (0.91)	0.24 (<.001)	0.44	0.03	0.59	291	6977
Early awakening	0.44 (<.001)	−0.003 (0.41)	0.13 (<.001)	0.47	0.03	0.59	291	6977
Awaken at Night	0.43 (<.001)	−0.002 (0.50)	0.11 (<.001)	0.47	.03	0.59	291	6977

[a] β_1, β_2, β_3 are the fixed effects (group averages) for the intercept, slope and covariate
[b] σ_1, σ_2, σ_ϵ are the random effects (variability) for the intercept, slope and residual error

greatest treatment effects on hot flashes for women who had higher depression scores at baseline. Further analyses examining treatment effects on depressed mood are in process (McCurry, personal communication).

Perceived stress and stressful life events during MT have been associated with depressed mood in other cohorts [14, 23, 56]. SWAN investigators studied women's experiences of stressful and very stressful life events. Using a scale of 18 items women rated as most stressful, they found that women in the MT experiencing two or more very stressful life events since the last study visit (usually a one year period) reported the highest depressive mood score [23]. More recently Gordon and colleagues found that reports of very stressful life events experienced by women in the MT during the six months before study baseline were associated with depressive symptoms (CES-D) over a year later [56]. Very stressful life events included only the following six events: divorce or separation from a partner, serious illness or death of a close family member or close friend, a major worsening in one's financial status or major chronic financial

problems, being physically attacked or having one's life threatened, being sexually abused or assaulted, and being arrested for a serious crime or having a mate or close relative arrested for a serious crime [57]. Gordon and colleagues proposed that estradiol variability may have enhanced emotional sensitivity to these very stressful events that influenced depressed mood in this sample of midlife women 45–60 years of age [56, 58, 59].

The experience of sexual abuse has been included among very stressful life events in earlier studies and also associated with depressive symptoms in an earlier SMWHS investigation using the CES-D [25] as well as in the analyses of reports of depressed mood severity reported here. Sexual abuse history has not been associated with depressed mood in other cohorts of women during the MT. Nonetheless, Allsworth and colleagues found that history of sexual abuse or physical violence was associated with the timing of the MT [60] and violence history with high FSH and low estradiol during the perimenopause (MT), suggesting a plausible relationship of sexual abuse to endocrine perturbation [61].

Table 4 Final random effects model for depressed mood (diary) with age as predictor and significant psychosocial and hormonal covariates entered simultaneously ($N = 234$; Observations = 6766)

	Beta Coefficient	Standard Error/ Standard Deviation	p value
Fixed effects			
β_1 intercept	0.05	0.05	0.34
β_2 Age (-47.7) years	0.01	0.004	0.02
β_3 Menopausal Transition Stage			
Early Stage	0.02	0.03	0.57
Late Stage	-0.01	0.04	0.77
Early PM	-0.10	0.05	0.03
B_4 Perceived Stress	0.16	0.008	<.001
B_5 History sexual abuse	0.18	0.06	0.002
B_6 Amount exercise	$-<0.001$	0.0002	0.004
B_7 Problem getting to sleep	0.19	0.01	<.001
B_8 Early Awakening	0.05	0.01	<.001
B_9 Awakening at night	0.02	0.01	0.09
B_{10} If partnered	-0.11	0.03	0.001
Random effects			
b_1 Intercept σ_1		0.39	
b_2 Age (-47.7) years σ_2		0.02	
b_ε residual σ_ε		0.57	

Factors that protect women from experiences of depressed mood include those considered part of one's health promotion practices, such as engaging in physical activity and being in positive relationships. Sternfield and colleagues found that midlife women participating in an exercise trial experienced less severe depressive symptoms than controls when measured by PHQ-8 [62]. Being in a relationship with a partner may serve as either a risk or protective factor depending on the nature of the relationship [25, 63]. In analyses reported here, being partnered had protective effects on depressive symptoms. It is likely that the nature of the relationship influences the experience of depressed mood: SWAN participants who reported stressful relationships with partners were likely to experience more depressive symptoms [63].

Limitations of this study include relatively small numbers of women who provided urine specimens for hormonal assays ($N = 131$) compensated for in part by the intensive measurement on multiple occasions, yielding over 4,900 data points. SWAN provided data from a larger number of women from multiple sites in the US with annual measures for most variables, including a daily hormone study involving nearly 1,000 women. In addition, the proportion of women in SMWHS with low levels of education and income and a low proportion of women of color limit our ability to generalize the results broadly. SWAN and the POAS included a much more representative population of women.

Conclusions

In conclusion, given the frequent and coincident measures of depressed mood and endocrine levels available for our analyses, it is likely that estrone and FSH did not play a major role in depressed mood severity reported for the same 24 h period. Nonetheless, others have found relationships when analyses were focused on the MT stages or endocrine values and when using measures of MDD or more severe depressive symptoms such as those included in the CES-D and a longer reference period. In addition, the results reported here afforded an examination of the relationships among depressed mood, urinary estrone and FSH levels, and perceived stress, hot flashes and sleep symptoms obtained for the same 24 h time period as recorded in a health diary, conditions that have not been available to many other investigators. We conclude that it is important for clinicians to consider the relationship of depressed mood to everyday life, even during the MT when it is tempting to attribute depressed mood to endocrine variability. These findings bear replication in larger populations of women and those in which ethnic/racial variability is maximized.

Abbreviations
FMP: final menstrual period; FSH: follicle-stimulating hormone; MT: menopausal transition; PM: Postmenopause; SMWHS: Seattle Midlife Women's Health Study; STRAW: Staging Reproductive Aging Workshop

Funding
National Institute of Nursing Research R01-NR 04141; NINR P30 NR 04001; University of Washington Research Intramural Funding Program.

Authors' contributions
NFW and ESM both contributed to writing the manuscript and both authors read and approved the final manuscript.

Authors' information
NFW and ESM: Study design and principal investigator of the Seattle Midlife Women's Health Study. Over the course of the entire study NFW and ESM rotated roles as principal investigator.

Competing interests
The authors declare they have no competing interests.

Author details
[1]Family and Child Nursing, University of Washington, Seattle, USA.
[2]Biobehavioral Nursing and Health Informatics, University of Washington, Seattle, USA.

References
1. Pratt LA, Brody DJ. Depression in the U. S. household population, 2009–2012. NCHS Data Brief. 2014;172:1–8.
2. Deecher D, Andree TH, Sloan D, Schechter LE. From menarche to menopause: exploring the underlying biology of depression in women experiencing hormonal changes. Psychoneuro. 2008;33:3–17.
3. Harlow SD, Cain K, Crawford S, Dennerstein L, Little R, Mitchell ES, Nan B, Randolph JF Jr, Taffe J, Yosef M. Evaluation of four proposed bleeding criteria for the onset of late menopausal transition. J Clin Endocrinol Metab. 2006;91:3432–8.
4. Harlow SD, Mitchell ES, Crawford S, Nan B, Little R, Taffe J, ReSTAGE Collaboration. The ReSTAGE collaboration: defining optimal bleeding criteria for onset of early menopausal transition. Fertil Steril. 2008;89:129–40.
5. Harlow SD, Crawford S, Dennerstein L, Burger HG, Mitchell ES, Sowers MF, ReSTAGE Collaboration. Recommendations from a multi-study evaluation of proposed criteria for staging reproductive aging. Climacteric. 2007;10:112–9.
6. Soules MR, Sherman S, Parrott E, Rebar R, Santoro N, Utian W, Woods NF. Executive summary: stages of reproductive aging workshop (STRAW). Fertil Steril. 2001;76:874–8.
7. Harlow SD, Gass M, Hall JE, Lobo R, Maki P, Rebar RW, Sherman S, Sluss PM, de Villiers TJ. Executive summary of STRAW+10: addressing the unfinished agenda of staging reproductive aging. Climacteric. 2012;15:105–14.
8. Dennerstein L, Dudley EC, Hopper JL, Guthrie JR, Burger HG. A prospective population-based study of menopausal symptoms. Obstet Gynecol. 2000;96:351–8.
9. Sowers M, Crawford S, Sternfeld B, Morganstein D, Gold E, Greendale G, Evans D, Neer R, Matthews K, Sherman S, Lo A, Weiss G, Kelsye J. SWAN: a multicenter, multiethnic community-based cohort study of women and the menopausal transition. In: Lobo R, Kelsey J, Marcus R, editors. Menopause: biology and pathobiology. San Diego: Academic Press; 2000. p. 175–88.
10. Freeman EW, Sammel MD, Lin H, Gracia ER, Pien GW, Nelson DB, Sheng L. Symptoms associated with menopausal transition and reproductive hormones in midlife women. Obstet Gynecol. 2007;110:230–40.
11. Mitchell ES, Woods NF, Mariella A. Three stages of the menopausal transition from the Seattle midlife Women's health study: toward a more precise definition. Menopause. 2000;7:334–49.
12. Avis NE, Brambilla D, McKinlay SM, Vass K. A longitudinal analysis of the association between menopause and depression. Ann Epidemiol. 1994;4:214–20.
13. Bromberger JT, Assmann SF, Avis NE, et al. Persistent mood symptoms in a multiethnic community cohort of pre-and perimenopausal women. Am J Epidemiol. 2003;158(4):347–56.
14. Soares CN, Almeida OP. Depression during the perimenopause. Arch Gen Psychiatry. 2001;58:306.
15. Freeman EW, Sammel MD, Liu L, Gracia CR, Nelson DB, Hollander L. Hormones and menopausal status as predictors of depression in women in transition to menopause. Arch Gen Psychiatry. 2004;61:62–70.
16. Freeman EW, Sammel MD, Lin H, Nelson DB. Associations of hormones and menopausal status with depressed in mood in women with no history of depression. Arch Gen Psychiatry. 2006;63:375–82.
17. Dennerstein L, Guthrie JR, Clark M, Leher P, Henderson VW. A population-based study of depressed mood in middle-aged, Australian-born women. Menopause. 2004;11:563–8.
18. Freeman EW, Sammel MD, Boorman DW, Zhang R. Longitudinal pattern of depressive symptoms around natural menopause. JAMA Psychiatr. 2014;71:36–43.
19. Bromberger JT, Kravitz HM, Chang YF, Cyranowski JM, Brown C, Matthews KA, et al. Major depression during and after the menopausal transition: Study of Women's Health Across the Nation (SWAN). Psychol Med. 2011;41:1879–88.
20. Bromberger JT, Kravitz HM, Matthews K, Youk A, Brown C, Feng W, et al. Predictors of first lifetime episodes of major depression in midlife women. Psychol Med. 2009;39:55–64.
21. Freeman EW. Depression in the menopause transition: risks in the changing hormone milieu as observed in the general population. Women's Midlife Health. 2015;1:2. https://doi.org/10.1186/s40695-015-002-y.
22. Bromberger JT, Schott LL, Kravitz HM, Sowers M, Avis NE, Gold EB, et al. Longitudinal change in reproductive hormones and depressive symptoms across the menpausal transition: results from the study of Women's health across the nation (SWAN). Arch Gen Psychiatry. 2010;67:598–607.
23. Bromberger JT, Matthews KA, Schott LL, Brockwell S, Avis NE, Kravitz HM, et al. Depressive symptoms during the menopausal transition: the study of Women's health across the nation (SWAN). J Affect Disord. 2007;103:267–72.
24. Ryan J, Burger HG, Szoeke C, Lehert P, Ancelin ML, Henderson VW, et al. A prospective study of the association between endogenous hormones and depressive symptoms in postmenopausal women. Menopause. 2009;16:509–17.
25. Woods NF, Smith-DiJulio K, Percival DB, Tao EY, Mariella A, Mitchell ES. Depressed mood during the menopausal transition and early postmenopause: observations from the Seattle midlife Women's health study. Menopause. 2008;15:223–32.
26. Woods NF, Smith-DiJulio K, Percival DB, Tao EY, Taylor HJ, Mitchell ES. Symptoms during the menopausal transition and early postmenopause and their relation to endocrine levels over time: observations from the Seattle midlife Women's health study. J Women's Health. 2007;110:230–40.
27. Judd FK, Hickey M, Bryant C. Depression and midlife: are we overpathologising the menopause? J Affect Disord. 2012;136:199–211.
28. Moore R, Depp CA, Wetherell JL, Lenze E. Ecological momentary assessment versus standard assessment instruments for measuring mindfulness, depressed mood, and anxiety among older adults. J Psychiatr Res. 2016;75:116–23.
29. Woods NF, Mitchell ES. The Seattle midlife Women's health study: a longitudinal prospective study of women during the menopausal transition and early postmenopause. Women's Midlife Health. 2016;2:6. https://doi.org/10.1186/s40695-016-0019-x.
30. Bjorner J, Rose M, Gandek B, Stone A, Junghaenel D, Ware JJ. Difference in method of administration did not significantly impact item response: an IRT-based analysis from the patient-reported outcomes measurement information system (PROMIS) initiative. Qual Life Res. 2013;23:212–27.
31. Cella D, Yount S, Rothrock N, Gershon R, Cook K, Reeve B, et al. The Patient-Reported Outcomes Measurement Informatino System (PROMIS): progress of an NIH Roadmap cooperative group during its first two years. Med Care. 2007;45:S3e11.
32. Reeve B, Hays RD, Bjorner JB, Cook KF, Crane PK, Teresi JA, et al. Psychometric evelation and calibration of health-related quality of life item banks: plans for the Patient-Reported Outcomes Measurement Informatino System (PROMIS). Med Care. 2007;45:S22e31.
33. Taussky HH. A microcolorimetric determination of creatinine in urine by the Jaffe reaction. J Biol Chem. 1954;208:853–61.
34. Woods NF, Smith-DiJulio K, Percival DB, Tao EY, Taylor HJ, Mitchell ES. Symptoms during the menopausal transition and early post menopause and their relation to endocrine levels over time: observations from the Seattle midlife Women's health study. J Women's Health. 2007;16:667–77.
35. Denari JH, Farinati Z, Casas PR, Oliva A. Determination of ovarian function using first morning urine steroid assays. Obstet Gynecol. 1981;58:5–9.
36. Stanczyk FZ, Miyakawa I, Goebelsmann U. Direct radioimmunoassay of urinary estrogen and pregnanediol glucuronides during the menstrual cycle. Am J Obstet Gynecol. 1980;137:443–50.
37. O'Connor KA, Brindle E, Holman DJ, Klein NA, Soules MR, Campbell KL, Kohen F, Munro CJ, Shofer JB, Lasley BL, Woods JW. Urinary estrone conjugate and pregnanediol 3-glucuronide enzyme immunoassays for population research. Clin Chem. 2003;49:1139–48.

38. Baker TE, Jennison KIM, Kellie AE. The direct radioimmunoassay of oestrogen glucuronides in human female urine. Biochem J. 1979;177:729–38.

39. Ferrell RJ, O'Connor KA, Holman DJ. Monitoring the transition to menopause in a five year prospective study: aggregate and individual changes in steroid hormones and menstrual cycle lengths with age. Menopause. 2005;12:567–77.

40. O'Connor KA, Brindle E, Shofer JB, Miller RC, Klein NA, Soules MR, Campbell KL, Mar C, Handcock MS. Statistical correction for non-parallelism in a urinary enzyme immunoassay. J Immunoass Immunochem. 2004;25:259–78.

41. Woods NF, Mitchell ES. Pathways to depressed mood for midlife women: observations from the Seattle midlife Women's health study. Res Nurs Health. 1997;20:119–29.

42. Qui Q, Overstreet JW, Todd H, Nakajima ST, Steward DR, Lasley BL. Total urinary follicle stimulating hormone as a biomarker for detection of early pregnancy and peri implantation spontaneous abortion. Environ Health Perspect. 1997;105:862–6.

43. Brantley PJ, Waggoner CD, Jones GN, Rappaport NB. A daily stress inventory: development, reliability, and validity. J Behav Med. 1987;10:61–74.

44. Pinheiro J, Bates D, DebRoy S, Sarkar D, R Core Team. nlme: Linear and nonlinear mixed effects models, R package version 3.1. 2107:1–131. https://CRAN.R-project.org/package=nlme.

45. R Development Core Team. R: A Language and Environment for statistical computing. Vienna: R Foundation for Statistical Computing; 2005. http://www.R-project.org.

46. Sarkar D. Lattice: multivariate data visualization with R. http://lattice.r-forge.r-project.org/.

47. Pinheiro J, Bates D. Mixed-effects models in S and S-PLUS. NY: Springer; 2000.

48. Hox J. Multilevel analysis: techniques and applications. Mahwah: Lawrence Erlbaum Associates; 2002.

49. Gibson CJ, Thurston RC, Bromberger JT, Kamarck T, Matthews KA. Negative affect and vasomotor symptoms in the study of Women's health across the nation daily hormone study. Menopause. 2011;18:1270–7.

50. Woods NF, Mitchell ES. Patterns of depressed mood in midlife women: observations from the Seattle midlife Women's health study. Res Nurs Health. 1996;19:11–123.

51. Freeman EW, Sammel MD, Lin H. Tempral association of hot flashes and depression in the transition to menopause. Menopause. 2009;16:728–34.

52. Woods N, Mitchell ES. Sleep symptoms during the menopausal transition and early menopause: observations from the Seattle midlife Women's health study. Sleep. 2010;33(4):539–49.

53. Burleson MH, Todd M, Trevathan WR. Daily vasomotor symptoms, sleep problems, and mood: using daily data to evaluate the domino hypothesis in middle-aged women. Menopause. 2010;17:87–95.

54. Shaver JL, Woods NF. Sleep and menopause: a narrative review. Menopause. 2015;22:899–915.

55. Kahn M, Sheppes G, Sadeh A. Sleep and emotions: bidirectional links and underlying mechanisms. Int J Psychophysiol. 2013;89:218–28.

56. Gordon JL, Rubinow DR, Eisenlohr-Moul TA, Leserman J, Girdler SS. Estradiol variability, stressful life events, and the emergence of depressive symptomatology during the menopausal transition. Menopause. 2016;23:257–66.

57. Mugavero MJ, Raper JL, Reif S, Whetten K, Leserman J, Thielman NM, Pence BW. Overload: impact of incident stressful events on antiretroviral medication adherence and virologic failure in a longitudinal, multisite human immunodeficiency virus cohort study. Psychosom Med. 2009;71:920–6.

58. Woods NF, Mitchell ES, Percival DB, Smith-DiJulio K. Is the menopausal transition stressful? Observations of perceived stress from the Seattle midlife Women's health study. Menopause. 2009;16(1):90–7.

59. Freeman WE, Sammel MD, Boorman DW, Zhang R. Longitudinal pattern of depressive symptoms around natural menopause. JAMA Psychiatry. 2014;71:36–43.

60. Allsworth JE, Zierler S, Krieger N, Harlow BL. Ovarian function in late reproductive years in relation to lifetime experiences of abuse. Epidemiology. 2001;12(6):676–81.

61. Allsworth JE, Zierler S, Lapane KKL, Krieger N, Hogan JW, Harlow BL. Longitudinal study of the inception of perimenopasue in relation to lifetime history of sexual or physical violence. J Epidemiol Community Health. 2004;58:938–43.

62. Sternfeld B, Guthrie KA, Ensrud KE, et al. Efficacy of exercise for menopausal symptoms: a randomized controlled trial. Menopause. 2014;21:330–8. PMCID: PMC3353828

63. Lanza di Scalea T, Matthews KA, Avis NE, Thurston RC, Brown C, Harlow S, Bromberger JT. Role stress, role reward, and mental health in a multiethnic sample of midlife women: results from the study of Women's health across the nation (SWAN). J Women's Health (Larchmt). 2012;21(5):481–9.

5

Perceived stress across the midlife: longitudinal changes among a diverse sample of women, the Study of Women's health Across the Nation (SWAN)

Elizabeth Hedgeman[1]* , Rebecca E. Hasson[2], Carrie A. Karvonen-Gutierrez[1], William H. Herman[3] and Siobán D. Harlow[1]

Abstract

Background: In women, midlife is a period of social and physiological change. Ostensibly stressful, cross-sectional studies suggest women experience decreasing stress perceptions and increasing positive outlook during this life stage. The aim of this paper was to describe the longitudinal changes in perceived stress as women transitioned through the midlife.

Methods: Premenopausal women ($n = 3044$) ages 42–52 years at baseline, were recruited from seven sites in the Study of Women's Health Across the Nation, and followed approximately annually over 13 visits with assessment of perceived stress and change in menopausal status. Longitudinal regression models were used to assess the effects of age, menopausal status and baseline sociodemographic variables on the trajectory of perceived stress over time.

Results: At baseline, mean age was 46.4 ± 2.7 years; participants were white (47%), black (29%), Hispanic (7%), Japanese (9%), or Chinese (8%). Hispanic women, women with lesser educational attainment, and women reporting financial hardship were each more likely to report high perceived stress levels at baseline (all $p < 0.0001$). After adjustment for baseline sociodemographic factors, perceived stress decreased over time for most women ($p < 0.0001$), but increased for both Hispanic and white participants at the New Jersey site ($p < 0.0001$). Changing menopausal status was not a significant predictor of perceived stress.

Conclusions: Self-reported stress decreased for most women as they transitioned across the midlife; changing menopausal status did not play a significant role after adjustment for age and sociodemographic factors. Future studies should explore the stress experience for women by racial / ethnic identity and demographics.

Keywords: Women's health, Stress, Minority health/disparities/SES, Aging, Menopausal transition, Epidemiology

Background

The midlife, bounded by young adulthood and old age, has heretofore received only limited scientific attention. Modern social scientists place the beginning of midlife at 35 or 40 years of age, to highlight the period when most adults have finished schooling, entered the workforce, and embarked into marriage with childbearing and rearing [1] – a period of "life past the initial putting together [2]." Clinically this life phase coincides with the age at which chronic conditions begin to appear, an age that can vary by cultural and sociodemographic identity [3]. When asked themselves, adults cite midlife as beginning anywhere from 35 to 45 and ending around 55–60 years of age [2, 4, 5].

For modern women 40–65 years of age, these middle years are marked by the potential for profound social and physiological changes [6]. Households are changing, with children leaving and "boomerang" children returning [7, 8]. Aging parents may require more care as their health and functioning decline. Workplace stress may

* Correspondence: ehedgeman@gmail.com; hedgeman@umich.edu
[1]Department of Epidemiology, School of Public Health, University of Michigan, 6610B SPH I, 1415 Washington Heights, Ann Arbor, MI 48109-2029, USA
Full list of author information is available at the end of the article

increase with the attainment of seniority, additional job strain, and concomitantly increasing time demands [9, 10]. The menopausal transition – a period beginning in the early forties, marking reproductive senescence, changing estrogen levels, and ultimate cessation of the menstrual cycle – can bring vasomotor and genitourinary symptoms, disrupted sleep cycles and mood changes [2, 11–14]. Though the 'midlife crisis' has been largely debunked [15], the midlife years appear to be a period ripe for stress. Previous work has demonstrated that positive affect – a measure of positive mood and outlook – was significantly lower in midlife women (ages 35–64 years in 1995–1996) as compared to younger and older women, with relationship stress and occupational stress found to be strong drivers of the observed dissatisfaction [16, 17].

And yet, perhaps contrary to expectation, research suggests that perceived stress – a self-reported, subjective measure of individual control and coping – decreases, and quality of life increases, through midlife in some populations. Among nearly 14,000 women ages 40–55 years, contacted in 1994 for the Study of Women's Health Across the Nation (SWAN) cross-sectional screening study, increased age was positively associated with quality of life for white and black women, though not for Chinese, Hispanic or Japanese women [18]. Similar cross-sectional results from the first wave of the Midlife Development in the United States (MIDUS; 1995–1996) study suggest that overall quality of life reaches a nadir in the late 30s to early 40s, only to increase through the remaining midlife and beyond [19]. Cross-sectional studies from both the United States (1983) and United Kingdom (circa 2006) suggest that levels of perceived stress decrease over the entire lifespan for all race / ethnicities [20, 21]. Corresponding with these cross-sectional findings of lower stress perception with age, the longitudinal Melbourne Women's Midlife Health Project of Australian-born midlife women (ages 45–55 in 1991) found that negative moods – feelings of tension, confusion, helplessness, loneliness, insignificance – decreased significantly over the 11 years of follow-up [22]. However, missing from this literature is a longitudinal assessment of perceived stress, particularly across the midlife.

The aim of this study was to describe the longitudinal reports of perceived stress as women transitioned through the midlife in the SWAN cohort. Specific hypotheses, based on the findings from prior research, were that perceived stress (i) would decrease over time for some, but not all women, due to differing racial / ethnic experiences of aging, and (ii) would increase as women progressed through perimenopause, but generally decrease with age. Socioeconomic factors were included in models as modifying factors expected to influence perceived stress. Secondary data were obtained from this large, sociodemographically diverse cohort of women, with individual perceived stress assessed at multiple points over 15 years and 13 visits. Potential differences in the experience of perceived stress by race / ethnicity, adjusted for socioeconomic status, and whether stress profiles were influenced by stage of the menopausal transition, considered a key biological hallmark of this lifestage, were assessed for longitudinal differences over time.

Methods

Study population

A full description of the Study of Women's Health Across the Nation (SWAN) longitudinal cohort and methodology has been published in detail elsewhere [23]. Briefly, SWAN was instituted in 1996 as an observational cohort study of women, their lifestyles, and their health through the menopausal transition with longitudinal follow-up to determine outcomes over time. Eligibility was based on age (42–52 years), self-reported race / ethnicity, and reproductive status (not pregnant or lactating; at least one menstrual cycle in previous three months; uterus and at least one ovary intact; not taking exogenous hormones affecting ovarian function at time of enrollment). Study sites – located in Boston, Massachusetts (MA); Chicago, Illinois (IL); Southeast Michigan (MI); Los Angeles, California (CA); Newark, New Jersey (NJ); Pittsburgh, Pennsylvania (PA); and Oakland, CA – invited recruitment from white, black, Hispanic, Chinese and Japanese communities. All sites recruited white participants, four sites recruited black participants (MA, MI, IL, PA) and one site each recruited Chinese (Oakland, CA), Japanese (Los Angeles, CA) or Hispanic (NJ) participants. At baseline, the full study included 3302 women. Women were followed approximately annually for 13 visits with study participation at 74.5% by visit 13.

For this analysis, women were excluded if they had fewer than two perceived stress scores ($n = 253$) or experienced a pregnancy ($n = 5$) over follow-up. The final analytical sample included 3044 women. Data from the NJ site were truncated at visit five due to an interruption in site operations, affecting 108 white and all 212 Hispanic women.

Variables

Age, self-reported race / ethnicity, educational attainment (less than high school, high school degree [or equivalent], college degree, post-college training) and smoking status (current smoker yes or no) were ascertained by questionnaire at baseline for all participants. Baseline financial hardship was estimated by self-report to the question: "How hard is it for you to pay for the very basics like food, housing, medical care, and heating". Available responses were 'Very Hard', 'Somewhat Hard' and 'Not very hard at all'. Baseline physical measures including height (centimeters), weight (kilograms) and lightly-clothed waist circumference (in centimeters) were assessed by trained staff during the clinic visit. Body mass index (BMI) was calculated as weight (kg) divided by height (cm) squared.

Perceived stress was self-reported at each visit using the four-item Perceived Stress Scale questionnaire (PSS4) developed and validated by Cohen et al. [20, 24]. PSS4 questions included:

1. In the past two weeks, how often have you felt you were unable to control the important things in your life?
2. In the past two weeks, how often have you felt confident about your ability to handle your personal problems?
3. In the past two weeks, how often have you felt that things were going your way?
4. In the past two weeks, how often have you felt difficulties were piling up so high that you could not overcome them?

Participants indicated the frequency they experienced each of the four stressful situations using a 5-point Likert scale (1 = never, 2 = almost never, 3 = sometimes, 4 = fairly often, 5 = very often). For scoring total perceived stress, responses to negative questions were summed with the reverse of the responses to positive questions, yielding a composite score ranging from 4 to 20. Larger PSS4 scores indicated increased time experiencing stressful situations in the prior two weeks. Perceived stress questions were asked at baseline (year 0) and each follow-up visit, for a total of 13 possible measurements. The mean number of available perceived stress scores per woman was 10.2 (median: 12, range: 2–13); 15.6% had five or fewer perceived stress scores.

Menopausal status was assessed at each visit based on participant's report of menstrual irregularity [25] or complete cessation of cycles, plus self-reported information on hysterectomy and / or oophorectomy and current hormone use. Menopausal status was coded as premenopausal (menses has occurred in previous 3 months with no change in predictability over past 12 months), early perimenopausal (menses has occurred in previous 3 months, but with less predictability), late perimenopausal (menses has occurred in previous 12 months, but without menses in previous 3 months) or postmenopausal (no menses in past 12 months and / or both ovaries removed). Unknown menopausal status due to hormone use or hysterectomy was collapsed into a single 'unknown' category.

Statistical analysis

Baseline descriptive information was compared for all participants and by baseline reported perceived stress level (categorized as low [≤ 25th percentile], moderate, high [≥ 75 percentile]). Women without a baseline PSS score ($n = 86$) were not included in analyses focused on stress at baseline, but were included in the longitudinal models of perceived stress. Logistic regression, adjusting for age, was used to assess the association of sociodemographic variables with high (versus low + moderate) perceived stress at baseline. To assess for potential bias due to selective loss of participants reporting higher baseline perceived stress, linear regression, adjusting for age, was used to test the difference in baseline perceived stress by loss to follow-up status over the 13 visits.

To guide modeling, change in mean perceived stress was first explored graphically by age, stratified by selected sociodemographic variables expected to contribute to perceived stress (race / ethnicity, educational attainment, baseline financial hardship, site of recruitment). For graphing crude means, age was truncated at 65 years (55 years for Hispanic women) to prevent leverage in slope estimation due to cohort attrition and the smaller numbers of women at the upper tail of the age distribution.

A linear mixed model was examined to understand the contribution of sociodemographic variables and menopausal status to change in perceived stress over time. Variables of interest were first reviewed individually for their effects on perceived stress. Model building was performed sequentially, using a forward stepwise approach, with statistical significance of added variables assessed by variable significance and model fit tested by Likelihood Ratio with alpha set to 0.05. Appropriateness of random effects in models were tested using restricted maximum likelihood and mixed effects were tested using maximum likelihood. An unstructured variance-covariate matrix was assumed. All models incorporated race / ethnicity and age, centered at 42 years, as a time-varying variable and included a random slope for age. Potential interactions of longitudinal age with sociodemographic variables were evaluated to assess differences in slope. Additional interactions with race / ethnicity and socio-economic variables were assessed in separate models, but small cell sizes resulted in model instability.

Final models were assessed for appropriate specification by review of the errors from the random effects (age) as well as the conditional errors for the fixed effects. All errors were assessed for normality graphically. All graphing and statistics were performed using SAS version 9.4 (SAS Institute, Cary, NC).

Results

Baseline characteristics

At baseline, the 3044 women eligible for this analysis were a mean age of 46.4 years (range: 42.0–53.0 years) with a racial / ethnic distribution of 47.4% white, 28.7% black, 8.9% Japanese, 8.0% Chinese and 7.0% Hispanic (Table 1). The majority of the cohort (> 90%) had obtained at least a high school degree while 44.1% had attained a college degree or higher. Financial difficulty was reported by nearly 40% of women, with 8.7% reporting that it was 'very hard' to pay for the basics of living. Among the 2958 women reporting perceived stress at baseline, mean perceived stress score was 8.5 (median: 8.0, range: 4–19). Characteristics of 86 women without a baseline perceived stress score are available in Additional file 1: Table S1.

At baseline, Hispanic women were significantly more likely to report high perceived stress as compared to any other race / ethnicity (all comparisons $p < 0.0001$), while Chinese women were significantly less likely to report high stress ($p < 0.0001$ for white, black and Hispanic women, $p = 0.0185$ for Japanese women) (Table 1). Women reporting higher levels of financial hardship were more likely to report high perceived stress than

Table 1 Population characteristics by baseline perceived stress score

| | N | Overall (n = 3044) | Category of Baseline Perceived Stress[a][b] | | |
			Low (n = 844)	Moderate (n = 1352)	High (n = 762)
Perceived Stress[c]	2958	8.5 ± 2.9	5.1 ± 0.8	8.5 ± 1.1	12.4 ± 1.5
Age[c]	3044	46.4 ± 2.7	46.3 ± 2.7	46.4 ± 2.7	46.2 ± 2.7
Race / Ethnicity (%)					
White	1443	–	29.1	48.1	22.8
Black	874	–	32.3	39.0	28.7
Hispanic	212	–	18.0	31.0	51.0
Japanese	272	–	22.7	54.6	22.7
Chinese	243	–	26.3	59.4	14.3
Education (%)					
Less than High School	191	–	15.4	35.1	49.5
High School	1496	–	26.6	44.0	29.3
College Degree	627	–	30.0	48.5	21.5
Post-College	705	–	34.5	49.9	15.6
Difficulty paying for Basics (%)					
Very Hard	263	–	10.0	38.6	51.4
Somewhat Hard	899	–	17.4	44.2	38.5
Not hard	1865	–	36.5	47.3	16.2
Site of Recruitment (%)					
PA	439	–	29.9	42.8	27.3
MI	503	–	30.7	40.0	29.3
MA	424	–	25.1	51.6	23.4
IL	433	–	34.4	41.8	23.8
Oakland, CA	442	–	27.1	54.9	18.1
Los Angeles, CA	483	–	30.4	50.7	18.9
NJ	320	–	18.7	36.0	45.3
Smoking Status (%)					
Non-Smoker	2522	–	29.0	47.6	23.4
Smoker	498	–	26.6	36.5	36.9
BMI (kg/m^2)[c]	3009	28.2 ± 7.2	27.9 ± 6.8	27.9 ± 7.1	29.3 ± 7.8
Waist Circumference (cm)[c]	3012	86.1 ± 16.1	85.4 ± 15.6	85.6 ± 15.7	88.7 ± 17.2

[a]Categorical variable *rows* sum to 100%. Numbers may not sum to 100 due to rounding
[b]Note that 86 women had missing baseline PSS4 scores
[c]Mean ± SD

women reporting some or no financial hardship (p = 0.0003 and < 0.0001, respectively); and women without a high school diploma were significantly more likely to report high perceived stress than women with a high school diploma, college or other advanced degree (all p < 0.0001). Likewise, women who were current smokers were more likely to report high levels of perceived stress as compared to women who were not (p < 0.0001), and women with increased BMI or waist circumference were also more likely to report high perceived stress (p < 0.0001 for each).

Perceived stress and increasing age

Mean cohort age increased to 62.0 years at the 13th follow-up visit while unadjusted mean perceived stress scores declined by − 0.06 ± 0.00 points with each increased year of age. No difference was seen in baseline perceived stress between women retained and those who died or were lost to follow-up (8.4 ± 2.9 vs 8.5 ± 3.0, respectively, p = 0.38). Trajectories for change in perceived stress with age are displayed in Fig. 1a-d, by race / ethnicity, educational attainment, financial hardship, and site of recruitment. Corresponding with the baseline results, women with less educational attainment, women reporting increased financial hardship and women recruited from NJ had higher mean reported levels of perceived stress than their counterparts. In addition, mean perceived stress was observed to decline with age across all sociodemographic categories with the exception of Hispanic women.

Unadjusted regressions for each variable and the final multivariable regression model evaluating the effects of age, menopausal status, race / ethnicity, educational attainment, baseline financial hardship and site of recruitment on longitudinal change in perceived stress are displayed in Table 2. In the final multivariate regression model, women reporting financial hardship and with lesser attained education reported significantly higher levels of perceived stress at baseline as compared to women reporting no financial hardship or training beyond a college degree. Only Japanese race / ethnicity remained as a statistically significant predictor of higher perceived stress after adjustment for financial hardship and educational attainment. Interactions between financial strain and age suggested that moderate and severe baseline financial hardship were associated with a steeper decline in perceived stress over time as compared to no financial hardship. Though mean reported perceived stress decreased over time for most women, for white and Hispanic women located in NJ, perceived stress increased (0.07 ± 0.03 points with each increased year of age) over the five available visits for this site. For interpretation purposes, within this cohort a 42-year-old white woman living near Pittsburgh, with a high school

diploma and no reported baseline financial hardship (the 'reference category') had a perceived stress score of 7.93, that decreased by 0.10 points over each increasing year of age. In comparison, a Japanese woman of the same age, living near Los Angeles, with a high school education and no baseline financial hardship, reported a perceived stress of 8.17 that decreased by 0.01 points each year, and a Hispanic woman of the same age, living near New Jersey, without a high school education and no baseline financial hardship had a mean perceived stress score of 8.05 that increased by 0.11 points each year.

When menopausal status was added to the final adjusted model with longitudinal age, model fit increased significantly (Likelihood Ratio p < 0.00001). Results suggested that progression through each stage of the menopausal transition (from pre-menopause onward) was associated with a further decrease in perceived stress, however the menopausal status variable did not reach statistical significance (p = 0.5203; data not shown) and thus was omitted from the final model.

Discussion

This study is one of the first to describe longitudinal change in perceived stress levels in a multi-ethnic sample of midlife women in the United States. Mean levels of self-reported stress, as measured annually by Cohen's Perceived Stress Scale, decreased for most women as they transitioned across the midlife. Compared to similar black, white and Chinese women within SWAN, mean levels of perceived stress decreased in a more attenuated fashion for Japanese women, but increased over time for white and Hispanic women living in New Jersey. In addition, women with lower educational attainment, and in particular, baseline financial hardship, consistently reported higher levels of perceived stress, though this difference diminished with time. After adjustment for other sociodemographic variables, race / ethnicity was a significant predictor of increased perceived stress for only Japanese women. Changing menopausal status did not play a significant role in change in perceived stress after adjustment for age and sociodemographic factors.

Cross-sectional studies performed both in the United States and the United Kingdom have suggested that perceived stress decreases with age. A 1983 population-based survey of adults in the United States reported a mean PSS4 of 4.9 ± 3.0 for adults ages 18−29 years, 4.4 ± 2.9 for adults ages 45−54 years and 4.0 ± 3.0 for adults ages 65 years and older using a 0−15 scale (corresponding to mean PSS4 scores of 8.9, 8.4 and 8.0, respectively, on the 4−20 scale used here) [20]. Reported perceived stress was higher among women compared to men, Hispanics and blacks as compared to whites, and increased with lower annual income and educational attainment. Similarly, a more recent cross-sectional review

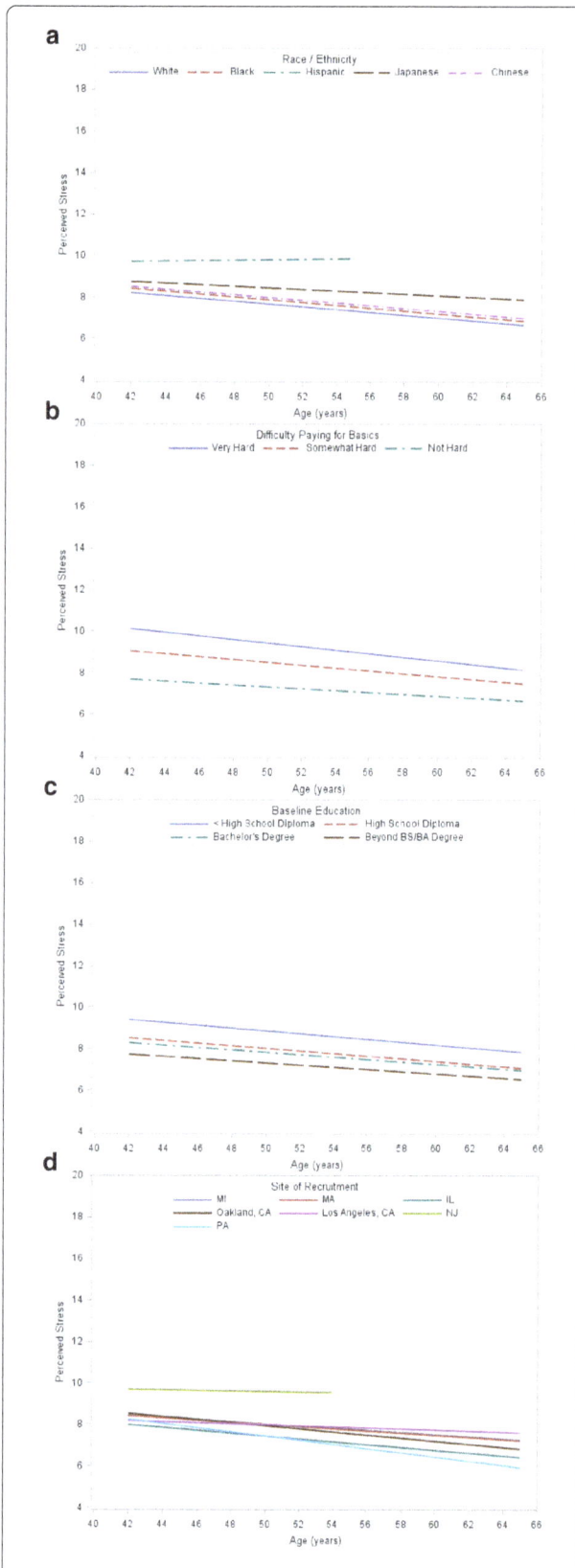

a Race / Ethnicity

b Difficulty Paying for Basics

c Baseline Education

d Site of Recruitment

of reported perceived stress from individuals ages 16–85 years living in the United Kingdom indicated that younger age, female sex, reduced social support and black, Asian (Indian, Pakistani, Bangladeshi, other) or mixed (as compared to white) race were associated with higher PSS4 scores [21].

While the unadjusted results indicated that women of non-white ethnicity or with lower socioeconomic means tended to report higher perceived stress, supporting the findings from the above referenced studies, the *adjusted* analyses presented here indicated that black women and Hispanic women reported lower perceived stress at baseline as compared to similar white, Japanese and Chinese women in SWAN. Although these differences did not reach statistical significance, our findings are in contrast to studies of SWAN participants that indicate that black women (in particular) and Chinese women report higher levels of perceived discrimination and unfair treatment than their peers, and that these reports are tied to increased biological stress reactivity and decreased mental and physical health [26–28]. This paradox – lower perceived stress reports among subgroups showing higher biological response to stressors – may be explained by a tendency for women with lower social standing to internalize and normalize stressors that are experienced frequently [29–31]. For example, Lee and Bierman found that, in older adults experiencing discrimination, decreased social status was associated with fewer outward expressions of anger, but more suppressed or internalized experiences of anger; the authors theorized that anger suppression was a coping mechanism and a method to de-escalate potentially dangerous situations [30]. These finding with the SWAN cohort are intriguing and warrant further investigation.

In further comparison to the cross-sectional studies, the work presented here indicates that there are variations in the rate of change of perceived stress in some subgroups of women and, moreover, that not all individuals experience decreases over time. The faster rate of decrease in perceived stress scores for women initially in the higher categories of baseline financial hardship may be due to alleviation of the stressor as women age into retirement [32] or may reflect acute baseline financial stressors associated with only temporary increases in perceived stress. Conversely, the results may reflect selective cohort loss over time among women reporting

Table 2 Unadjusted and fully adjusted random effects model explaining perceived stress over increasing age

	Unadjusted Parameters		Fully Adjusted Model*	
	β (95% CI)	P (Type 3)	β (95% CI)	P (Type 3)
Intercept	–	–	7.93 (7.65, 8.20)	–
Age	−0.06 (− 0.07, − 0.06)	< 0.0001	−0.10 (− 0.12, − 0.08)	< 0.0001
Race / Ethnicity		< 0.0001		< 0.0001
White	REF		REF	
Black	0.16 (−0.02, 0.35)		−0.06 (− 0.26, 0.14)	
Hispanic	2.06 (1.73, 2.39)		−0.33 (− 0.86, 0.20)	
Japanese	0.71 (0.43, 0.99)		0.84 (0.47, 1.21)	
Chinese	0.31 (0.01, 0.61)		0.28 (−0.11, 0.67)	
Difficulty paying for Basics (%)		< 0.0001		< 0.0001
Not hard	REF		REF	
Somewhat Hard	1.26 (1.09, 1.43)		1.28 (1.06, 1.51)	
Very Hard	2.20 (1.92, 2.48)		2.37 (2.00, 2.74)	
Education		< 0.0001		0.0016
Less than High School	1.37 (1.03, 1.71)		0.34 (−0.02, 0.69)	
High School	REF		REF	
College Degree	−0.23 (− 0.43, − 0.02)		−0.02 (− 0.22, 0.18)	
Post-College Degree	−0.79 (− 0.99, − 0.60)		−0.32 (− 0.52, − 0.12)	
Site of Recruitment		< 0.0001		0.0487
PA	REF		REF	
MI	0.67 (0.40, 0.95)		−0.20 (−0.54, 0.15)	
MA	0.59 (0.3, 0.87)		0.01 (−0.34, 0.37)	
IL	0.02 (−0.27, 0.31)		−0.04 (− 0.40, 0.32)	
Oakland, CA	0.44 (0.15, 0.72)		0.03 (−0.39, 0.44)	
Los Angeles, CA	0.61 (0.33, 0.89)		−0.59 (− 0.99, − 0.18)	
NJ	2.21 (1.89, 2.53)		0.11 (−0.47, 0.70)	
Menopausal Status		< 0.0001	–	–
Pre	REF		–	–
Early peri	−0.20 (−0.29, − 0.10)		–	–
Late peri	−0.30 (− 0.42, − 0.17)		–	–
Post	− 0.67 (− 0.76, − 0.58)		–	–
Unknown	−0.33 (− 0.47, − 0.20)		–	–
Age * Difficulty paying for Basics Interaction	–	–		< 0.0001
Age*Not hard	–	–	REF	
Age*Somewhat Hard	–	–	−0.02 (− 0.04, − 0.01)	
Age*Very Hard	–	–	− 0.05 (− 0.08, − 0.02)	
Age * Site Interaction	–	–		
Age*PA	–	–	REF	< 0.0001
Age*MI	–	–	0.08 (0.05, 0.10)	
Age*MA	–	–	0.06 (0.03, 0.08)	
Age*IL	–	–	0.02 (− 0.00, 0.05)	
Age*Oakland, CA	–	–	0.04 (0.02, 0.07)	
Age*Los Angeles, CA	–	–	0.09 (0.06, 0.11)	
Age*NJ	–	–	0.21 (0.16, 0.26)	

*The multivariate model includes all variables listed; menopausal status was not statistically significant (*p* > 0.05) in the final model higher financial hardship, although mean baseline perceived stress scores did not vary by attrition status. Curiously, while our results indicate that perceived stress decreased for all women to some varying degree as they aged across the midlife, Hispanic and white women living in or near Newark, NJ reported increasing perceived stress over the course of their five visits from baseline. Due to the interruption of activities at the NJ site, it is impossible to determine whether the observed perceived stress trajectory would have continued to increase or reverse course over the remaining 8 visits. Notably, the fifth follow-up occurred primarily in 2001/2002, and results may have been influenced by the World Trade Center bombing in September 2001 [33]. Moreover, as Hispanic women were recruited only from this site, it is impossible to disentangle the site effect from the experience of being a midlife Hispanic woman in the United States.

Our results found no increase in perceived stress associated with changing menopausal status after adjustment for aging and sociodemographic characteristics. These findings are in contrast to existing cross-sectional work and some longitudinal work suggesting that the menopausal transition is associated with higher stress and depression. Freeman et al. found that higher perceived stress was independently associated with higher menopausal symptom severity including: hot flushes, poor sleep quality, depression and general aches and stiffness [34]. Though these findings are intriguing, they excluded assessment of general socioeconomic status – obscuring the role of general life stressors during the experience of menopause [35]. More recently, when adjusting for study visit, Falconi et al. found that early and late perimenopause were significantly associated with increases in perceived stress [36], but they did not adjust for age or sociodemographic indicators. Prior publications have indicated that women who proceed through menopause at an earlier age are socioeconomically disadvantaged [37–39] and already prone to increased life stress [40]. Woods et al., in longitudinal analyses from the Seattle Midlife Women's Study, which included predominately white women but adjusted for age, found that factors such as employment and health status, but also preexisting mood disturbances, were the only significant predictors of perceived stress over a decade, and not the menopausal transition itself [41]. Our findings are consistent with Woods et al. as we found that the role of socioeconomic factors such as educational attainment, employment and financial hardship were stronger predictors of perceived stress over midlife than the menopausal transition itself in this larger, more diverse sample of midlife women. These findings may suggest that women experience the menopausal transition as a series of acute stressors (e.g., hot flashes, sleep disturbances) that

can be attenuated by chronic, socioeconomic-based life stressors, however further work would be necessary to substantiate this theory.

Explanations for the observed decreases in perceived stress with age are suggestive yet incomplete. Research suggests that older adults show more maturity and regulation of emotion [42, 43], leading to increased feelings of optimism and fewer symptoms of psychological distress than younger adults [44, 45], however the cross-sectional nature of most extant studies can not rule out a cohort effect based on era of birth. Beyond changes in the appraisal and regulation of stress, changing life roles with age, such as retirement or the relinquishment of parenting, may lead to the occurrence of fewer stressful events even as individual health may be declining [46]. Focus groups performed with women in the United States suggest that the midlife is a time of reduced childrearing responsibilities leading to role restructuring, more control over one's time, and an increased sense of personal power and freedom [47–50] – concepts embedded in Cohen's Perceived Stress Scale. Finally, recent longitudinal work performed by Lachman et al. for the Midlife in the United States (MIDUS) study shows that life satisfaction significantly increases across the midlife decades (4th to 5th, 5th to 6th decades) [5], again corresponding with the decreases in perceived stress seen in this work.

Despite the decreasing perception of stress with age, individuals who report relatively greater stress at the start of the midlife continue to report higher stress levels as they age, an important finding given that more highly stressed individuals are at greater health risk than their less-stressed peers. Arnold et al. found that high or moderate baseline perceived stress increased mortality risk for adults hospitalized with acute myocardial infarction (high/moderate vs. low PSS4 score: aHR = 1.42 [95% CI = 1.15–1.76]) [51]. Investigators for the REGARDS study found that, for individuals with household incomes < \$35,000/ yr., baseline PSS4 score was associated with all-cause mortality risk (high vs. no stress: aOR = 1.55 [95%CI: 1.31–1.82]), and marginally associated with incident coronary heart disease (high vs. no stress: aOR = 1.29 [95%CI: 0.99–1.69]) [52]. Similarly, Aggarwal et al. identified increased baseline perceived stress, as measured by a modified 'PSS6' score, to be predictive of future cerebral infarct in older adults (high vs. low PSS6 score: aOR = 1.94, 95% CI = 1.11–3.40) [53]. As individuals in lower socioeconomic and sociocultural strata are more at risk of adverse health outcomes such as diabetes, stroke and myocardial infarct [54–59], it is plausible that individual perception and internal assimilation of stress is one of many factors directly influencing health [60]. Future work will assess whether the women of SWAN who report higher perceived stress, and lower socioeconomic means, are more at risk of adverse outcomes.

The primary limitation of this study was our limited ability to understand perceived stress among women reporting the highest levels over time. Hispanic women, women reporting extreme financial hardship at baseline, and those with the least education, each comprised less than 10% of the study sample, limiting power and preventing analyses to disentangle potential interactions among these subgroups. Similarly, the disruption of operations at the NJ site, a site situated to recruit Hispanic women and women of lower socioeconomic means, prevented a complete review of change in reported perceived stress over time at that site. Only baseline financial hardship was assessed in these models as it was not measured at every follow-up visit. Fluctuating hardship levels may explain additional variability over time. It is also worth noting that we are ascribing self-reports of perceived stress over a two-week period to women's perceptions over the course of a year, ruling out a detailed assessment of stress that women may feel on a day-to-day basis. This broader view of stress, in addition to our exploration of menopausal *stages* versus menopausal *symptoms*, may have precluded the assessment of the impact of stressors that fluctuate on a daily basis, such as from vasomotor symptoms. Finally, we have chosen to review and model mean change over time, which may obscure subtle differences in trajectories of stress that are non-linear; a subject worth further exploration. Nonetheless, the analyses presented, incorporating the diverse cohort from the SWAN longitudinal study, provide important information about stress over the midlife and menopausal transition.

Conclusion

In conclusion, this study found that the perception of stress decreased over time for the majority of this diverse set of midlife women in the United States. Perceived stress increased for the Hispanic and white women recruited from New Jersey, and was consistently greater among women with lesser education attainment and women experiencing financial difficulty. Concomitant with the increased reporting of stress, those with higher stress were more likely to smoke and have higher BMIs at baseline. While we are limited to observing the change in stress over the thirteen years of study – and solely within women – our results add credence to the original surveys performed by Cohen et al. [20, 24], and provide further evidence that decreases in stress are truly age-related and not related to era of birth. Future work is necessary to further explore the stress experience for women in the United States, especially as it varies by racial / ethnic identity, but also to assess longitudinal trajectories of stress that are non-linear or unchanging over time, change with changing life roles, and to tie the observed perceived stress differences with adverse mental and clinical outcomes.

Acknowledgements

We thank all the women who participated in SWAN and the study personnel at each site.
Clinical Centers: University of Michigan, Ann Arbor – Siobán Harlow, PI 2011 – present, MaryFran Sowers, PI 1994-2011; Massachusetts General Hospital, Boston, MA – Joel Finkelstein, PI 1999 – present; Robert Neer, PI 1994 – 1999; Rush University, Rush University Medical Center, Chicago, IL – Howard Kravitz, PI 2009 – present; Lynda Powell, PI 1994 – 2009; University of California, Davis/Kaiser – Ellen Gold, PI; University of California, Los Angeles – Gail Greendale, PI; Albert Einstein College of Medicine, Bronx, NY – Carol Derby, PI 2011 – present, Rachel Wildman, PI 2010 – 2011; Nanette Santoro, PI 2004 – 2010; University of Medicine and Dentistry – New Jersey Medical School, Newark – Gerson Weiss, PI 1994 – 2004; and the University of Pittsburgh, Pittsburgh, PA – Karen Matthews, PI.
NIH Program Office: National Institute on Aging, Bethesda, MD – Chhanda Dutta 2016- present; Winifred Rossi 2012–2016; Sherry Sherman 1994 – 2012; Marcia Ory 1994 – 2001; National Institute of Nursing Research, Bethesda, MD – Program Officers.
Central Laboratory: University of Michigan, Ann Arbor – Daniel McConnell (Central Ligand Assay Satellite Services).
SWAN Repository: University of Michigan, Ann Arbor – Siobán Harlow 2013 - Present; Dan McConnell 2011 - 2013; MaryFran Sowers 2000 – 2011.
Coordinating Center: University of Pittsburgh, Pittsburgh, PA – Maria Mori Brooks, PI 2012 - present; Kim Sutton-Tyrrell, PI 2001 – 2012; New England Research Institutes, Watertown, MA - Sonja McKinlay, PI 1995 – 2001.
Steering Committee: Susan Johnson, Current Chair; Chris Gallagher, Former Chair.

Funding

The Study of Women's Health Across the Nation (SWAN) has grant support from the National Institutes of Health (NIH), DHHS, through the National Institute on Aging (NIA), the National Institute of Nursing Research (NINR) and the NIH Office of Research on Women's Health (ORWH) (Grants U01NR004061; U01AG012505, U01AG012535, U01AG012531, U01AG012539, U01AG012546, U01AG012553, U01AG012554, U01AG012495). The content of this article is solely the responsibility of the authors and does not necessarily represent the official views of the NIA, NINR, ORWH or the NIH. SDH gratefully acknowledge use of the services and facilities of the Population Studies Center at the University of Michigan, funded by NICHD Center Grant R24 HD041028.
The National Institute of Aging and National Institute of Nursing Research program officers participated in the design of the SWAN study. They were not involved in the data analysis, interpretation of data or writing of this manuscript.

Authors' contributions

EH conducted the literature review and data analyses, and had primary responsibility for the drafting the manuscript. SDH and CKG made substantial contributions to the design and oversaw the data analyses. All authors contributed to the critical review and revision of the manuscript for intellectual content. All authors read and approved the final manuscript.

Competing interests

The authors declare that they have no competing interests.

Author details
[1]Department of Epidemiology, School of Public Health, University of Michigan, 6610B SPH I, 1415 Washington Heights, Ann Arbor, MI 48109-2029, USA. [2]School of Kinesiology, School of Public Health, University of Michigan, Ann Arbor, USA. [3]Department of Internal Medicine, School of Public Health, University of Michigan, Ann Arbor, USA.

References
1. Lachman ME. Development in Midlife. Annu Rev Psychol. 2004;55:305–31.
2. Woods NF, Mitchell ES. Women's images of midlife: observations from the Seattle midlife women's health study. Health Care Women Int. 1997;18:439–53.
3. Ward BW, Schiller JS, Goodman RA. Multiple chronic conditions among US adults: a 2012 update. Prev Chronic Dis. 2014;11 https://doi.org/10.5888/pcd11.130389.
4. Brim OG, Ryff CD, Kessler RC, editors. How healthy are we?: a national study of well-being at midlife. Chicago: University of Chicago Press; 2004.
5. Lachman ME, Teshale S, Agrigoroaei S. Midlife as a pivotal period in the life course: balancing growth and decline at the crossroads of youth and old age. Int J Behav Dev. 2015;39:20–31.
6. Williams K, Kurina LM. The social structure, stress, and women's health. Clin Obstet Gynecol. 2002;45:1099–118.
7. Jacobsen L, Mather M, Dupuis G. Household change in the United States. Popul Bull. 2012;67 http://www.prb.org/Publications/Reports/2012/us-household-change.aspx. Accessed 23 Oct 2016
8. Fry R. For first time in modern era, living with parents edges out other living arrangements for 18- to 34-year-olds. Washington, D.C: Pew Research Center; 2016. http://www.pewsocialtrends.org/2016/05/24/for-first-time-in-modern-era-living-with-parents-edges-out-other-living-arrangements-for-18-to-34-year-olds/. Accessed 27 Sep 2016
9. Amick BC, Kawachi I, Coakley EH, Lerner D, Levine S, Colditz GA. Relationship of job strain and iso-strain to health status in a cohort of women in the United States. Scand J Work Environ Health. 1998;24:54–61.
10. Lundberg U, Frankenhaeuser M. Stress and workload of men and women in high-ranking positions. J Occup Health Psychol. 1999;4:142–51.
11. Woods NF, Mitchell ES. Symptoms during the perimenopause: prevalence, severity, trajectory, and significance in women's lives. Am J Med. 2005; 118(Suppl 12B):14–24.
12. Davis SR, Castelo-Branco C, Chedraui P, Lumsden MA, Nappi RE, Shah D, et al. Understanding weight gain at menopause. Climacteric J Int Menopause Soc. 2012;15:419–29.
13. Hall JE. Endocrinology of the menopause. Endocrinol Metab Clin N Am. 2015;44:485–96.
14. Santoro N, Epperson CN, Mathews SB. Menopausal symptoms and their management. Endocrinol Metab Clin N Am. 2015;44:497–515.
15. Freund AM, Ritter JO. Midlife crisis: a debate. Gerontology. 2009;55:582–91.
16. Mroczek DK, Kolarz CM. The effect of age on positive and negative affect: a developmental perspective on happiness. J Pers Soc Psychol. 1998;75:1333–49.
17. Mroczek D. Positive and negative affect at midlife. In: Brim OG, Ryff CD, Kessler RC, editors. How healthy are we?: a national study of well-being at midlife. Chicago, IL: University of Chicago Press; 2004. p. 205–26.
18. Avis NE, Assmann SF, Kravitz HM, Ganz PA, Ory M. Quality of life in diverse groups of midlife women: assessing the influence of menopause, health status and psychosocial and demographic factors. Qual Life Res Int J Qual Life Asp Treat Care Rehabil. 2004;13:933–46.
19. Fleeson W. The quality of American life at the end of the century. In: Brim O, Ryff C, Kessler R, editors. How healthy are we?: a National Study of well-being at midlife. Chicago, IL: University of Chicago Press; 2004. p. 252–72.
20. Cohen S. Perceived stress in a probability sample of the United States. In: The social psychology of health. Newbury Park, Calif: sage publications; 1988. p. 31–67.
21. Warttig SL, Forshaw MJ, South J, White AK. New, normative, English-sample data for the short form perceived stress scale (PSS-4). J Health Psychol. 2013;18:1617–28.
22. Dennerstein L, Guthrie JR, Clark M, Lehert P, Henderson VW. A population-based study of depressed mood in middle-aged. Australian-born women Menopause N Y N. 2004;11:563–8.
23. Sowers M, Crawford SL, Sternfeld B, Morganstein D, Gold E, Greendale G, et al. SWAN: a multicenter, multiethnic, community-based cohort study of women and the menopausal transition. In: Lobo RA, Kelsey JL, Marcus R, editors. Menopause: biology and pathobiology. San Diego, CA: Academic Press; 2000. p. 175–88.
24. Cohen S, Kamarck T, Mermelstein R. A global measure of perceived stress. J Health Soc Behav. 1983;24:385–96.
25. Brambilla DJ, McKinlay SM, Johannes CB. Defining the perimenopause for application in epidemiologic investigations. Am J Epidemiol. 1994;140:1091–5.
26. Guyll M, Matthews KA, Bromberger JT. Discrimination and unfair treatment: relationship to cardiovascular reactivity among African American and European American women. Health Psychol Off J Div Health Psychol Am Psychol Assoc. 2001;20:315–25.
27. Brown C, Matthews KA, Bromberger JT, Chang Y. The relation between perceived unfair treatment and blood pressure in a racially/ethnically diverse sample of women. Am J Epidemiol. 2006;164:257–62.
28. Pascoe EA, Smart Richman L. Perceived discrimination and health: a meta-analytic review. Psychol Bull. 2009;135:531–54.
29. Thomas SA, González-Prendes AA. Powerlessness, anger, and stress in African American women: implications for physical and emotional health. Health Care Women Int. 2009;30:93–113.
30. Lee Y, Bierman A. A longitudinal assessment of perceived discrimination and maladaptive expressions of anger among older adults: does subjective social power buffer the association? J Gerontol. Series B, Psychol Sci Soc Sci. 2016.
31. Krieger N. Discrimination and health inequities. Int J Health Serv Plan Adm Eval. 2014;44:643–710.
32. van der Heide I, van Rijn RM, Robroek SJ, Burdorf A, Proper KI. Is retirement good for your health? A systematic review of longitudinal studies. BMC Public Health. 2013;13 https://doi.org/10.1186/1471-2458-13-1180.
33. Silver RC, Holman EA, McIntosh DN, Poulin M, Gil-Rivas V. Nationwide longitudinal study of psychological responses to September 11. JAMA. 2002;288:1235–44.
34. Freeman EW, Sammel MD, Lin H, Gracia CR, Pien GW, Nelson DB, et al. Symptoms associated with menopausal transition and reproductive hormones in midlife women. Obstet Gynecol. 2007;110(2 Pt 1):230–40.
35. Nosek M, Kennedy HP, Beyene Y, Taylor D, Gilliss C, Lee K. The effects of perceived stress and attitudes toward menopause and aging on symptoms of menopause. J Midwifery Womens Health. 2010;55:328–34.
36. Falconi AM, Gold EB, Janssen I. The longitudinal relation of stress during the menopausal transition to fibrinogen concentrations: results from the study of Women's health across the nation. Menopause N Y N. 2016;23:518–27.
37. Stanford JL, Hartge P, Brinton LA, Hoover RN, Brookmeyer R. Factors influencing the age at natural menopause. J Chronic Dis. 1987;40:995–1002.
38. Gold EB. Factors associated with age at natural menopause in a multiethnic sample of midlife women. Am J Epidemiol. 2001;153:865–74.
39. Gold EB, Crawford SL, Avis NE, Crandall CJ, Matthews KA, Waetjen LE, et al. Factors related to age at natural menopause: longitudinal analyses from SWAN. Am J Epidemiol. 2013;178:70–83.
40. Bromberger JT, Matthews KA, Kuller LH, Wing RR, Meilahn EN, Plantinga P. Prospective study of the determinants of age at menopause. Am J Epidemiol. 1997;145:124–33.
41. Woods NF, Mitchell ES, Percival DB, Smith-DiJulio K. Is the menopausal transition stressful? Observations of perceived stress from the Seattle midlife Women's health study. Menopause N Y N. 2009;16:90–7.
42. Boeninger DK, Shiraishi RW, Aldwin CM, Spiro A. Why do older men report low stress ratings? Findings from the veterans affairs normative aging study. Int J Aging Hum Dev. 2009;68:149–70.
43. Brummer L, Stopa L, Bucks R. The influence of age on emotion regulation strategies and psychological distress. Behav Cogn Psychother. 2014;42:668–81.
44. Lawton MP, Kleban MH, Rajagopal D, Dean J. Dimensions of affective experience in three age groups. Psychol Aging. 1992;7:171–84.
45. Chang E. Optimism–pessimism and stress appraisal: testing a cognitive interactive model of psychological adjustment in adults. Cogn Ther Res. 2002;26:675–90.
46. Aldwin CM, Sutton KJ, Chiara G, Spiro A. Age differences in stress, coping, and appraisal: findings from the normative aging study. J Gerontol B Psychol Sci Soc Sci. 1996;51:P179–88.

47. Berg JA, Taylor DL. Symptom responses of midlife Filipina Americans. Menopause N Y N. 1999;6:115–21.

48. Sampselle CM, Harris V, Harlow SD, Sowers M. Midlife development and menopause in African American and Caucasian women. Health Care Women Int. 2002;23:351–63.

49. Kagawa-Singer M, Wu K, Kawanishi Y, Greendale GA, Kim S, Adler SR, et al. Comparison of the menopause and midlife transition between Japanese American and European American women. Med Anthropol Q. 2002;16:64–91.

50. Villarruel AM, Harlow SD, Lopez M, Sowers M. El cambio de Vida: conceptualizations of menopause and midlife among urban Latina women. Res Theory Nurs Pract. 2002;16:91–102.

51. Arnold SV, Smolderen KG, Buchanan DM, Li Y, Spertus JA. Perceived stress in myocardial infarction: long-term mortality and health status outcomes. J Am Coll Cardiol. 2012;60:1756–63.

52. Redmond N, Richman J, Gamboa CM, Albert MA, Sims M, Durant RW, et al. Perceived stress is associated with incident coronary heart disease and all-cause mortality in low- but not high-income participants in the reasons for geographic and racial differences in stroke study. J Am Heart Assoc. 2013;2: e000447.

53. Aggarwal NT, Clark CJ, Beck TL, Mendes de Leon CF, DeCarli C, Evans DA, et al. Perceived stress is associated with subclinical cerebrovascular disease in older adults. Am J Geriatr Psychiatry Off J Am Assoc Geriatr Psychiatry. 2014; 22:53–62.

54. Salomaa V, Niemela M, Miettinen H, Ketonen M, Immonen-Raiha P, Koskinen S, et al. Relationship of socioeconomic status to the incidence and prehospital, 28-day, and 1-year mortality rates of acute coronary events in the FINMONICA myocardial infarction register study. Circulation. 2000;101:1913–8.

55. Gerber Y, Benyamini Y, Goldbourt U, Drory Y. For the Israel study group on first acute myocardial infarction. Neighborhood socioeconomic context and long-term survival after myocardial infarction. Circulation. 2010;121:375–83.

56. Krishnan S, Cozier YC, Rosenberg L, Palmer JR. Socioeconomic status and incidence of type 2 diabetes: results from the black Women's health study. Am J Epidemiol. 2010;171:564–70.

57. Addo J, Ayerbe L, Mohan KM, Crichton S, Sheldenkar A, Chen R, et al. Socioeconomic status and stroke: an updated review. Stroke. 2012;43: 1186–91.

58. Hasson RE, Adam TC, Pearson J, Davis JN, Spruijt-Metz D, Goran MI. Sociocultural and socioeconomic influences on type 2 diabetes risk in overweight/obese African-American and Latino-American children and adolescents. J Obes. 2013; 2013:1–9.

59. Schneiderman N, Llabre M, Cowie CC, Barnhart J, Carnethon M, Gallo LC, et al. Prevalence of diabetes among Hispanics/Latinos from diverse backgrounds: the Hispanic community health study/study of Latinos (HCHS/SOL). Diabetes Care. 2014;37:2233–9.

60. Marshall IJ, Wang Y, Crichton S, McKevitt C, Rudd AG, Wolfe CDA. The effects of socioeconomic status on stroke risk and outcomes. Lancet Neurol. 2015;14: 1206–18.

6

Chronic vulvar pain in a cohort of post-menopausal women: Atrophy or Vulvodynia?

Susanna D. Mitro[1], Siobán D. Harlow[1*], John F. Randolph[2] and Barbara D. Reed[2]

Abstract

Background: Although postmenopausal vulvar pain is frequently attributed to vaginal atrophy, such symptoms may be due to vulvodynia, a chronic vulvar pain condition. Given the limited research on vulvodynia in postmenopausal women, the objective of this study was to provide preliminary population-based data on the associations of vaginal symptoms, serum hormone levels and hormone use with chronic vulvar pain in a multiethnic sample of post-menopausal women.

Methods: We used data from 371 participants at the Michigan site of the Study of Women's Health Across the Nation (SWAN) who participated in the 13th follow-up visit. Women completed a validated screening instrument for vulvodynia and provided information on additional vaginal symptoms as well as demographic characteristics, and hormone use by questionnaire. Blood samples were obtained to assess hormone levels. We compared women who screened positive for vulvodynia and women with past or short-duration vulvar pain to women without vulvar pain, using Chi-squared and Fisher's Exact tests. Relative odds ratios and 95 % confidence intervals were calculated using multinomial logistic regression models adjusting for age, body mass index, and race/ethnicity.

Results: Current chronic vulvar pain consistent with vulvodynia was reported by 4.0 % of women, while 13.7 % reported past but not current chronic vulvar pain or short-duration vulvar pain symptoms. One quarter of women who reported current chronic vulvar pain did not report vaginal dryness. Women with current chronic and with past/short duration vulvar pain symptoms were more likely to have used hormones during the preceding year than women without vulvar pain symptoms (13.3 %, 17.6 %, 2.0 %, respectively; $p < .01$). Increased relative odds of current vulvar pain symptoms were associated with each log unit decrease in serum dehydroepiandrosterone-sulfate, estradiol and testosterone levels at the previous year's visit.

Conclusion: Some women who experience chronic vulvar pain symptoms do not report vaginal dryness, and others report continued or first onset of pain while using hormones. Vulvodynia should be considered in the differential diagnosis of postmenopausal women presenting with vulvar pain symptoms.

Background

Although vulvar pain symptoms can occur at any time over the life span, it is not uncommon for symptoms to begin for the first time after menopause [1–3]. In fact, the prevalence of chronic vulvar pain in mid-life women has been estimated to be 8.9-38 % percent, making chronic vulvar pain a major health concern for women in this age group [4, 5]. However, despite recognition of

the burden of chronic vulvar pain symptoms in the mid-life, research on vulvodynia, a chronic pain condition characterized by pain in the vulva, has mainly focused on premenopausal women [1, 2].

Until recently, research on postmenopausal vulvar pain symptoms has largely focused on vaginal dryness and vulvar atrophy, secondary to estrogen deprivation. However, evidence indicates that postmenopausal vulvar pain may occur for other reasons as well [6–9]. Additionally, women with atrophy do not all experience pain [7], episodes of postmenopausal vulvar pain are not all successfully treated using estrogen therapy [8, 9], and in a

* Correspondence: harlow@umich.edu
[1]Department of Epidemiology, School of Public Health, 1415 Washington Heights, Ann Arbor, MI 48109, USA
Full list of author information is available at the end of the article

recent study serum estradiol, estrone, and progesterone levels of postmenopausal women were not tightly correlated with vulvar pain [3]. These findings suggest that some vulvar pain reported by postmenopausal women may be a condition other than atrophy, such as vulvodynia, and present independent of estrogen-or atrophy-related changes.

This paper evaluates chronic vulvar pain reported by African American and white women participating in the Michigan site of the longitudinal, multiethnic Study of Women's Health Across the Nation (SWAN). Although the sample size is limited, prospective measurements of age at final menstrual period, symptoms of vaginal dryness, and hormone therapy (HT) use, as well as serum hormone levels obtained prior to the assessment of current pain status, provide preliminary data on the estimated prevalence of chronic vulvar pain, consistent with vulvodynia in post-menopausal women and its association with hormones, HT use and vaginal dryness in this population-based sample of postmenopausal women.

Methods

This study used data from the Michigan site of SWAN, a multiethnic prospective cohort study addressing health-related changes in the midlife and menopausal transition. The cohort has been described in detail previously [10]. Briefly, in 1996, each SWAN clinic site enrolled white women and one targeted minority population. The Michigan SWAN population, established using a community census, was composed of women aged 42–52 years at baseline, who were not using exogenous hormones at the time of enrollment, had an intact uterus and at least one ovary and had had a menstrual period in the three months before enrollment, were not pregnant or lactating, and self-identified as either white or African American. At baseline and each follow-up visit a blood sample was collected, height and weight measures were taken while demographic characteristics, medication use, and symptoms of vaginal dryness were ascertained by questionnaire. Over the next 17 years women participated in follow-up visits approximately annually. At the 13th follow-up visit in 2012, the Michigan site added several screening instruments for chronic pain conditions including a validated screening instrument for vulvodynia [11].

At baseline, the Michigan SWAN cohort was composed of 543 women, 60 % of whom were African American by design. In 2012, 32 (5.9 %) women had died and 411 (80.4 % of the non-deceased cohort) were still active, 380 (92.5 %) of whom participated in follow-up Visit 13. Nine women who did not answer any questions pertaining to vulvar pain were excluded, leaving 371 womeN (61.7 % African American) eligible for this analysis. For analyses including endogenous serum hormone levels, we evaluated hormone levels at Visit 12, to ensure hormone levels preceded the report of vulvar pain status at Visit 13. These analyses include 319 women as we excluded the 37 women who did not have blood drawn and the 15 women who reported HT use at Visit 12.

Ethics and consent

This study was approved by Health Sciences and Behavioral Sciences Institutional Review Board of the University of MichigaN (HUM00083308). Women provided informed consent at baseline and each follow-up interview.

In Visit 13, Michigan participants completed a validated screening questionnaire for vulvodynia [11] that obtained information on symptoms of vulvar pain or discomfort, including date of pain onset, duration of pain, and whether pain continues. We interpret a positive screen in this postmenopausal population to be consistent with vulvodynia but acknowledge that this screening tool may not adequately differentiate vulvodynia from atrophy in this postmenopausal cohort. Therefore we use the term "chronic vulvar pain" in lieu of vulvodynia when presenting the results.

Based on responses to the vulvodynia questionnaire, each participant was categorized into one of three groups: women with current chronic (lasting 3 months or longer) vulvar pain, women who reported ever having chronic vulvar pain in the past or reported having short-duration (less than 3 months duration) vulvar pain symptoms, and women reporting no current or past vulvar pain symptoms. Current chronic vulvar pain was defined by a history of vulvar pain or discomfort at the opening to the vagina that had lasted for at least three months and had been experienced in the preceding three months. The past chronic vulvar pain/short-duration vulvar pain symptom group included women who had a history of vulvar pain lasting for at least three months but who had not experienced pain in the preceding three months and women with current vulvar pain lasting for less than three months. This group represents a heterogeneous symptomatic group who, based on prior work [12], are more likely than the non-symptomatic group to develop vulvodynia, and hence we categorize them separately from the no pain group.

Age was modeled as a continuous variable. Race/ethnicity was self-reported as either white or African American. Measured height and weight were used to calculate body mass index (BMI) (weight in kilograms (kg) divided by height in meters (m) squared). BMI was further categorized as normal weight, overweight, or obese (<25, $25\text{-} < 30$, and $> = 30$ kg/m^2). Socioeconomic status was assessed by self-reported difficulty paying for basics (very hard versus somewhat or not hard) and education at baseline (high school or less versus at least some college). Marital status was categorized as either married or not married.

In addition to questions about vulvar pain, we asked about other specific vulvovaginal symptoms at Visit 13 including self-reported number of days in the past 2 weeks of vaginal dryness, soreness, and irritation categorized into three duration levels (0 days, 1–5 days, or >6 days). In addition, we created variables to reflect whether women ever reported vaginal dryness before, and after, the final menstrual period (FMP) or hysterectomy (yes/no) based on responses at each follow-up visit. Although women were not eligible to enroll in SWAN ff they were using HT, women who began using HT after enrollment remained in the study. Two HT variables were considered: current HT use (yes/no), and ever used HT during the study (yes/no).

At each visit, a fasting blood sample was collected, refrigerated for 1–2 h after collection, and then centrifuged. Serum hormone levels of estradiol (E2), dehydro-epiandrosterone-sulfate (DHEA-S), follicle stimulating hormone (FSH), sex hormone-binding globuliN (SHBG), and testosterone (T) were determined.

All assays were performed on the ACS-180 automated analyzer (Bayer Diagnostics Corporation, Tarrytown, NY) at the CLASS laboratory at the University of Michigan, utilizing a double-antibody chemiluminescent immunoassay with a solid phase anti-IgG immunoglobulin conjugated to paramagnetic particles, anti-ligand antibody, and competitive ligand labeled with dimethylacridinium ester (DMAE). The FSH assay is a modification of a manual assay kit (Bayer Diagnostics) utilizing two monoclonal antibodies directed to different regions on the beta subunit, with a lower limit of detection (LLD) of 1.05 mIU/mL. Inter-and intra-assay coefficients of variation were 12.0 % and 6.0 %, respectively. The E2 assay modifies the rabbit anti-E2-6 ACS-180 immunoassay to increase sensitivity, with a LLD of 1.0 pg/mL and inter- and intra-assay coefficients of variation averaging 10.6 % and 6.4 %, respectively. The T assay modifies the rabbit polyclonal anti-T ACS-180 immunoassay, with a LLD of 2.19 ng/dL and inter-and intra-assay coefficients of variation of 10.5 % and 8.5 %, respectively. The DHEA-S and SHBG assays were developed using rabbit anti-DHEA-S and anti-SHBG antibodies, with LLDs of 1.52 mcg/dL and 1.95 nM, respectively. For DHEA-S, the inter- and intra-assay coefficient of variation were 11.3 % and 8.0 %, respectively. For SHBG, the inter- and intra-assay coefficient of variation were 9.9 % and 6.1 %, respectively. Duplicate E2 assays were conducted, with results reported as the arithmetic mean for each subject, with a CV of 3-12 %. All other assays were single determinations. Hormone levels below the lower limit of detection were assigned a random number between 0 and the lower limit of detection.

The prevalence of vulvar symptoms overall and stratified by demographic characteristics were calculated and compared using Chi-squared and Fisher's Exact tests as appropriate. Hormone levels were log-transformed for regression analyses. The median values of the log-transformed E2, DHEA-S, SHBG, FSH, and T at Visit 12 were compared overall and across symptoms groups using Kruskal-Wallis tests. Relative odds ratios (OR) and 95 % confidence intervals (CI) comparing the current chronic vulvar pain and past/short-duration vulvar pain groups to the no vulvar pain group were calculated using multinomial logistic regression models appropriate for outcomes with more than two categories [13]. These models compare odds for reporting current chronic vulvar pain symptoms in relation to the no pain category and odds for reporting past/short-term vulvar pain symptoms in relation to the no pain category. In addition to an unadjusted model, models adjusted for race, BMI, and age were also assessed. Analyses were performed using SAS 9.3 (Cary, NC).

Results

At follow-up Visit 13, participants ranged in age from 56 to 68 years (median 61.3 years). Of the 371 women eligible for this analysis, 15 women (4.0 %; 95 % CI: 2.5 %, 6.6 %) reported current chronic vulvar pain, 51 (13.7 %; 95 % CI: 10.6 %, 17.6 %) reported past chronic or short-duration vulvar pain, and 305 (82.2 %; 95 % CI: 78.0 %, 85.8 %) reported no vulvar pain. Of the 15 women reporting current chronic vulvar pain, one did not provide an age of symptom onset, four experienced symptom onset before age 45, two experienced onset between age 46 and 55, and the remaining 8 experienced onset between ages 56 and 64 years. Five of the 15 women reported first onset since their previous follow-up visit, representing an incidence of 1.3 %.

Median age, marital status, and proportion sexually active in the previous 6 months did not differ by chronic vulvar pain status (Table 1). However, women with current chronic vulvar pain were more likely to be white, less likely to be obese, and more likely to have completed at least some college compared to women in the other vulvar pain groups (Table 1).

Although few women reported current HT use, both the current chronic and past/short-duration vulvar pain groups were more likely than women with no vulvar pain symptoms to report having used HT during the preceding year (Table 1). Women with past/short-duration vulvar pain were more likely to have ever used HT and more likely to have had a hysterectomy than women in the other two groups (Table 1). Two of the 15 women with current symptoms (13.3 %) began HT after pain onset but did not report remission while 3 of the 32 women with current or past chronic vulvar pain

Table 1 Demographic and clinical characteristics of women in the MI SWAN population, by self-reported vulvar pain

Variable	Total N (%)	Current Chronic Vulvar Pain n (%)	Past/Short-term Vulvar Pain n (%)	No Vulvar Pain n (%)	p-value[6]
Race					< .01
White	142 (38.3 %)	10 (66.7 %)	27 (52.9 %)	105 (34.4 %)	
African American	229 (61.7 %)	5 (33.3 %)	24 (47.1 %)	200 (65.5 %)	
Education at Baseline[1]					.05
High School or less	108 (30.1 %)	2 (15.4 %)	9 (18.0 %)	97 (32.8 %)	
At least some college	251 (69.9 %)	11 (84.6 %)	41 (82.0 %)	199 (67.2 %)	
Marital Status[2]					.65
Married	188 (55.8 %)	10 (66.7 %)	27 (57.5 %)	151 (54.9 %)	
Not Married	149 (44.2 %)	5 (33.3 %)	20 (42.5 %)	124 (45.1 %)	
Sexually Active in Last 6 Months [3]					.40
Yes	120 (39.7 %)	7 (58.3 %)	18 (40.0 %)	95 (38.8 %)	
No	182 (60.3 %)	5 (41.7 %)	27 (60.0 %)	150 (61.2 %)	
BMI[4]					.02
<25 kg/m^2	47 (14.2 %)	3 (21.4 %)	12 (26.7 %)	32 (11.7 %)	
25 - <30 kg/m^2	81 (24.4 %)	6 (42.9 %)	9 (20.0 %)	66 (24.2 %)	
> = 30 kg/m^2	204 (61.4 %)	5 (35.7 %)	24 (53.3 %)	175 (64.1 %)	
Currently Use HT					< .01
Yes	17 (4.6 %)	2 (13.3 %)	9 (17.6 %)	6 (2.0 %)	
No	354 (95.4 %)	13 (86.7 %)	42 (82.4 %)	299 (98.0 %)	
Ever Used HT					< .01
Yes	137 (36.9 %)	7 (46.7 %)	30 (58.8 %)	100 (32.8 %)	
No	234 (63.1 %)	8 (53.3 %)	21 (41.2 %)	205 (67.2 %)	
History of Hysterectomy					.21
Yes	63 (17.0 %)	2 (13.3 %)	13 (25.5 %)	48 (15.7 %)	
No	308 (83.0 %)	13 (86.7 %)	38 (74.5 %)	257 (84.3 %)	
Urogenital Symptoms in previous 2 weeks					
Dryness					< .01
0 days	272 (73.3 %)	4 (26.7 %)	33 (64.7 %)	235 (77.1 %)	
1-5 days	53 (14.3 %)	3 (20.0 %)	9 (17.6 %)	41 (13.4 %)	
6-14 days	46 (12.4 %)	8 (53.3 %)	9 (17.6 %)	29 (9.5 %)	
Soreness[2]					< .01
0 days	318 (94.4 %)	10 (66.7 %)	44 (93.6 %)	264 (96.0 %)	
1-5 days	15 (4.4 %)	3 (20.0 %)	3 (6.4 %)	9 (3.3 %)	
6-14 days	4 (1.2 %)	2 (13.3 %)	0 (0.0 %)	2 (0.7 %)	
Irritation[2]					< .01
0 days	280 (83.1 %)	8 (53.3 %)	35 (74.5 %)	237 (86.2 %)	
1-5 days	43 (12.8 %)	3 (20.0 %)	10 (21.3 %)	30 (10.9 %)	
6-14 days	14 (4.2 %)	4 (26.7 %)	2 (4.3 %)	8 (2.9 %)	
History of Reported Dryness					
Dry Before FMP/Hysterectomy[5]					.46
Yes	126 (46.7 %)	7 (63.6 %)	16 (50.0 %)	103 (45.4 %)	
No	144 (53.3 %)	4 (36.4 %)	16 (50.0 %)	124 (54.6 %)	

Table 1 Demographic and clinical characteristics of women in the MI SWAN population, by self-reported vulvar pain *(Continued)*

Dry After FMP/Hysterectomy[5]				.01
Yes	232 (62.5 %)	10 (90.9 %)	23 (71.9 %)	124 (54.6 %)
No	139 (37.5 %)	1 (9.1 %)	9 (28.1 %)	103 (34.3 %)

Missing observations: [1]12, [2] 34, [3]69, [4]39 , [5]101.
[6]All p-values calculated using Chi-squared tests except BMI, Difficulty Paying for Basics, Currently Use HT, Vaginal Dryness, Vaginal Soreness, and Vaginal Irritation, which were calculated using Fisher's Exact test

symptoms (9.4 %) reported first onset of vulvar pain while taking HT.

Prevalences of self-reported dryness, soreness, and/or irritation were lowest in the no vulvar pain symptoms group and highest in the current chronic vulvar pain group (Table 1). However, although over half of women with current vulvar pain indicated they had "dryness" for over 6 days in the past 2 weeks, approximately a quarter (26.7 %) of women with current vulvar pain did not report vaginal dryness. Similarly, although reporting of "soreness" or "irritation" was most frequent in women with current chronic vulvar pain, over half of the women with current chronic vulvar pain did not report soreness or irritation.

In the multinomial logistic regression models adjusted for race, odds of having current chronic vulvar pain symptoms were significantly elevated in white women, current HT users, and individuals reporting dryness, soreness, or irritation for 6 or more days in the preceding 2 weeks (Table 2). Odds of past/short-duration vulvar pain symptoms were significantly elevated in white women, current and past HT users, women who had had a hysterectomy, and individuals reporting vaginal irritation 1–5 days in the previous 2 weeks. Adjusting the logistic models for age or BMI did not substantially alter results (data not shown).

At Visit 12, median serum hormone levels of E2 and DHEA-S tended to be lower ($p = 0.06$) in women who subsequently reported current chronic vulvar pain symptoms at Visit 13 compared to those who reported no vulvar symptoms (Table 3). The unadjusted relative odds of current chronic vulvar pain symptoms versus no vulvar symptoms at Visit 13 were elevated with each log unit decrease in Visit 12 E2, DHEA-S, and T levels (Table 4). After adjustment for age, race and BMI, the odds remained elevated only for DHEA-S and T. FSH and SHBG levels were not associated with chronic vulvar pain. In an exploratory analysis we evaluated longitudinal endocrine patterns prior to pain onset in the five women reporting new onset chronic pain symptoms at visit 13. From Visit 10 to Visit 12, three of the five experienced a sharp drop in E2 levels (defined < =15 % of the Visit 10 level at Visit 12) as did only 12 of 256 women without symptoms.

Discussion

Postmenopausal women are as likely as younger women to report chronic vulvar pain consistent with vulvodynia

[4, 14, 15]. This study is one of the first population-based studies to examine the association between symptoms of vaginal dryness, serum hormone levels, hormone use and chronic vulvar pain symptoms in postmenopausal women. We found that women with current chronic vulvar pain symptoms often experienced pain onset prior to menopause. Women with current chronic pain were more likely than women without such pain symptoms to be using HT, and some reported the onset of vulvar pain symptoms while already taking HT. Despite the possibility of inadequate hormonal treatment in some cases, vulvar pain unresponsive to HT further supports the presence of a chronic pain condition such as vulvodynia that is likely to require alternative, non-hormonal, treatment modalities. Notably, more than a quarter of women who reported current chronic vulvar pain did not report vaginal dryness, a common complaint associated with vaginal atrophy. Lower average DHEA-S, and T levels prior to ascertainment of vulvar pain symptoms were associated with elevated odds of subsequently reporting chronic vulvar pain, further supporting that for some, hormonal levels may contribute to symptoms experienced. These results provide additional evidence that chronic vulvar pain in postmenopausal women has a heterogeneous etiology and, in many women, may not be explained by estrogen deficiency-related atrophy alone [6, 14, 15].

In this sample of postmenopausal women, the prevalence and incidence of chronic vulvar pain was somewhat lower than that observed in other studies. One previous study reported prevalences in women age 40–65 years of 13.9 % and 8.9 % among women who had and had not used HT, respectively [4, 5], and an incidence of approximately 3.3 per 100 person-years in women age 50 and older [16]. A second paper reported a prevalence of vulvovaginal symptoms suggestive of atrophy in 38 % of women aged 45–65 [5]. The low prevalence of chronic vulvar pain reported in this study reflects the large proportion of African Americans who have been shown to be less likely than white women to report chronic vulvar pain. Vulvodynia is more prevalent in white women than African American women in most [2, 4, 16], although not all studies [17]. The low prevalence reported here also reflects the older average age of the study population, as previous reports have indicated that vulvodynia prevalence and incidence decline with

Table 2 Relative odds ratios (OR) and 95 % confidence intervals (CI) for selected variables, adjusted for race

Variable	Current Chronic Vulvar Pain vs none OR (95 % CI)	P	Past/Short-term Vulvar Pain vs none OR (95 % CI)	P
Categorical BMI				
<25 kg/m^2	REF	–	REF	–
25-<30 kg/m^2	0.96 (0.22, 4.13)	0.34	0.36 (0.14, 0.95)	.21
>= 30 kg/m^2	0.30 (0.07, 1.35)	0.12	0.36 (0.16, 0.81)	.01
Currently Use HT				
Yes	7.12 (1.27, 39.94)	0.03	10.24 (3.42, 30.68)	< .01
No	REF	–	REF	–
Ever Use HT				
Yes	1.79 (0.63, 5.13)	0.28	2.93 (1.59, 5.40)	< .01
No	REF	–	REF	–
Sexually Active in Last 6 months.				
Yes	2.17 (0.66, 7.11)	0.20	1.04 (0.54, 2.01)	.90
No	REF	–	REF	–
Hysterectomy				
Yes	0.91 (0.20, 4.23)	0.91	1.95 (0.96, 3.97)	.07
No	REF	–	REF	–
Vaginal Dryness				
0 days	REF	–	REF	–
1-5 days	5.47 (1.14, 26.12)	0.03	1.79 (0.78, 4.07)	.17
6-14 days	16.34 (4.53, 58.85)	<0.01	2.22 (0.96, 5.16)	.06
Vaginal Soreness				
0 days	REF	–	REF	–
1-5 days	14.43 (2.95, 70.56)	<0.01	2.46 (0.63, 9.68)	.20
6-14 days	28.28 (2.99, 267.5)	<0.01	(Insufficient data)	.99
Vaginal Irritation				
0 days	REF	–	REF	–
1-5 days	3.30 (0.81, 13.42)	0.09	2.40 (1.07, 5.41)	< .01
6-14 days	12.60 (3.00, 52.86)	0.03	1.53 (0.31, 7.65)	.60

Table 3 Serum hormone levels (median and interquartile range (IQR)) at Visit 12 for all women not using hormonal therapy, by self-reported vulvar pain symptoms at Visit 13

Variable	Total Median (IQR)	Current Chronic Vulvar Pain Median (IQR)	Past/Short-term Vulvar Pain Median (IQR)	No Vulvar Pain Median (IQR)	p-value
Age (yr)	61.3 (59.4-63.7)	59.3 (58.6-60.4)	61.4 (60.0-63.7)	61.3 (59.4-63.7)	.23
Hormones (log transformed)					
	N = 319	n = 12	n = 38	n = 264	
E2 (average, pg/mL)	19.8 (12.0-27.2)	15.2 (3.7-24.4)	23.2 (18.8-26.9)	19.4 (12.0-27.3)	0.06
DHEA-S (ug/dL)	63.7 (36.8-88.6)	28.5 (8.0-73.1)	62.0 (49.3-83.2)	65.0 (37.7-90.1)	0.06
FSH (mIU/mL)	52.2 (36.8-70.7)	55.4 (38.7-64.6)	52.7 (31.5-79.6)	51.5 (36.9-70.6)	0.92
SHBG (nM)	48.8 (35.7-68.7)	56.4 (31.8-94.1)	53.1 (34.8-68.5)	48.8 (35.8-67.8)	0.83
T (ng/dL)	49.8 (38.5-61.8)	45.2 (22.5-54.9)	54.7 (41.7-65.4)	49.8 (38.7-61.6)	0.22

Table 4 Relative odds ratios (OR) and 95 % confidence intervals (CI) for having chronic vulvar pain by log-transformed serum hormone levels at Visit 12 among women not using hormones

Hormone (log)	Unadjusted Model		Adjusted Model*	
	Current Chronic Vulvar Pain vs none	Past/Short-term Chronic Pain vs none	Current Chronic Vulvar Pain vs none	Past/Short-term Vulvar Pain vs none
	OR (95 % CI)	OR (95 % CI)	OR (95 % CI)	OR (95 % CI)
Visit 12 (N = 319)				
E2 (average, pg/mL)	0.49 (0.28, 0.86)**	1.37 (0.86, 2.19)	0.58 (0.32, 1.04)	1.52 (0.92, 2.50)
DHEA-S (ug/dL)	0.46 (0.29, 0.75) ***	1.09 (0.69, 1.73)	0.45 (0.28, 0.72)***	1.07 (0.66, 1.74)
FSH (mIU/mL)	1.13 (0.39, 3.28)	1.11 (0.60, 2.05)	0.76 (0.28, 2.10)	1.15 (0.56, 2.39)
SHBG (nM)	1.45 (0.49, 4.31)	0.99 (0.52, 1.89)	1.00 (0.29, 3.47)	0.99 (0.47, 2.11)
T (ng/dL)	0.13 (0.04, 0.48) ***	1.38 (0.55, 3.47)	0.14 (0.04, 0.56)***	1.39 (0.53, 3.68)

* adjusted for age, categorical BMI, and race
** $p = .01$; *** $p < .01$

age, especially if those not having sexual intercourse are included in the analysis [4, 16].

Previous research has suggested that a drop in estrogen may be associated with onset of chronic vulvar pain that will not necessarily be reversed by subsequent estrogen supplementation [8]. We observed that lower levels of E2, DHEA-S, and T were associated with increased odds of reporting current chronic vulvar pain, although only DHEA-S and T remained significant after adjustment. When we evaluated longitudinal endocrine patterns prior to pain onset only in the five women reporting new onset chronic pain symptoms at visit 13, three of the five had experienced a prior sharp drop in E2 levels compared to just five percent of women with no symptoms. Although consistent with the theory that a variable hormonal environment may contribute to chronic vulvar pain, we observed only a small number of new onset cases. Further study of the relationship between longitudinal endocrine patterns and risk for chronic vulvar pain is warranted.

Lower DHEA-S levels at visit 12 were associated with higher odds of reporting current chronic vulvar pain symptoms, a finding that should be explored in future studies. An association between low DHEAS and sexual dysfunctioN (as measured by the Female Sexual Function Index) [18] and a weak association of serum androgens and sexual well-being in women with premature ovarian failure have been reported [19]. However, a mechanism to explain a direct relationship between DHEAS and vulvar symptoms is unclear. The topical application of DHEA to the vagina in women with severe atrophy has been reported to improve all domains of sexual function, including pain with sexual activity, in controlled clinical trials [20–22], potentially due to local conversion to androgens and estrogens. Future studies are needed to confirm and further assess these findings.

This study adds to the literature indicating that postmenopausal vulvar pain may be caused by factors other than vulvovaginal atrophy [6–9, 14, 15]. Hormone use did not always prevent symptom onset and was not associated with symptom remission in all women. However, as the vulvodynia screening instrument was administered at only Visit 13, timing of vulvar pain onset was ascertained by retrospective report. Also, information on details of HT such as dose, route of administration, indication and duration of use was limited or unavailable; thus, we are not able to assess adequacy of treatment for presumed estrogen deficiency. However, those with vulvar pain symptoms secondary to atrophy who had been adequately treated with estrogen would not be included in the chronic vulvar pain group–hence only those with persistent symptoms despite hormone therapy, and those with persistent symptoms who have not taken HT, were included in the chronic vulvar pain group.

This analysis was constrained by the limited sample size, particularly the small number of women with current vulvar pain symptoms meeting our screening criteria. As a categorization of chronic pain requires a minimum duration of three months and categorization as a past case depends on participant recall, it is possible that some participants forgot to report past episodes, thus attenuating the findings. Nonetheless, a unique strength of this study is the availability of longitudinal data on HT use, serum hormone levels, and self-reports of vaginal dryness in postmenopausal women within a defined timeframe after the final menstrual period permitting a more detailed, though preliminary, look at the relationship between vaginal symptoms, hormone levels and vulvar pain in a population-based, multi-ethnic sample of midlife women. Future studies might consider evaluation of additional pain symptoms such as dyspareunia in relation to reporting of chronic vulvar pain.

Conclusion

This preliminary but rich longitudinal population-based study adds to the growing literature suggesting that vulvar atrophy may not be the sole cause of postmeno-pausal vulvar pain. Postmenopausal women may be experiencing new onset, exacerbated and/or long-term chronic vulvar pain consistent with a diagnosis of vulvodynia. Health care providers should consider and evaluate for vulvodynia when treating postmenopausal women with chronic vulvar pain, especially those women who fail to respond to HT. The best tool for distinguishing if chronic vulvar pain consistent with both atrophy and vulvodynia will respond to HT is to give a trial of HT, followed by alternative vulvodynia treatments in those not responding. Future research should focus on the diagnosis and treatment of women who do not respond to this intervention.

Abbreviations

BMI, body mass index; DHEA-S, dehydroepiandrosterone-sulfate; E2, estradiol; FSH, follicle stimulating hormone; HT, hormone therapy; Kg, kilograms; M, meters; SHBG, steroid hormone binding globulin; SWAN, Study of Women's Health Across the Nation; T, testosterone

Acknowledgements

Clinical Centers: *University of Michigan, Ann Arbor—Siobán Harlow, PI 2011 –present, MaryFran Sowers, PI 1994–2011; Massachusetts General Hospital, Boston, MA—Joel Finkelstein, PI 1999–present; Robert Neer, PI 1994–1999; Rush University, Rush University Medical Center, Chicago, IL—Howard Kravitz, PI 2009 –present; Lynda Powell, PI 1994–2009; University of California, Davis/Kaiser –Ellen Gold, PI; University of California, Los Angeles—Gail Greendale, PI; Albert Einstein College of Medicine, Bronx, NY—Carol Derby, PI 2011–present, Rachel Wildman, PI 2010–2011; Nanette Santoro, PI 2004–2010; University of Medicine and Dentistry–New Jersey Medical School, Newark—Gerson Weiss, PI 1994–2004; and the University of Pittsburgh, Pittsburgh, PA—Karen Matthews, PI.* NIH Program Office: *National Institute on Aging, Bethesda, MD—Winifred Rossi 2012-present; Sherry Sherman 1994–2012; Marcia Ory 1994–2001; National Institute of Nursing Research, Bethesda, MD—Program Officers.* Central Laboratory: *University of Michigan, Ann Arbor—Daniel McConnell* (Central Ligand Assay Satellite Services). Coordinating Center: *University of Pittsburgh, Pittsburgh, PA –Maria Mori Brooks, PI 2012-present; Kim Sutton-Tyrrell, PI 2001–2012; New England Research Institutes, Watertown, MA-Sonja McKinlay, PI 1995–2001.* Steering Committee: Susan Johnson, Current Chair, Chris Gallagher, Former Chair. We thank the study staff at each site and all the women who participated in SWAN.
The Study of Women's Health Across the NatioN (SWAN) has grant support from the National Institutes of Health (NIH), DHHS, through the National Institute on Aging (NIA), the National Institute of Nursing Research (NINR) and the NIH Office of Research on Women's Health (ORWH) (Grants U01NR004061; U01AG012505, U01AG012535, U01AG012531, U01AG012539, U01AG012546, U01AG012553, U01AG012554, U01AG012495). The content of this article is solely the responsibility of the authors and does not necessarily represent the official views of the NIA, NINR, ORWH or the NIH. SDH gratefully acknowledges use of the services and facilities of the Population Studies Center at the University of Michigan, funded by NICHD Center Grant R24 HD041028.

Authors' contributions

SM contributed to the literature review, conducted the data analysis and had primary responsibility for drafting the manuscript. SDH, JFR, and BDR made substantial contributions to conception, design, and acquisition and interpretation of the data. SDH oversaw the data analysis, contributed to the drafting and critical revisions of the manuscript. BDR and JFR contributed to the critical revision of the manuscript for important intellectual content. All authors have read and approved the final manuscript.

Competing interests

The authors have no competing interests.

Author details

[1]Department of Epidemiology, School of Public Health, 1415 Washington Heights, Ann Arbor, MI 48109, USA. [2]School of Medicine, University of Michigan Ann Arbor, Ann Arbor, MI, USA.

References

1. Harlow BL, Stewart EG. A population-based assessment of chronic unexplained vulvar pain: have we underestimated the prevalence of vulvodynia? JAMWA. 2003;58:82–8.
2. Harlow BL, Wise LA, Stewart EG. Prevalence and predictors of chronic lower genital tract discomfort. Am J Obstet Gynecol. 2001;185(3):545–50.
3. Kao A, Binik YM, Amsel R, Funaro D, Leroux N, Khalife S. Biopsychosocial predictors of postmenopausal dyspareunia: the role of steroid hormones, vulvovaginal atrophy, cognitive-emotional factors, and dyadic adjustment. J Sex Med. 2012;9:2066–76.
4. Reed BD, Harlow SD, Sen A, Legocki LJ, Edwards RM, Arato N, et al. Prevalence and demographic characteristics of vulvodynia in a population-based sample. Am J Obstet Gynecol. 2012;206:170.e1–9.
5. Kingsberg SA, Wysocki S, Magnus L, Krychman ML. Vulvar and vaginal atrophy in postemenopausal women: findings from the REVIVE (REal women's Views of treatment options for menopausal Vaginal changEs) survey. J Sex Med. 2013;10:1790–9.
6. Kao A, Binik K, Amsel R, Funaro D, Leroux N, Khalife S. Challenging atrophied perspectives on postmenopausal dyspareunia: a systematic description and synthesis of clinical pain characteristics. J Sex Marital Ther. 2012;38:128–50.
7. Goetsch MF. Unprovoked vestibular burning in late estrogen-deprived menopause: a case series. J Low Genit Tract Di. 2012;16(4):442–6.
8. Leclair CM, Goetsch MF, Li H, Morgan TK. Histopathologic characteristics of menopausal vestibulodynia. Obstet Gynecol. 2013;122:787–93.
9. McKay M. Dysesthetic ("essential") vulvodynia: treatment with amitriptyline. J Reprod Med. 1993;38(1):9–13.
10. Sowers MF, Crawford S, Sternfeld B, Morganstein D, Gold E, Greendale G, Evans D, Neer R, Matthews KA, Sherman S, Lo A, Weiss G, Kelsey J. SWAN: A multi-center, multi-ethnic, community-based cohort study of women and the menopausal transition. In: Lobo RA, Kelsey J, Marcus R, editors. Menopause. New York: Academic; 2000. p. 175–88.
11. Reed BD, Haefner HK, Harlow SD, Gorenflo DW, Sen A. Reliability and validity of self-reported symptoms for predicting vulvodynia. Obstet Gynecol. 2006;108:906–13.
12. Reed BD, Haefner HK, Sen A, Gorenflo DW. Vulvodynia incidence and remission rates among adult women: a 2-year follow-up study. Obstet Gynecol. 2008;112:231–7.
13. Agresti A. Categorical Data Analysis. 3rd ed. New York, NY: John Wiley & Sons; 2012.
14. Phillips N, Bachmann G. Vulvodynia: An often overlooked cause of dyspareunia in the menopausal population. Menopausal Medicine. 2010; 18(S1):S3–5.
15. Phillips NA, Brown C, Foster D, Bachour C, Rawlinson L, Wan J, Bachman G. Presenting symptoms among premenopausal and postmenopausal women with vulvodynia: a case series. Menopause. 2015;22:1296–300.
16. Reed BD, Legocki LJ, Plegue MA, Sen A, Haefner HK, Harlow SD. Factors associated with vulvodynia incidence. Obstet Gynecol. 2014;123:225–31.
17. Bachmann G, Rosen R, Arnold L, Burd I, Rhoads GG, Leiblum SR, et al. Chronic vulvar and other gynecologic pain: prevalence and characteristics in a self-reported survey. J Reprod Med. 2006;51:3–9.
18. Gracia CR, Freeman EW, Sammel MD, Lin H, Mogul M. Hormones and sexuality during transition to menopause. Obstet Gynecol. 2007;109: 831–40.
19. van der Stege JG, Groen H, Van Zadelhoff SJ, Lambalk CB, Braat DD, Van Kasteren YM, et al. Decreased androgen concentrations and diminished general and sexual well-being in women with premature ovarian failure. Menopause. 2008;15:23–31.
20. Labrie F, Archer D, Bouchard C, Fortier M, Cusan L, Gomez JL, Girard G, Baron M, Ayotte N, Moreau M, Dubé R, Côté I, Labrie C, Lavoie L, Berger L, Gilbert L, Martel C, Balser J. Effect of intravaginal dehydroepiandrosterone (Prasterone) on libido and sexual dysfunction in postmenopausal women. Menopause. 2009;16:923–31.

21. Labri F, Archer DF, Bouchard C, Fortier M, Cusan L, Gomez JL, Girard G,
     Baron M, Ayotte N, Moreau M, Dubé R, Côté I, Labrie C, Lavoie L, Berger L,
     Gilbert L, Martel C, Balser J. Intravaginal dehydroepiandrosterone
     (prasterone), a highly efficient treatment of dyspareunia. Climacteric. 2011;
     14(2):282–8.
22. Archer D, Larie F, Bouchard C, Portman DJ, Koltun W, Cusan L, Labrie C,
     Cote I, Lavoie L, Martel C, Balser J and the VVA Prasterone Group.
     Treatment of pain at sexual activity (dyspareunia) with intravaginal
     dehydroepiandrosterone (prasterone). Menopause 2015; 22, DOI:
     10.1097/gme.0000000000000428.

7

Work outcomes in midlife women: the impact of menopause, work stress and working environment

Claire Hardy[1], Eleanor Thorne[1], Amanda Griffiths[2] and Myra S. Hunter[1]* ⓘ

Abstract

Background: There is growing research interest in the question of whether menopause impacts upon mid-aged women's work outcomes, but the evidence to date is inconclusive. This paper examines whether: (i) menopausal status, and experience of hot flushes and night sweats (HFNS), and whether (ii) work stress and work environment, are associated with work outcomes (absenteeism, job performance, turnover intention, and intention to leave the labor force).

Methods: An online survey (sociodemographic, menopause, health, well-being and aspects of work) was completed by 216 (pre-, peri- and postmenopausal) women aged 45–60 years.

Results: Work outcomes were not associated with menopausal status but were significantly associated with job stress and aspects of the work environment, such as demand, control and support. HFNS presence, frequency and problem-rating were not significantly associated with work outcomes. HF problem rating at work was significantly associated with intention to leave the labor force, after controlling for age (F(2,101), 6.742, $p = .002$).

Conclusions: The main predictors of work outcomes in this sample of mid-aged women were aspects of the working environment (particularly role clarity and work stress). Menopausal status was not associated with work outcomes but having problematic hot flushes at work was associated with intention to stop working. These results challenge assumptions about the menopause transition by providing evidence that the menopause does not impact on women's self-reported work performance and absence. However, support for women with problematic HFNS at work may be beneficial, as might addressing working environment issues for mid-aged women.

Keywords: Menopausal status, Absenteeism, Job performance, Turnover intention, Intention to leave the labor force, Job stress, Working environment

Background

The increasing age of the working population in most European countries means that more women will be working during their menopausal transition than ever before [1]. The menopause - the last menstrual cycle - generally occurs on average between the ages of 50 and 51 in western cultures [2]. The perimenopause or menopause transition is the time from the onset of menstrual cycle changes until one year after the final menstrual period [3]. Although highly variable between women, the menopausal transition can last on average two to four years, but can last up to ten years [4, 5].

It has been estimated that between 20 and 40% of menopausal women experience hot flushes and night sweats (HFNS), also referred to as vasomotor symptoms, which can impact negatively on quality of life, including personal and work life [6]. Women tend to report that these symptoms are more difficult to manage in the work place, due to embarrassment and concern about the reactions of others [7–9]. Menopausal status and HFNS are often kept hidden [10] and not disclosed to managers at work [11]; consequently menopause taboos are not challenged and women may not obtain practical support that could be helpful. This has led to various

* Correspondence: myra.hunter@kcl.ac.uk
[1]Department Psychology (at Guy's), Institute of Psychiatry, Psychology and Neuroscience, Kings College London, 5th Floor Bermondsey Wing, Guy's Campus, London SE1 9RT, UK
Full list of author information is available at the end of the article

guidance and recommendations that menopause at work warrants attention and support for women. For example, the UK Faculty of Occupational Medicine of the Royal College of Physicians has published guidance on how employers can best support menopausal women in the workplace [12].

Recent research on this topic has focused on two main areas: (i) that menopause can have negative effects at work and (ii) that certain working environments negatively impact on experience of menopausal symptoms. A recent systematic review by Jack and colleagues [13] explored menopause at work and found a number of studies suggesting that women with problematic menopausal symptoms may experience impairments on a range of work outcomes. For example, in an Australian survey of approximately 1000 women aged 40–70 years, HFNS frequency was significantly associated with reduced job satisfaction, work engagement, organizational commitment, and a higher intention to quit their job [14]. In the US, a significant relationship was found between night sweat severity and impaired worker productivity on a large sample of over 3000 mid-aged women [15]. Overall, however, the systematic review concluded that evidence was still inconclusive in terms of the impact of menopause on work outcomes. It is important to note that almost without exception, evidence relating to performance at work is based on self-perceived measures.

Since the review's publication, a further cross-sectional study of 1274 female workers aged 40–65 years in Australia found that having HFNS were associated with a greater likelihood of poor self-rated work ability [16]. In another recent study Hickey and colleagues [17] examined relationships between work outcomes and stage of menopause, in a study of over 1000 women in Australia. Self-reported work engagement, job satisfaction, organizational commitment, or work limitations did not differ with menopausal status. Postmenopausal women were less likely to report intention to leave their employing organization (turnover intention) than pre- or peri-menopausal women. However, the study did not control for the potential impact of age on these variables, which the authors noted may have been important to consider.

Finally, a recent report published in 2017 systematically reviewed the economic evidence of possible impact of menopause upon work outcomes, i.e. whether the menopause transition is a problem for UK working women and, in turn, workplaces and the wider labor market [18]. Both positive and negative effects were found for women transitioning whilst in employment, and some evidence suggested that menopausal women were unable to seek employment, were reducing their working hours, leaving or losing their job whilst in

transitions, and identifying negative impact on their career. However, they, like Jack and colleagues [13], stated that evidence for the menopause having an economic impact remains inconclusive. It is also important to note that evidence relating to women's performance is based on self-perceived performance not objective measures.

A key aspect of the workplace is job or work stress. Work-related stress is one of the main reasons reported for sickness absence in many developed countries; for example in the UK work stress has been the focus of much research over the last several decades [19]. Job stress is generally understood as a result of an employee's cognitive appraisal that their working environment may be imposing greater demands (stressors) on them than they can cope with. The relationships between these cognitive appraisals and psychosocial environmental stressors has been largely influenced by Lazarus's transactional model [20], which posits that stress results when person/environment transactions lead the individual to perceive a discrepancy between the demands of a situation and his/her resources or ability to cope with those demands. Stress has been examined in many populations and occupations, yet, mid-aged women have been largely overlooked.

Researchers have attempted to identify aspects of the work environment that might result in job stress and work outcomes. For example, early work was influenced by role stress theory [21] and the Person-Environment fit theory [22]. These theories proposed that the employee's role was key and that if the employee did not fit the working environment appropriately then stress would occur. More recently this field has been more heavily influenced by Karasek's jobs demands-control model [23] and the spin-off job demands-resources (JDR) model [24]. Within these theories, if an employee has insufficient control or resources or lack of support to be able to meet the demands of their job, then stress would occur. The JDR model [24] refers to control as a resource, specifically, but also suggests that other resources are available in the employee's physical, psychological, social, or organizational domains.

In the context of female employees at midlife, there is a need for more research exploring job stress in menopausal women as well as the possible impact of menopausal status on work outcomes. This paper attempts to contribute by addressing the following research questions: (i) are menopausal status and the experience of menopausal symptoms – hot flushes and night sweats – associated with key work outcomes, including absenteeism, job performance, turnover intention (leaving the current employing organization), intention to leave the labor force, and (ii) what is the association of job stress and the working environment on these work outcomes?

Method

An electronic survey was sent via email to female members of a trade union and professional association for family court and probation staff in England, Wales and Northern Ireland in June 2016. The workforce had undergone organizational change during the past three years and was considered a suitable population to explore job stress. Self-report data was collected on demographic and health-related questions, including age, ethnicity, educational level, general health, work-related variables included: employment status (full-time, part-time), working hours, flexible working, manual working, and managerial/supervisory responsibilities.

Job stress was measured using a single-item asking women how stressful they find their jobs (1 = not stressful to 4 = extremely stressful, [25]). The working environment was measured using the Health and Safety Executive's Management Standards Indicator Tool (MSIT) which includes 35 items to measure six aspects of work which if badly managed are known to be associated with the experience of stress; demands, control, support (manager and peer), relationships, role and change [26]. Responses are given using a 5-point Likert-scale (1 = never to 5 = always) and were all shown to have acceptable levels of reliability (α = .68–.87).

Menopausal status was determined according to menstrual criteria: regular periods (regular for them), changes in menstrual periods but had menstruated in the last 6 months, or had not menstruated for a least 1 year. Participants were grouped as pre, peri-, and post-menopausal, respectively; perimenopause or menopause transition being the time from the onset of menstrual cycle changes until one year after the final menstrual period [3]. HFNS were assessed using the Hot Flush Rating Scale [7] including the presence of HFNS, HFNS frequency in the past week, HFNS problem rating (3 ten point scales items assessing interference, distress and problem ratings of HFNS α = .87), and an additional single item 10 point scale assessing HFNS problem rating specifically when at work.

Dependent variables were: number of days affected by work absence in the last 4 weeks (summed total number of full days, arriving to work late, and leaving early), a self-rated job performance item (a single item, 1 = poor-5 = excellent, [27, 28]), turnover intention was measured using an existing 4-item measure, with 5-point Likert scales, to assess the employee's intention to leave the organization (α = 0.78) [29]), and intention to leave the work force was measured using a single-item (1 = no, 2 = sometimes, 3 = yes).

Univariate regression analyses were conducted to determine any significant associations between sociodemographic variables and the outcomes. Only age was significantly related to intention to leave the labor force

only (r = .36, p = .000) and was controlled for in the main analyses. ANOVA was used to determine if there were menopausal group differences in the outcome variable absence; Kruskal-Wallis H Tests were used to determine if there were differences in perceived job performance and turnover intentions between the menopausal groups, and ANCOVAs were conducted to determine whether there were group differences in the outcome intention to stop working, controlling for age. Mann-Whitney U tests were used to determine whether there was an association between HFNS presence and the work outcomes. Bivariate linear regression analyses were conducted to determine whether experience of HFNS was associated with the outcome variables, and multiple regression analyses were used to determine the relative associations between significant univariate variables with the outcomes variable.

Ethical approval was given by King's College London, Ethical Review Committee (reference number: HR-15/16–2492) and all participants gave their consent to participate and publish the results.

Results
Sample characteristics

Two hundred and sixteen women aged 40–65 years were included in this study. Table 1 shows the characteristics of the sample. Women were on average 53 years, white (88.7%), mostly educated to at least degree or professional qualification level (85.6%) and were generally healthy. Over half exercised a minimum of 2 times per week (55.1%). The sample's mean BMI score (29.30) is considered at the upper end of being overweight.

Fifty-eight per cent of the women were postmenopausal, with the remainder divided roughly equally between peri- or pre-menopausal. 62% were experiencing HFNS, on average, 19 times in the past week. Apart from one participant, none were taking HRT. A small proportion of women were taking non-prescribed medication for the menopause (7.7%) and fewer were taking prescribed medication (4.8%).

The majority of women worked full-time, for an average of 36 h per week in non-manual jobs (97.7%), within a public sector organization. Most of the women in the sample had degree level education and were employed in non-manual work. The majority (81.5%) were experiencing moderate to severe levels of job stress with only 2.3% reporting no job stress.

Women had been affected by absence, on average, for 4 days in the last 4 weeks. Specifically, they took an average of 2.37 (sd = 5.59) full days, arrived late to work 1.26 (sd = 3.56) times in the past 4 weeks, and left work early 1.13 (sd = 2.90) times in the past 4 weeks.

Self-rated work performance was generally perceived as high with three-quarters (74.9%) rating their performance

Table 1 Sample characteristics

Characteristic		Mean (SD) or N (%)
Age (n = 216)	Mean (sd)	52.51 (5.75)
Ethnicity (n = 212)	White	188 (88.7%)
	Black	19 (9.0%)
	Asian	5 (2.4%)
Menopausal status (n = 216)	Pre (regular periods)	48 (22.2%)
	Peri (irregular periods for last 6 months)	42 (19.4%)
	Post (no period for 12 months)	126 (58.3%)
HFNS frequency in past week (n = 102)	Mean (sd)	19.45 (17.90)
		range: 0–89
HFNS problem rating (n = 104)	Mean (sd)	4.77 (2.11)
HFNS Problem rating at work (n = 104)	Mean (sd)	5.03 (2.71)
General health (n = 216)	Mean (sd)	2.81 (1.07)
BMI (n = 199)	Mean (sd)	29.30 (7.39)
Education level (n = 215)	'O' Grade/ 'O' Level/ Standard Grade	17 (7.9%)
	Higher/ 'A' Level/ National Grade	14 (6.5%)
	Degree or professional qualification	106 (49.3%)
	Post-graduate qualification	78 (36.3%)
Relationship status (n = 214)	Single/Divorced/ Separated/Widowed	63 (29.4%)
	Married/With partner	151 (70.6%)
Work full-time (n = 212)		155 (73.1%)
Working hours (n = 211)	Mean (SD)	36.44 (9.68)
Flexible working (n = 212)		148 (69.8%)
Non-manual job (n = 215)		210 (97.7%)
Managerial/supervisory responsibilities (n = 212)		59 (27.8%)
Sector (n = 216)	Public	131 (60.6%)
	Private	85 (39.4%)
How stressful do you find your job? (n = 216)	Not stressful	5 (2.3%)
	Mildly stressful	35 (16.2%)
	Moderately stressful	95 (44%)
	Extremely stressful	81 (37.5%)

as very good/excellent compared to others in a similar role. Approximately half of the women (52.3%) indicated that they have considered leaving the labor force altogether.

Menopause and work outcomes

Table 2 shows the scores for the menopausal status groups on the key work outcomes.

No significant differences were found between menopausal status and any work outcome, i.e. number of days affected by absence (total number of days taken off, arrived late, left early), job performance, turnover intention. Intention to leave the labor force was significantly different between the menopausal groups, $H = 19.300$, $p = .001$, with post-menopausal women showing a significantly higher intention than pre- or peri-menopausal women. However, this difference became non-significant after controlling for age.

Job stress and work environment

Relationships between job stress and work environment were considered as possible predictors of work outcomes. To improve normality of the job stress variable, responses were recoded to combine the lower two response options and create a 3-point scale (i.e. low, moderate, high stress) for use in the following analyses. Higher perceived job stress was significantly associated with lower self-rated job performance, $F(1, 209) = 22.317$, $p = .0001$, higher turnover intention, $F(1, 214) = 37.016$, p = .0001, and higher intention to leave the labor force controlling for age, $F(2, 213) = 23.012$, $p = .0001$. Job stress was not associated with number of days affected by absence.

Regarding the working environment, higher self-rated job performance was associated with lower demands, $F(1, 209) = 11.59$, $p = .001$, clearer job role, $F(1, 209) = 30.53$, $p = .0001$, and having more control at work, $F(1, 209) = 7.771$, $p = .006$.

Higher turnover intention was associated with higher demands at work, $F(1, 214) = 18.575$, $p = .000$, lower role clarity, $F(1, 214) = 41.683$, $p = .0001$, low control, $F(1, 214) = 21.611$, $p = .000$, better relationships, $F(1, 214) = 4.019$, $p = .046$, lower manager support, $F(1, 214) = 23.99$, $p = .000$, lower peer support, $F(1, 214) = 10.155$, $p = .002$, and poor change management, $F(1, 214) = 24.467$, $p = .0001$.

Higher intention to leave the labor force, controlling for age, was associated with higher demands, $F(2, 213) = 20.307$, $p = .0001$, poor role clarity, $F(2, 213) = 5.826$, $p = .017$, lower control, $F(2, 213) = 16.199$, $p = .022$, lower peer support, $F(2, 213) = 19.766$, $p = .014$, and poorer change management, $F(2, 213) = 19.639$, $p = .015$.

Absence (more days/part days off work) in the last four weeks were associated with lower perceived levels of control, $F(1, 214) = 5.826$, $p = .017$, and better relationships, $F(1, 214) = 9.256$, $p = .003$.

The role of HFNS

A subsample (n = 168) of peri and post-menopausal women provided data relating to HFNS, and relationships between HFNS and work outcomes were examined. Neither the presence of vasomotor symptoms (HFNS) nor

Table 2 Total sample and pre, peri, and postmenopausal status groups on work outcomes

	Number	Pre-menopause M (SD)	Number	Peri-menopause M (SD)	Number	Post-menopause M (SD)	Number	Total M (SD)
Absence (Number of days affected by absence in last 4 weeks)	48	5.49 (6.59)	42	4.60 (6.13)	126	3.89 (6.20)	216	4.38 (6.28)
Job performance	47	3.00 (0.75)	39	2.87 (0.73)	125	2.86 (0.75)	211	2.89 (0.75)
Turnover intention	48	3.19 (0.99)	42	3.11 (0.99)	126	3.18 (1.04)	211	3.17 (1.02)
Intention to leave the labor force	48	0.48 (0.80)	42	0.64 (0.88)	126	1.07 (0.87)	216	0.84 (0.89)

HFNS frequency or Problem-rating were associated with work outcomes. However, reporting more problematic hot flushes *at work* was significantly associated with intention to stop working, $F(2, 101) = 6.742$, $p = .002$. Specifically, higher problem ratings were associated with a greater intention to leave ($B = .082$).

Relationships between age, job stress, working environment, HFNS, and work outcomes

Significant variables in univariate analyses were entered into stepwise linear regression analyses to determine the strongest predictors of each work outcome (see Table 3). Overall, the number of days affected by work absence was predicted by (better) relationships at work and (lower) control at work, but together these variables only accounted for a small (6%) amount of the variance. Job performance was best predicted by the working environment subscales, (higher) job role and (lower) job stress, which accounted for 16.1% of the variance. Intention to leave the employing organization was best predicted by (poorer) role clarity, (higher) job stress, and (poorer) managerial support, which accounted for 24.9% of the

variance. Intention to stop working was best predicted by (older) age, (poorer) role clarity, and (higher) problematic hot flushes at work, which account for 22.5% of the variance.

Discussion

This study contributes to the evidence regarding the potential impact of menopausal experience, and of work stress and work environment on work outcomes. The sample was highly educated and generally healthy, but reported moderate and severe levels of work stress and fairly high levels of work absence (2.37 full days absence in past 4 weeks), compared with a national average for annual sickness absence in the UK of 4.3 days [30]. There was not a particularly strong intention to leave their employing organization, but approximately half of the women had considered leaving the labor force altogether. Despite this, their subjective ratings of their own work performance were relatively high. The organization had recently undergone substantial change, which is known to be associated with a high report of stress. The results also suggest that performance

Table 3 Predictors of work outcomes: step-wise linear regression analyses

Work outcome	Variable	Regression statistics
Number of days affected by absence (n = 216)	Relationships	B = 2.667, 95% CI = .746–4.587, p = .007
	Control	B = −1.498, 95% CI = −2.957–.040, p = .044
		$R^2 = .060$
Job performance (n = 211)	Role	B = .324, 95% CI = .189–.459, p = .0001
	Job stress	B = −.206, 95% CI = −.346–.066, p = .004
		$R^2 = .161$
Turnover intention (n = 216)	Role	B = −.342, 95% CI = −.529–.156, p = .0001
	Job stress	B = .344, 95% CI = .164–.524, p = .0001
	Managerial support	B = −.184, 95% CI = −.317–.051, p = .0001
		$R^2 = 249$
Intention to leave the labor force (n = 104)	Age	B = .072, 95% CI = .037–.107, p = .0001
	Role	B = −.264, 95% CI = −.475–.054, p = .014
	HF Problem rating at work	B = .065, 95% CI = .006–124, p = .031
		$R^2 = .225$

remained high despite considerable work stress, absence and intention to leave the labor force. There is some evidence from qualitative data that women might work harder in order that their performance is not affected [11].

We found that there were no differences between pre, peri, and post-menopausal women with respect to work absence, job performance, turnover intention, and intention to leave the labor force. Neither were dimensions of HFNS reporting (prevalence, frequency and problem-rating) associated with work outcomes. However, having problematic hot flushes, specifically at work, was associated with a higher intention to leave the labor force. These results suggest that any impact of menopause or menopausal symptoms on work outcomes is likely to be minimal and quite specific. Interestingly, it is the problematic nature of HFNS, not their frequency that had an impact on the work outcomes studied here. This supports previous findings that it is how bothersome or problematic that HFNS are that is associated with quality of life, rather than their frequency [6].

Overall, our results support those of Hickey and colleagues [17] who found few differences between reproductive status on a range of work outcomes. Women rated their work performance positively in both studies. Hickey and colleagues found one significant association - that postmenopausal women had a lower intention to leave the labor force than pre- and peri-menopausal women. However, age was not controlled for in this study. In contrast we found that post-menopausal women reported a higher intention to leave the labor force than pre- or peri-menopausal women. However, this difference became non-significant after controlling for age.

The impact of work stress and the work environment was also examined and found to be significantly associated with key work outcomes. Successive Health and Safety Executive Labour Force Surveys on self-reported work-related illness have revealed that mid-life women (aged 45–54) are the group reporting most work-related stress [19]. We did not find an association between work stress and menopausal status. However, levels of work stress were relatively high across these stages. The results are similar to those reported by professionals in a similar occupational field (i.e. the police, [25]). In the UK, public service industries show the highest levels of stress and it is the main reason for absence from work [19].

Work stress and the working environment appeared to play a greater role in the work outcomes than menopausal status or experience. Specifically, job stress was associated with job performance, and turnover intention, although not significantly for days affected by absence. The working environment appeared to be more strongly associated with absence, especially having better relationships at work and less control over work. Job role clarity was also a key influence on these work outcomes, especially for intention to leave the employing organization and labor force. Managerial support was associated with turnover intention but none of the other outcomes. Intention to leave the labor force was additionally influenced by age and problematic hot flushes at work, which was the only outcome to be associated with the menopausal experience.

With regards to the menopause transition, there is guidance [1, 12] that encourages managers to be informed about the menopause and to foster a culture where women feel empowered to speak up about any difficulties. Increased flexibility, attention to workplace temperatures and access to information and advice are also recommended [11]. In a recent study of how mid-aged women wanted to be treated in the workplace [31] most women mentioned that employers/managers should not consider the menopause in an overly negative light, for example, as an 'affliction' or a 'condition' affecting all older female employees. They believed that employers/managers should be aware that the menopause is a normal process and one that is highly variable between women.

It is also important to mention other symptoms that may be associated with the menopause that we did not examine. These include tiredness, poor concentration and memory, and low confidence, and sleep disturbance [9, 11, 15]. Hickey et al. [17] found that sleep problems were most commonly reported by peri-menopausal women, while for postmenopausal women it was joint and muscular discomfort. Only hot flushes and vaginal dryness were significantly more frequent in peri- and post, compared to premenopausal women. Whitely and colleagues [9] concluded, from a study examining the effects of menopausal symptoms on work impairment, that whilst women with menopausal symptoms reported significantly higher work impairment, there was no specific symptom that significantly predicted work productivity losses.

In this context and in the light of the current findings and those of Hickey et al. [17], we suggest that specific symptoms or physical changes, such as HFNS, are considered since menopausal status does not appear to be associated with most work outcomes. This is likely to reduce general stereotyping of 'menopausal women' and address women's concerns about being perceived as 'not good at their jobs' because they are going through the menopause. In addition, work outcomes, such as performance and work intentions, appear to differ markedly in their relationship to HFNS, so future studies might usefully include a broad range of work outcomes. It is also important to report positive findings, for example in the current study work performance was highly rated in this sample of working mid-aged women.

Attempts to retain women in the labor force might focus on providing support to those women who are having problematic HFNS specifically at work, as well as modifying aspects of the work environment that can exacerbate experience and women's ability to cope with symptoms [1, 11, 12]. Information and advice on managing symptoms using a cognitive behavioural approach is available [32, 33], including a self-help approach for working women with problematic symptoms [28], and may be offered as needed. The results also suggest that steps need to be taken to help employees to have clarity of roles, feel supported, and have more control over their work.

Future research might investigate changes at work and their impact on menopause experience: for example, providing information and training about the menopause to all staff. Such enquiries might compare different delivery methods (face to face, paper or online). Research might explore attempts to improve workplace culture regarding health-related issues for women. The effectiveness of risk assessment and risk management initiatives could be explored, where key factors affecting women are identified and interventions designed to reduce them.

Some limitations should also be noted. The overall sample size was relatively small and also derived from one job sector (i.e. the probation service) that had undergone organizational change in the past 3 years. This may influence the generalizability of the findings, and further research exploring a range of different job sectors is recommended.

The women appeared to be experiencing relatively high levels of stress, but we did not explore non-work sources of stress, which are commonly reported during midlife, such as caring roles and family responsibilities [34].

Conclusion

This study presents evidence that menopausal status does not appear to be associated with work outcomes (absence, performance, turnover intention and intention to leave the labor force) and most women maintained high levels of self-rated performance at work despite menopause and high levels of work stress. The results therefore challenge the assumptions that the menopause has a negative impact on work performance and levels of absence from work. The findings suggest implications for possible changes to workplace practices and policy that may benefit those mid-aged women experiencing difficulties during mid-life and/or the menopause. In particular, providing support for women with problematic HFNS at work, as well as addressing working environment issues. Investigations examining the impact of such workplace changes and tailored interventions are needed.

Acknowledgements
We would like to thank Sarah Friday and colleagues for their feedback and input to the study.

Funding
This research was funded by the charity Wellbeing of Women RG1701.

Authors' contributions
CH and MSH designed the study, drafted the manuscript; ET contributed to data collection and the statistical analysis; AG contributed to the final draft; all authors read and approved the manuscript.

Competing interests
The authors declare that they have no competing interests.

Author details
[1]Department Psychology (at Guy's), Institute of Psychiatry, Psychology and Neuroscience, Kings College London, 5th Floor Bermondsey Wing, Guy's Campus, London SE1 9RT, UK. [2]Division of Psychiatry & Applied Psychology, School of Medicine, University of Nottingham, Nottingham, UK.

References
1. Griffiths A, Ceausu I, Depypere H, Lambrinoudaki I, Mueck A, Pérez-López FR, van der Schouw YT, Senturk LM, Simoncini T, Stevenson JC, Stute P. EMAS recommendations for conditions in the workplace for menopausal women. Maturitas. 2016;85:79–81.
2. Freeman EW, Sammel MD, Lin H, Gracia CR. Anti-mullerian hormone as a predictor of time to menopause in late reproductive age women. J Clin Endocrinol. 2012;97(5):1673–80.
3. Harlow SD, Gass M, Hall JE, Lobo R, Maki P, Rebar RW, Sherman S, Sluss PM, De Villiers TJ. STRAW+ 10 Collaborative Group. Executive summary of the Stages of Reproductive Aging Workshop+ 10: addressing the unfinished agenda of staging reproductive aging. J Clin Endocrinol Metab. 2012 Apr 1;97(4):1159–68.
4. Hunter MS, Gentry-Maharaj A, Ryan A, Burnell M, Lanceley A, Fraser L, Jacobs I, Menon U. Prevalence, frequency and problem rating of hot flushes persist in older postmenopausal women: impact of age, body mass index, hysterectomy, hormone therapy use, lifestyle and mood in a cross-sectional cohort study of 10 418 British women aged 54–65. BJOG: An International Journal of Obstetrics & Gynaecology. 2012;119(1):40–50.
5. Avis NE, Crawford SL, Greendale G, Bromberger JT, Everson-Rose SA, Gold EB, Hess R, Joffe H, Kravitz HM, Tepper PG, Thurston RC. Duration of menopausal vasomotor symptoms over the menopause transition. JAMA Intern Med. 2015;175(4):531–9.
6. Ayers B, Hunter MS. Health-related quality of life of women with menopausal hot flushes and night sweats. Climacteric. 2013;16(2):235–9.
7. Hunter MS, Liao K. A psychological analysis of menopausal hot flushes. Br J Clin Psychol. 1995;34(4):589–99.
8. Smith MJ, Mann E, Mirza A, Hunter MS. Men and women's perceptions of hot flushes within social situations: are menopausal women's negative beliefs valid? Maturitas. 2011;69(1):57–62.
9. Woods NF, Mitchell ES. Symptoms during the perimenopause: prevalence, severity, trajectory, and significance in women's lives. Am J Med. 2005;118(12):14–24.

10. Sergeant J, Rizq R. 'Its all part of the big CHANGE': a grounded theory study of women's identity during menopause. J Psychosom Obstet Gynecol. 2017;6:1–6.

11. Griffiths A, MacLennan SJ, Hassard J. Menopause and work: an electronic survey of employees' attitudes in the UK. Maturitas. 2013;76(2):155–9.

12. Faculty of Occupational Medicine. http://www.fom.ac.uk/health-at-work-2/information-for-employers/dealing-with-health-problems-in-the-workplace/advice-on-the-menopause. Accessed 12th September 2017.

13. Jack G, Riach K, Bariola E, Pitts M, Schapper J, Sarrel P. Menopause in the workplace: what employers should be doing. Maturitas. 2016;85:88–95.

14. Jack G, Bariola E, Riach K, Schnapper J, Work PM. Women and the menopause: an Australian exploratory study. Climacteric. 2014;17(Suppl 2):34.

15. Whiteley J, DiBonaventura MD, Wagner JS, Alvir J, Shah S. The impact of menopausal symptoms on quality of life, productivity, and economic outcomes. J Women's Health. 2013;22(11):983–90.

16. Gartoulla P, Worsley R, Bell RJ, Davis SR. Moderate to severe vasomotor and sexual symptoms remain problematic for women aged 60 to 65 years. Menopause. 2015;22(7):694–701.

17. Hickey M, Riach K, Kachouie R, Jack G. No sweat: managing menopausal symptoms at work. J Psychosom Obstet Gynecol. 2017;22:1–8.

18. Brewis J, Beck V, Davies A, Matheson J. The effects of menopause transition on women's economic participation in the UK. Research Report. 2017. https://www.gov.uk/government/publications/menopause-transition-effects-on-womens-economic-participation

19. Health and Safety Executive. http://www.hse.gov.uk/statistics/causdis/stress/stress.pdf. Accessed 12th September.

20. Lazarus RS. Psychological stress and the coping process. New York: McGraw-Hill.

21. Kahn RL, Wolfe DM, Quinn RP, Snoek JD. Rosenthal RA. Organizational stress: Studies in role conflict and ambiguity; 1964.

22. Harrison RV. The person-environment fit model and the study of job stress', Human Stress and Cognition in Organizations: An Integrated Perspective, ed. by TA Beehr and RS Bhagat.1985.

23. Karasek Jr RA. Job demands, job decision latitude, and mental strain: implications for job redesign. Adm Sci Q. 1979:285–308.

24. Demerouti E, Bakker AB, Nachreiner F, Schaufeli WB. The job demands-resources model of burnout. J Appl Psychol. 2001;86(3):499.

25. Houdmont J, Kerr R, Randall R. Organisational psychosocial hazard exposures in UK policing: management standards Indicator tool reference values. Policing: An Int J Police Strateg & Manage. 2012;35(1):182–97.

26. Health and Safety Executive (HSE). Management Standards Indicator Tool. http://www.hse.gov.uk/stress/standards/pdfs/indicatortool.pdf. Accessed 12th September 2017.

27. Hunter MS, Hardy C, Norton S, Griffiths A. Study protocol of a multicenter randomized controlled trial of self-help cognitive behavior therapy for working women with menopausal symptoms (MENOS@work). Maturitas. 92:186–92.

28. Hardy C, Griffiths A, Norton S, Hunter MS. Self-help cognitive behavior therapy for working women with problematic hot flushes and night sweats (MENOS@ Work): a multicenter randomized controlled trial. Menopause. 2018;25,(5) on line DOI: https://doi.org/10.1097/GME.0000000000001048.

29. Shore LM, Martin HJ. Job satisfaction and organizational commitment in relation to work performance and turnover intentions. Human relations. 1989;42(7):625–38.

30. Office of National Statistics (ONS). Table A05: Labour market by age group: Women by economic activity and age (seasonally adjusted). https://www.ons.gov.uk/employmentandlabourmarket/peopleinwork/employmentandemployeetypes/datasets/employmentunemploymentandeconomicinactivitybyagegroupseasonallyadjusteda05sa. Accessed 12th September 2017.

31. Hardy C, Griffiths A, Hunter MS. What do working menopausal women want? A qualitative investigation into women's perspectives on employer and line manager support. Maturitas. 2017;101:37–41.

32. Women's Health Concern. https://www.womens-health-concern.org/help-and-advice/factsheets/cognitive-behaviour-therapy-cbt-menopausal-symptoms. Accessed 12th September 2017.

33. Hunter MS, Smith M. Managing hot flushes and night sweats: a cognitive behavioural self-help guide to the menopause: Routledge; 2014.

34. Woods NF, Mitchell ES, Percival DB, Smith-DiJulio K. Is the menopausal transition stressful? Observations of perceived stress from the Seattle midlife Women's health study. Menopause. 2009;16:90–7.

8

The role of smoking in the relationship between intimate partner violence and age at natural menopause: a mediation analysis

Gita D. Mishra[1]* ⓘ, Hsin-Fang Chung[1], Yalamzewod Assefa Gelaw[1] and Deborah Loxton[2]

Abstract

Background: Age at natural menopause (ANM) is considered as a biologic marker of health and ageing. The relationship between intimate partner violence (IPV) and ANM is currently unknown, and whether smoking plays a role in this relationship is unclear. The aim of this study was to examine the association between IPV and ANM and to quantify the effect mediated through smoking.

Methods: Data were drawn from the 1946–51 cohort of the Australian Longitudinal Study on Women's Health, a prospective cohort study first conducted in 1996. History of IPV (yes or no) was self-reported at baseline. ANM was confirmed by at least 12 months of cessation of menses where this was not a result of medical interventions such as bilateral oophorectomy or hysterectomy and categorised as <45 (early menopause), 45–49, 50–51, 52–53, and ≥54 years. Regression models and mediation analyses based on the counterfactual framework were performed to examine the relationship between IPV and ANM and to quantify the proportion mediated through smoking (never, past, current <10, 10–19 and ≥20 cigarettes/day).

Results: Of 6138 women in the study with natural menopause, 932 (15%) reported a history of IPV and 429 (7.0%) had an early ANM (before age 45 years). Women with IPV were more likely to smoke and be heavy smokers (Odds Ratio: 2.77, 95% CI 2.19–3.51). Women with IPV were also at increased risk of early menopause (ANM <45 years) (Relative Risk Ratio: 1.36, 95% CI 1.03–1.80) after accounting for education level, income difficulties, age at menarche, parity, body mass index, and perceived stress, compared to the reference group (women without IPV and ANM at 50–51 years). This relationship was attenuated after adjusting for smoking (Relative Risk Ratio: 1.20, 95% CI 0.90–1.59). Mediation analysis showed that cigarette smoking explained 36.7% of the association between IPV and early menopause (ANM <45 vs. ≥45 years).

Conclusion: Cigarette smoking substantially mediated the relationship between IPV and early menopause. Findings suggest that as part of addressing the impact of IPV, timely interventions that result in cessation of smoking will partly mitigate the increased risk of early menopause.

Keywords: Age at natural menopause, Intimate partner violence, Mediation, Smoking

Background

While the exact definition of intimate partner violence (IPV) varies between countries, the World Health Organization (WHO) defines IPV as physical violence, sexual violence, stalking and psychological aggression (including coercive acts) by a current or former intimate partner [1]. In 2013, the WHO multi-country study

report documented the global prevalence of physical and/or sexual IPV was 30.0% (95% CI 27.8–32.2%), with the highest levels (approximately 37%) reported in the WHO African, Eastern Mediterranean and South-East Asia Regions [2, 3]. However, IPV against women can occur in all settings, age and socioeconomic groups [4] and is increasingly recognised as a pattern of behaviour that has both immediate and long term consequences for health and well-being [2, 5, 6]. The impact related to reproductive health for women who have experienced some form of IPV includes unintended and/or unwanted

* Correspondence: g.mishra@uq.edu.au
[1]School of Public Health, The University of Queensland, Herston Road, Herston, Brisbane, QLD 4006, Australia
Full list of author information is available at the end of the article

pregnancy, abortion, sexually transmitted diseases, cervical cancer and vaginal discharge [2, 6, 7]. The prevalence of smoking is also more likely to be higher among women who have experienced IPV [8–10].

Findings from Australia suggests that IPV is responsible for 8% of overall disease burden for women discussed as selected risks to health [11, 12]. An 11-year population-based study of mid-aged Australian-born women showed IPV was significantly associated with poorer mental and sexual health status [13], and analysis of data from the Australian Longitudinal Study on Women's Health (ALSWH) demonstrated mental and physical health deficits attributable to IPV that lasted the length of the 16 year study period [14]. A study in Victoria measuring the impact of IPV on the health of women reported that IPV accounted for 2.9% of the total disease and burden for women of all ages [15].

The age at natural menopause (ANM), which marks the cessation of menses, acts as a biomarker for reproductive ageing. The timing of ANM is also linked to a range of cardiovascular and metabolic conditions in later life [16], such as earlier ANM and increased risk of ischemic stroke [17]. While a range of factors is linked to the timing of ANM, smoking is one of the most well-established risk factors for earlier menopause [18]. Our earlier cross-sectional analysis of baseline ALSWH data indicated that smoking and postmenopausal status were associated with IPV among women aged 45–50 years [7]. However, 41% of women in the sample had not yet reached menopause, and the nature of the data precluded longitudinal analysis. Furthermore, the underlying mechanism by which IPV might act to drive early menopause was not identified. To date, there have been no studies that clearly identify links between IPV and ANM. Given that cigarette smoking is associated with both IPV and ANM, the aim of this study is to examine if IPV is associated with ANM and to investigate the role of cigarette smoking as a potential mediator of ANM by using a counterfactual framework for mediation analyses.

Methods

Study design and population
The Australian Longitudinal Study on Women's Health (ALSWH) is an ongoing population-based cohort study of factors affecting the health and well-being of Australian women born in 1921–26, 1946–51, and 1973–78. Women were randomly selected from the national Medicare dataset, which covers all citizens and permanent residents of Australia. Women were first surveyed in 1996 and were followed every 2–4 years using self-completed questionnaires. Full details of the study design, recruitment and response rates have been reported elsewhere [19, 20]. The study protocols were approved by the Human Research Ethics Committees of the University of Newcastle and University of Queensland, Australia. Informed consent was obtained from all participants at each survey.

The present study focused on the 1946–51 cohort, which was first surveyed in 1996 when the women were aged 45 to 50 years (Survey 1, $n = 13,714$), and then in 1998 (Survey 2, $n = 12,338$), 2001 (Survey 3, $n = 11,226$), 2004 (Survey 4, $n = 10,905$), 2007 (Survey 5, $n = 10,638$), 2010 (Survey 6, $n = 10,011$) and 2013 (Survey 7, $n = 9151$). ANM was determined for 7635 women who reported to have natural menopause (not a result of medical interventions) and recorded their age at menopause over the study period. Among these women, 1497 were excluded due to missing baseline data on history of IPV ($n = 44$), smoking status ($n = 236$) and relevant covariates including education level ($n = 46$), income difficulties ($n = 36$), body mass index (BMI) ($n = 223$), perceived stress ($n = 26$), number of children ($n = 179$), and age at menarche ($n = 707$). Therefore, data from 6138 women were included in the analyses.

Main outcome and exposure variables
Age at menopause was determined from responses to the question "if you have reached menopause, at what age did your periods completely stop?" asked in Survey 2 to Survey 6. ANM was confirmed by at least 12 months of cessation of menses where this was not a result of medical interventions such as surgical menopause due to bilateral oophorectomy or hysterectomy. If the ANM was reported at multiple surveys, data reported at the last available survey were used. ANM was treated as a continuous variable and was categorised as <45 (early menopause), 45–49, 50–51, 52–53 and ≥54 years [21].

IPV was defined from responses to the question at baseline "have you ever been in a violent relationship with a partner/spouse?" and categorised women as with or without a history of IPV. Women were also asked a question at Survey 5 "if you have ever lived with a violent partner or spouse, in which years did you experience violence?" Nearly 90% of the women reported they had experienced IPV before 1996 (baseline), which would indicate that the majority of victims had their first IPV experience before midlife.

Smoking and covariates
Smoking status was reported at baseline and categorised as never, past smoker, and current smoker with <10, 10–19 and ≥20 cigarettes per day. Other baseline covariates included area of residence (categorised as urban and rural/remote), education level (no formal qualifications, less than high school/high school, trade/certificate/diploma and university or higher), difficulty on income management (easy/not bad/some difficult and difficult/

impossible), marital status (married/de facto, separated/divorced, widowed and single), age at menarche (≤11, 12, 13, 14 and ≥15 years) and number of children (parity) (0, 1, 2–3 and ≥4 children). BMI was computed as self-reported weight (kg) divided by the square of height (m) and categorised as underweight (<18.5 kg/m^2), normal weight (18.5–24.9 kg/m^2), overweight (25–29.9 kg/m^2) and obese (≥30 kg/m^2). Perceived stress levels at baseline were assessed by asking participants to rate how stressed they had been in the last 12 months for the following life domains: own health, health of other family members, work/employment, living arrangements, study, money, relationship with parents, relationship with partner/spouse, relationship with children, relationship with other family members. The performance of this preceived stress scale was demonstrated with internal reliability and construct validity [22, 23]. The range of summary stress scores was from 0 to 4. Higher scores indicate more perceived stress. The scores were categorised as not at all stressed (0), somewhat stressed (<1), moderately stressed (1 to <2), very stressed (2 to <3) and extremely stressed (3 to 4). In our analysis, we dichotomised stressed status as absence (scores <1) and presence (scores ≥1).

Statistical analysis

Participant characteristics at baseline were described according to the history of IPV (yes or no) and five categories of ANM (<45, 45–49, 50–51, 52–53 and ≥54 years). Descriptive statistics were presented as percentages for categorical data and the median (interquartile range) for continuous data. Chi-squared tests and regression models were used to examine the differences between groups.

To examine the contribution of smoking to the IPV and ANM relationship, the causal diagram presented in Fig. 1 was formulated. IPV was hypothesised to affect ANM both directly and indirectly, in which smoking acted as a mediator. Interactions between IPV and smoking categories on ANM were tested and taken into account if significant. Education level, income difficulties, and age at menarche were the background confounders. High parity, obesity, and stress could be the consequence of IPV [24, 25], thus they were not considered as confounders in the causal diagram. To test these hypotheses, two complementary approaches were used. First, a series of logistic and linear regression models were performed to examine the relationship between IPV and ANM. Multinomial logistic regression models with five categories of outcome for ANM were used to estimate relative risk ratio (RRR) and 95% confidence interval (CI) with age 50–51 as the reference. Linear regression models were used to examine the association with ANM as a continuous outcome. Sequential multivariable regression models were built following multiple adjustment plans by adjusting for education level (Model 1), income difficulties (Model 2), age at menarche (Model 3), parity (Model 4), BMI (Model 5), stress status (Model 6), and subsequently further adjusting for smoking status (Model 7). Attenuated associations between IPV and ANM were expected after adjustment for smoking status, which would indicate a potential mediating role of smoking. Factors that were associated with IPV but did not affect the association between IPV and ANM included area of residence and marital status, thus they were not included in our models.

Second, we performed a formal mediation analysis by using the counterfactual approach [26, 27]. Using the counterfactual framework allows for decomposition of the total effect of IPV on ANM into natural direct and indirect effects mediated through smoking, even in models with non-linearities (e.g. when ANM and smoking are considered as a binary variable) and interactions (e.g. when the effect of IPV is worsened by smoking) [26, 27]. The mediation analysis was performed by fitting a logistic regression model for the binary outcome (ANM <45 and ≥45 years) and a linear regression model for ANM as a continuous outcome; fitting a linear or logistic regression model for the continuous mediator

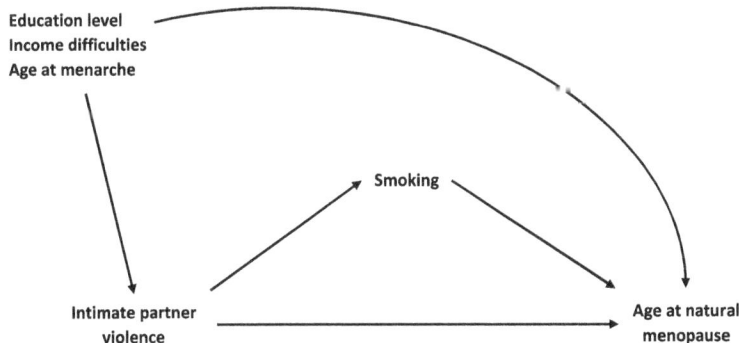

Fig. 1 Directed acyclic graph for mediation analysis of the relationships between intimate partner violence (exposure), smoking (mediator) and age at natural menopause (outcome)

(treating the ordinal variable for smoking status as continuous) or binary mediator (dicotomised as current and non-current smoking) [28]. Models were adjusted for education level, income difficulties, and age at menarche. Interactions between IPV and smoking were not statistically significant from our preliminary regression analyses (p for interaction >0.4), thus no exposure-mediator interaction was included in our models. From these combined models, we obtained odds ratios (ORs) of natural direct effect (OR^{NDE}), natural indirect effect (OR^{NIE}) and total effect (OR^{TE}) for the binary outcome, while for the linear outcome, we derived parameter estimates of β^{NDE}, β^{NIE} and β^{TE}. The proportion mediated through mediator was calculated on the risk difference scale. The proportion mediated was calculated as $[OR^{NDE} (OR^{NIE} - 1)] / [OR^{NDE} \times OR^{NIE} -1] \times 100\%$ for the binary outcome (assuming the outcome of early menopause <45 years is relatively rare) [29] or calculated as $(\beta^{NIE}/\beta^{TE}) \times 100\%$ for the continuous outcome.

Given that women who were excluded from the analysis due to incomplete data were more likely to be less educated, be stressed, be a current smoker, and have a history of IPV, we performed a sensitivity analysis using inverse probability weighting to account for this bias [30]. Logistic regression model was used to calculate propensity scores as the predicted probability of having data observed (i.e. not being missing). We performed a complete-case analysis but weighted the complete cases by the inverse of their probability of being a complete case. Statistical analyses were performed using SAS 9.4 (SAS Institute, Inc., Cary, North Carolina). The paramed program in STATA 14 (StataCorp LP, College Station, Texas) was used to perform the mediation analyses and estimate total, natural direct and natural indirect effects [28]. A 2-sided $p < 0.05$ was considered statistically significant.

Results

This study included 6138 women experiencing natural menopause. Compared with these women, those who were excluded due to incomplete data were more likely to have a lower level of education, have income difficulties, have a history of IPV, be stressed, be a current smoker and have an early ANM (Additional file 1: Table S1). For women included in the study, the mean ANM was 50.9 years (median 51.0 years, interquartile range: 49.0–54.0), with 7% of the women having early menopause (<45 years).

At baseline (when aged 45–50 years), almost one in six women (15%) reported that they had experienced IPV (Table 1). After adjusting for other factors, women with a history of IPV were more likely to live in rural/remote areas, to have lower education levels, to have income difficulties, to be single or separated/divorced, to have four or more children, and to be obese than women without IPV. Women who had suffered IPV were more

than twice as likely to report being stressed (OR 2.03, 95% CI 1.72–2.40) or be current smokers, with a markedly higher likelihood of being a heavy smoker (20 or more cigarettes per day) (OR 2.77, 2.19–3.51). This was also evident in the higher prevalence of heavy smokers (17%) among women with a history of IPV, compared with other women (7%).

Some similarities were evident in the characteristics of women and their time of ANM (Additional file 2: Table S2). Specifically, the risk factors for women associated with early ANM (before age 45 years) after adjusting for other factors and compared with ANM from 50 to 51 years (Table 2), included lower education levels, having income difficulties, and being a current smoker. The risk of early ANM also increased with the number of cigarettes smoked, such that heavy smokers were three times as likely (RRR 2.98, 95% CI 2.11–4.20) as having early ANM compared with those who had never smoked. Women who reported having an early menarche (at age 11 years or earlier) had an increased risk of having early ANM.

In terms of the relationship between IPV and the timing of menopause (Table 3), women who had a history of IPV were at 54% increased risk (RRR 1.54, 95% CI 1.17–2.01) of early ANM compared to the reference group (women without IPV and ANM at 50–51 years). This increased risk was attenuated (RRR 1.36, 1.03–1.80) after adjustment for education level, income difficulties, age at menarche, parity, BMI, and stress (Model 6). With further adjustment for smoking status (Model 7), the risk of early menopause was further attenuated and no longer significant (RRR 1.20, 0.90–1.59). IPV was still associated with an earlier ANM (effect size: –0.39 years, 95% CI -0.69 to –0.08) in the fully adjusted model that used continuous ANM as the outcome. In the sensitivity analysis which used inverse probability weighting to account for the bias caused by the complete-case analysis, we observed similar results that the risk of early menopause was attenuated from 1.37 (1.06–1.76) to 1.19 (0.92–1.55) after adjusting for smoking status.

The results of the multivariable mediation analysis are presented in Table 4. More than one-third (36.7%) of the association of IPV with increased risk of early menopause (ANM <45 years vs. ≥45 years) (OR 1.49, 95% CI 1.16–1.90) was mediated through the number of cigarettes smoked per day (five categories), after adjusting for education level, income difficulties, and age at menarche. The experience of IPV was also associated with having earlier ANM (–0.60 years, 95% CI -0.89 to –0.30) after full adjustment. As above, the number of cigarettes smoked per day accounted for 37.0% of the effect associated between IPV and the timing of ANM. For both early ANM and the timing of ANM, a similar proportion was mediated through smoking when smoking status was dichotomised as current and non-current smoking.

Table 1 Baseline characteristics of women according to their history of intimate partner violence ($n = 6138$)

	History of intimate partner violence (IPV)			
	No ($n = 5206$, 84.8%)	Yes ($n = 932$, 15.2%)	Crude OR (95% CI)	Adjusted[a] OR (95% CI)
Area of residence				
Urban	1913 (36.7)	307 (32.9)	Reference	Reference
Rural/remote	3293 (63.3)	625 (67.1)	1.18 (1.02–1.37)	1.25 (1.06–1.47)
Education level				
No formal qualifications	666 (12.8)	168 (18.0)	1.90 (1.48–2.44)	1.74 (1.32–2.30)
Less than high school/high school	2497 (48.0)	468 (50.2)	1.41 (1.14–1.74)	1.45 (1.15–1.82)
Trade/certificate/diploma	1102 (21.2)	171 (18.3)	1.17 (0.91–1.49)	1.21 (0.93–1.58)
University or higher	941 (18.1)	125 (13.4)	Reference	Reference
Difficulty on income management				
Easy/not bad/some difficult	4685 (90.0)	701 (75.2)	Reference	Reference
Difficult/impossible	521 (10.0)	231 (24.8)	2.96 (2.49–3.53)	1.66 (1.36–2.02)
Marital status				
Married/de facto	4548 (87.5)	606 (65.1)	Reference	Reference
Separated/divorced	399 (7.7)	272 (29.2)	5.12 (4.29–6.10)	4.29 (3.55–5.20)
Widowed	97 (1.9)	18 (1.9)	1.39 (0.84–2.32)	1.30 (0.76–2.23)
Single	156 (3.0)	35 (3.8)	1.68 (1.16–2.45)	2.27 (1.45–3.57)
Age at menarche (years)				
≤ 11	883 (17.0)	184 (19.7)	1.23 (1.00–1.52)	1.10 (0.88–1.38)
12	1109 (21.3)	178 (19.1)	0.95 (0.77–1.17)	0.92 (0.74–1.15)
13	1526 (29.3)	258 (27.7)	Reference	Reference
14	899 (17.3)	144 (15.5)	0.95 (0.76–1.18)	0.94 (0.74–1.19)
≥ 15	789 (15.2)	168 (18.0)	1.26 (1.02–1.56)	1.18 (0.94–1.48)
Number of children				
0	458 (8.8)	54 (5.8)	0.74 (0.55–1.00)	0.61 (0.43–0.86)
1	426 (8.2)	106 (11.4)	1.56 (1.24–1.97)	1.31 (1.02–1.69)
2–3	3586 (68.9)	571 (61.3)	Reference	Reference
≥ 4	736 (14.1)	201 (21.6)	1.72 (1.43–2.05)	1.55 (1.28–1.89)
Body mass index (kg/m^2)				
Underweight (<18.5)	90 (1.7)	16 (1.7)	1.03 (0.60–1.77)	0.79 (0.44–1.44)
Normal weight (18.5–24.9)	2802 (53.8)	482 (51.7)	Reference	Reference
Overweight (25–29.9)	1494 (28.7)	243 (26.1)	0.95 (0.80–1.12)	0.92 (0.77–1.10)
Obese (≥30)	820 (15.8)	191 (20.5)	1.35 (1.13–1.63)	1.24 (1.02–1.53)
Median BMI (Q1, Q3)	24.5 (22.1, 27.7)	24.6 (22.3, 28.7)		
Perceived stress				
No (stress scores <1)	4245 (81.5)	581 (62.3)	Reference	Reference
Yes (stress scores ≥1)	961 (18.5)	351 (37.7)	2.67 (2.30–3.10)	2.03 (1.72–2.40)
Median stress scores (Q1, Q3)	0.5 (0.2, 0.8)	0.7 (0.4, 1.2)		
Smoking status				
Never	3048 (58.5)	360 (38.6)	Reference	Reference
Ex-smoker	1469 (28.2)	316 (33.9)	1.82 (1.55–2.14)	1.73 (1.45–2.05)
Current smoker, <10 cigarettes/day	146 (2.8)	50 (5.4)	2.90 (2.07–4.07)	2.52 (1.75–3.63)
Current smoker, 10–19 cigarettes/day	178 (3.4)	47 (5.0)	2.24 (1.59–3.14)	1.80 (1.25–2.58)

Table 1 Baseline characteristics of women according to their history of intimate partner violence (*n* = 6138) *(Continued)*

	History of intimate partner violence (IPV)			
	No (*n* = 5206, 84.8%)	Yes (*n* = 932, 15.2%)	Crude OR (95% CI)	Adjusted[a] OR (95% CI)
Current smoker, ≥20 cigarettes/day	365 (7.0)	159 (17.1)	3.69 (2.97–4.58)	2.77 (2.19–3.51)

Data are presented as n (%), median (interquartile range) or odds ratio (OR) and 95% confidence interval (95% CI) using logistic regression models. Q1, 25th percentile; Q3, 75th percentile
[a]Adjusted model was adjusted for all the covariates listed in the table

Table 2 Adjusted associations of socioeconomic, reproductive and lifestyle factors with age at natural menopause (*n* = 6138)

	Age at natural menopause (ANM) (years)				
	<45 RRR (95% CI)	45–49 RRR (95% CI)	50–51 RRR (95% CI)	52–53 RRR (95% CI)	≥54 RRR (95% CI)
Education level					
No formal qualifications	1.72 (1.11–2.65)	1.36 (1.03–1.81)	Reference	0.95 (0.71–1.26)	0.71 (0.54–0.92)
Less than high school/high school	1.54 (1.08–2.20)	0.96 (0.77–1.20)	Reference	0.84 (0.67–1.04)	0.71 (0.58–0.86)
Trade/certificate/diploma	1.34 (0.90–2.01)	0.95 (0.74–1.23)	Reference	0.88 (0.69–1.13)	0.76 (0.60–0.95)
University or higher	Reference	Reference	Reference	Reference	Reference
Difficulty on income management					
Easy/not bad/some difficult	Reference	Reference	Reference	Reference	Reference
Difficult/impossible	1.47 (1.08–2.02)	1.14 (0.89–1.45)	Reference	0.91 (0.71–1.18)	1.10 (0.88–1.38)
Age at menarche (years)					
≤ 11	1.54 (1.10–2.16)	1.30 (1.03–1.64)	Reference	1.09 (0.86–1.37)	1.00 (0.80–1.24)
12	1.49 (1.10–2.03)	0.95 (0.76–1.18)	Reference	0.88 (0.71–1.09)	0.92 (0.76–1.13)
13	Reference	Reference	Reference	Reference	Reference
14	1.14 (0.80–1.62)	1.13 (0.90–1.43)	Reference	0.94 (0.74–1.18)	1.09 (0.88–1.35)
≥ 15	1.34 (0.94–1.91)	1.09 (0.86–1.39)	Reference	0.98 (0.77–1.25)	1.18 (0.95–1.46)
Number of children					
0	1.28 (0.87–1.89)	1.32 (1.00–1.73)	Reference	1.00 (0.76–1.34)	0.83 (0.63–1.08)
1	1.04 (0.71–1.52)	1.16 (0.89–1.51)	Reference	0.86 (0.65–1.14)	0.86 (0.66–1.11)
2–3	Reference	Reference	Reference	Reference	Reference
≥ 4	0.99 (0.73–1.35)	0.97 (0.78–1.20)	Reference	1.04 (0.84–1.29)	0.94 (0.77–1.15)
Body mass index (kg/m^2)					
Underweight (<18.5)	1.27 (0.57–2.83)	1.36 (0.77–2.40)	Reference	1.18 (0.65–2.14)	0.92 (0.51–1.65)
Normal weight (18.5–24.9)	Reference	Reference	Reference	Reference	Reference
Overweight (25–29.9)	1.10 (0.85–1.42)	1.06 (0.89–1.27)	Reference	1.12 (0.94–1.34)	1.34 (1.14–1.58)
Obese (≥30)	1.03 (0.75–1.41)	1.08 (0.87–1.34)	Reference	1.10 (0.88–1.37)	1.26 (1.03–1.55)
Perceived stress					
No (stress scores <1)	Reference	Reference	Reference	Reference	Reference
Yes (stress scores ≥1)	1.15 (0.88–1.50)	1.12 (0.93–1.36)	Reference	0.94 (0.77–1.14)	1.00 (0.83–1.19)
Smoking status					
Never	Reference	Reference	Reference	Reference	Reference
Ex-smoker	1.21 (0.93–1.57)	0.88 (0.74–1.05)	Reference	0.90 (0.76–1.07)	0.93 (0.80–1.09)
Current smoker, <10 cigarettes/day	1.69 (0.98–2.92)	0.84 (0.54–1.30)	Reference	0.86 (0.56–1.32)	0.73 (0.49–1.10)
Current smoker, 10–19 cigarettes/day	2.00 (1.22–3.27)	1.13 (0.77–1.67)	Reference	0.80 (0.53–1.23)	0.69 (0.46–1.03)
Current smoker, ≥20 cigarettes/day	2.98 (2.11–4.20)	1.71 (1.30–2.25)	Reference	0.82 (0.59–1.12)	0.81 (0.61–1.09)

Data are presented as relative risk ratio (RRR) and 95% confidence interval (CI) using multinomial logistic regression models, and all RRRs (95% CI) were adjusted for the covariates listed in the table

Table 3 Multivariable adjusted association between intimate partner violence and age at natural menopause (n = 6138)

| Intimate partner violence | Age at natural menopause (ANM) (years) | | | | | |
	<45 RRR (95% CI)	45–49 RRR (95% CI)	50–51 RRR (95% CI)	52–53 RRR (95% CI)	≥54 RRR (95% CI)	Continuous ANM β (95% CI)
Unadjusted model	1.54 (1.17–2.01)	1.06 (0.86–1.30)	Reference	0.87 (0.70–1.07)	0.83 (0.68–1.01)	−0.72 (−1.01 to −0.42)
Model 1: + education level	1.49 (1.14–1.95)	1.04 (0.84–1.28)	Reference	0.87 (0.70–1.08)	0.84 (0.69–1.02)	−0.66 (−0.95 to −0.36)
Model 2: Model 1 + income difficulties	1.39 (1.06–1.83)	1.01 (0.82–1.24)	Reference	0.88 (0.71–1.09)	0.82 (0.67–1.00)	−0.60 (−0.89 to −0.30)
Model 3: Model 2 + menarche	1.38 (1.05–1.82)	1.00 (0.81–1.23)	Reference	0.87 (0.70–1.09)	0.82 (0.67–1.00)	−0.60 (−0.89 to −0.30)
Model 4: Model 3 + parity	1.39 (1.05–1.83)	1.00 (0.81–1.24)	Reference	0.87 (0.70–1.09)	0.82 (0.67–1.00)	−0.62 (−0.92 to −0.32)
Model 5: Model 4 + BMI	1.39 (1.05–1.83)	1.00 (0.81–1.24)	Reference	0.87 (0.70–1.09)	0.82 (0.67–1.00)	−0.62 (−0.92 to −0.33)
Model 6: Model 5 + stress status	1.36 (1.03–1.80)	0.98 (0.80–1.22)	Reference	0.88 (0.71–1.10)	0.82 (0.67–1.00)	−0.60 (−0.90 to −0.29)
Model 7: Model 6 + smoking status	1.20 (0.90–1.59)	0.95 (0.76–1.17)	Reference	0.91 (0.73–1.13)	0.84 (0.68–1.03)	−0.39 (−0.69 to −0.08)

Multinominal logistic regression models were used to estimate relative risk ratio (RRR) and 95% confidence intervals (CI) for the categorical ANM. Linear regression models were used to estimate β (95% CI) for the continuous ANM

Discussion

Using data from a large population-based cohort, this study underscores that women with a history of IPV in midlife are at increased risk of obesity and are more likely to report having four or more children, being stressed and be current smokers, especially heavy smoking (20 or more cigarettes per day). To our knowledge, this is the first study to show that IPV is also associated with increased risk of early ANM (before age 45 years) after adjusting for other risk factors. This relationship was attenuated, however, after accounting for smoking, which is an established risk factor for early ANM. Findings from the mediation analyses using a counterfactual framework confirmed that a considerable part of the link between IPV and earlier ANM was mediated via current smoking status. Specifically, the number of cigarettes

smoked per day explained more than one third (36.7%) of the overall relationship of IPV with early ANM after adjusting for education level, income difficulties, and age at menarche. These findings are consistent with those from previous studies that have shown the strong links between IPV and higher rates of cigarette smoking [8–10] and between smoking and earlier ANM [18].

The association between IPV and tobacco use is well known and has repeatedly been reported in the literature [8–10]. While causality has not been demonstrated, the direct link approach such as that used in the current analysis is justified. A systematic review of IPV and tobacco use literature found the only factor that influenced the association between IPV and tobacco was pregnancy [31], a factor that is not relevant to the current analysis. The review authors propose that nicotine acts to both

Table 4 Natural direct and indirect effects of intimate partner violence on the age at natural menopause and the proportion mediated through smoking (n = 6138)[a]

	OR^{NDE} (95% CI)	OR^{NIE} (95% CI)	OR^{TE} (95% CI)	Proportion mediated by smoking (%)
Early menopause (ANM <45 vs. ≥45 years)				
Mediator: smoking				
Smoking status (5 categories)	1.31 (1.02–1.68)	1.14 (1.09–1.18)	1.49 (1.16–1.90)	36.7
Current vs. non-current smoking (2 categories)	1.34 (1.04–1.72)	1.13 (1.08–1.18)	1.51 (1.18–1.93)	33.7
	β^{NDE} (95% CI)	β^{NIE} (95% CI)	β^{TE} (95% CI)	Proportion mediated by smoking (%)
Continuous ANM				
Mediator: smoking				
Smoking status (5 categories)	−0.38 (−0.68 to −0.08)	−0.22 (−0.28 to −0.16)	−0.60 (−0.89 to −0.30)	37.0
Current vs. non-current smoking (2 categories)	−0.41 (−0.71 to −0.11)	−0.18 (−0.23 to −0.12)	−0.59 (−0.94 to −0.24)	29.8

ANM age at natural menopause, NDE natural direct effect, NIR natural indirect effect, TE total effect
[a]All estimates were adjusted for education level, income difficulties, and age at menarche. The mediation analysis was performed by fitting a logistic regression model for the binary outcome (ANM <45 vs. ≥45 years) and a linear regression model for the continuous ANM and fitting a linear or logistic regression model for the ordinal or binary mediator. The proportion mediated was calculated as [(OR^{NDE} (OR^{NIE} − 1)] / [OR^{NDE} × OR^{NIE} −1] × 100% for the binary outcome or (β^{NIE}/β^{TE}) × 100% for the continuous outcome

alleviate symptoms of depression that are caused by IPV and the symptoms of anxiety that accompany living with a violent partner [31]. More research is needed to allow for the development of effective smoking cessation interventions for women who have experienced IPV. It is possible that smoking cessation programs designed for those experiencing mental health disorders might be more effective than standard smoking cessation programs, given the much lower quit rates found among those with mental health problems [32]. It should be noted that while certain characteristics seem to cluster together (for example, cigarrette smoking, low education level, income difficulties, being stressed and being exposed to violence), cigarette smoking, by far, has been shown to be consistently linked with age at menopause. We also found that around 5% of the association between IPV and risk of early menopause was mediated through stress (without considering smoking status), but no significant joint effect between smoking status and stress status was observed (data not shown). Therefore, health promotion effort should be placed on smoking cessation programs.

IPV has been linked with sexually transmitted and reproductive disorders (e.g. cervical cancer, vaginal discharge) [2, 6, 7] but this is the first study to demonstrate a clear relationship with early reproductive ageing, which in turn has a known impact on cardiovascular disease [16]. Links have previously been shown between IPV and cardiovascular disease and metabolic syndrome disorder, with a strong focus on health behaviours (e.g. smoking, abdominal obesity) and mental distress as mechanisms that connect IPV with cardiovascular risk [33]. The current study adds to knowledge in this regard by highlighting the importance of reproductive ageing. Future research will need to take into account the multiple social and biological pathways through which IPV acts to influence health and well-being. Early life experience of violence may also affect ovarian function and reproductive ageing via stress response dysregulation [34, 35]. One cohort study found that women who experienced childhood or adolescent violence had more extreme levels of ovarian hormones during perimenopause, suggesting that early experience of violence may lead to neuroendocrine disruption, thereby affecting ovarian function [35]. However, this study found conflicting findings that early life violence was associated with delayed (rather than early) onset of perimenopause (measured by menstrual changes) [34]. Our previous cross-sectional analysis using baseline data found that IPV was associated with surgical menopause but not with postmenopause and perimenopause after adjustment for demographic and health behaviour variables [7]. A number of reasons may explain the conflicting results including different outcomes (hormones and menstrual cycle/status), different forms of violence (physical,

emotional, sexual), and different analytical approaches. Hence, more studies are needed to prove the link between the experience of all forms of violence and reproductive health.

The strengths of our study included large sample size and nationally representative study population, which improves the generalizability of our findings to other middle-aged women. Our study was strengthened by its prospective nature, particularly with respect to longitudinal data on the timing of menopause. This meant that reverse causation could be ruled out for the relationships observed between IPV at baseline and ANM. The extensive survey data collected from the women has also allowed adjustment for a wide range of confounders, including known risk factors for IPV and earlier ANM. However, there were some limitations that should be acknowledged. First, all the data were self-reported, which may have led to some under-reporting of IPV. It was also the case that women who were excluded from the analyses due to incomplete data were more likely to have a history of IPV, be a current smoker, and have an early ANM compared to those who were included. If this potential underestimation of the prevalence of IPV, current smoking, and early menopause were included, it seems likely that the observed associations would be strengthened. Second, since the study is limited to Australian women, these findings should be replicated in other populations. Further research is also needed to investigate potential mechanisms for the relationship between IPV and ANM that is not explained by smoking and other risk factors in this study.

Conclusions

Women who had a prior history of IPV were at increased risk of early menopause (<45 years), with this relationship substantially mediated through smoking. Our findings suggest that as part of addressing the issue of IPV and its subsequent consequences for women, smoking cessation interventions tailored for women who have lived with IPV will partly mitigate the links with earlier menopause, which is an established risk factor for a range of adverse health outcomes in later life in addition to the effects of smoking.

Abbreviations

ALSWH: Australian Longitudinal Study on Women's Health; ANM: Age at natural menopause; BMI: Body mass index; CI: Confidence interval; IPV: Intimate partner violence; NDR: Natural direct effect; NIR: Natural indirect effect; OR: Odds ratio; RRR: Relative risk ratio; TE: Total effect; WHO: World Health Organization

Acknowledgements
The research on which this paper is based was conducted as part of the Australian Longitudinal Study on Women's Health, the University of Newcastle, and the University of Queensland. We are grateful to the Australian Government Department of Health for funding and to the women who provided the survey data.

Funding
The Australian Longitudinal Study on Women's Health is funded by the Australian Government Department of Health. GDM is supported by the Australian National Health and Medical Research Council Principal Research Fellowship (APP1121844).

Authors' contributions
GDM conceptualized the study and drafted the manuscript; HFC performed the statistical analysis and contributed to interpretation of results; YAG performed the literature review; DL provided critical revision of the manuscript for important intellectual content. All authors read and approved the final manuscript.

Competing interests
The authors declare that they have no competing interests.

Author details
¹School of Public Health, The University of Queensland, Herston Road, Herston, Brisbane, QLD 4006, Australia. ²Research Centre for Generational Health and Ageing, The University of Newcastle, Callaghan, NSW, Australia.

References
1. Basile KC, Black MC, Breiding MJ, Chen J, Merrick MT, Smith SG, et al. National intimate partner and sexual violence survey. Atlanta: Centers for Disease Control and Prevention; 2011.
2. World Health Organization. Global and regional estimates of violence against women: prevalence and health effects of intimate partner violence and non-partner sexual violence. Geneva: WHO Press; 2013.
3. World Health Organization: Violence against women: Intimate partner and sexual violence against women (Fact Sheet No. 239). 2016. http://www.who.int/mediacentre/factsheets/fs239/en/. Accessed 8 Aug 2017.
4. Garcia-Moreno C, Jansen HA, Ellsberg M, Heise L, Watts CH, WHO Multi-country Study on Women's Health and Domestic Violence against Women Study Team. Prevalence of intimate partner violence: findings from the WHO multi-country study on women's health and domestic violence. Lancet. 2006;368:1260–9.
5. Moore M. Reproductive health and intimate partner violence. Fam Plan Perspect. 1999;31:302–6.
6. World Health Organization. Women and health: today's evidence tomorrow's agenda. Geneva: WHO Press; 2009.
7. Loxton D, Schofield M, Hussain R, Mishra G. History of domestic violence and physical health in midlife. Violence Against Women. 2006;12:715–31.
8. Cheng D, Salimi S, Terplan M, Chisolm MS. Intimate partner violence and maternal cigarette smoking before and during pregnancy. Obstet Gynecol. 2015;125:356–62.
9. Yoshihama M, Horrocks J, Bybee D. Intimate partner violence and initiation of smoking and drinking: a population-based study of women in Yokohama, Japan. Soc Sci Med. 2010;71:1199–207.
10. Jun HJ, Rich-Edwards JW, Boynton-Jarrett R, Wright RJ. Intimate partner violence and cigarette smoking: association between smoking risk and psychological abuse with and without co-occurrence of physical and sexual abuse. Am J Public Health. 2008;98:527–35.
11. Begg S, Vos T, Barker B, Stevenson C, Stanley L, Lopez AD. The burden of disease and injury in Australia 2003. Canberra: Australian Institute of Health and Welfare; 2007.
12. García-Moreno C, Zimmerman C, Morris-Gehring A, Heise L, Amin A, Abrahams N, et al. Addressing violence against women: a call to action. Lancet. 2015;385:1685–95.
13. Schei B, Guthrie J, Dennerstein L, Alford S. Intimate partner violence and health outcomes in mid-life women: a population-based cohort study. Arch Womens Ment Health. 2006;9:317–24.
14. Loxton D, Dolja-Gore X, Anderson AE, Townsend N. Intimate partner violence adversely impacts health over 16 years and across generations: a longitudinal cohort study. PLoS One. 2017;12:e0178138.
15. Vos T, Astbury J, Piers L, Magnus A, Heenan M, Stanley L, et al. Measuring the impact of intimate partner violence on the health of women in Victoria, Australia. Bull World Health Organ. 2006;84:739–44.
16. Mishra GD, Cooper R, Kuh D. A life course approach to reproductive health: theory and methods. Maturitas. 2010;65:92–7.
17. Lisabeth LD, Beiser AS, Brown DL, Murabito JM, Kelly-Hayes M, Wolf PA. Age at natural menopause and risk of ischemic stroke: the Framingham heart study. Stroke. 2009;40:1044–9.
18. Schoenaker DA, Jackson CA, Rowlands JV, Mishra GD. Socioeconomic position, lifestyle factors and age at natural menopause: a systematic review and meta-analyses of studies across six continents. Int J Epidemiol. 2014;43: 1542–62.
19. Dobson AJ, Hockey R, Brown WJ, Byles JE, Loxton DJ, McLaughlin D, et al. Cohort profile update: Australian longitudinal study on Women's health. Int J Epidemiol. 2015;44:1547a–f.
20. Lee C, Dobson AJ, Brown WJ, Bryson L, Byles J, Warner-Smith P, et al. Cohort profile: the Australian longitudinal study on Women's health. Int J Epidemiol. 2005;34:987–91.
21. Mishra GD, Pandeya N, Dobson AJ, Chung HF, Anderson D, Kuh D, et al. Early menarche, nulliparity and the risk for premature and early natural menopause. Hum Reprod. 2017;32:679–86.
22. Bell S, Lee C. Development of the perceived stress questionnaire for young women. Psychol Health Med. 2002;7:189–201.
23. Bell S, Lee C. Perceived stress revisited: the Women's health Australia project young cohort. Psychol Health Med. 2003;8:343–53.
24. Gee RE, Mitra N, Wan F, Chavkin DE, Long JA. Power over parity: intimate partner violence and issues of fertility control. Am J Obstet Gynecol. 2009;201:148. e141-7
25. Bosch J, Weaver TL, Arnold LD, Clark EM. The impact of intimate partner violence on women's physical health: findings from the Missouri behavioral risk factor surveillance system. J Interpers Violence. 2017;32:3402–19.
26. Robins JM, Greenland S. Identifiability and exchangeability for direct and indirect effects. Epidemiology. 1992;3:143–55.
27. Pearl J. Direct and Indirect Effects. Proceedings of the Seventeenth conference on Uncertainty in Artificial Intelligence. Seattle, WA, 2001. 411–20.
28. Valeri L, Vanderweele TJ. Mediation analysis allowing for exposure-mediator interactions and causal interpretation: theoretical assumptions and implementation with SAS and SPSS macros. Psychol Methods. 2013;18:137–50.
29. Vanderweele TJ, Vansteelandt S. Odds ratios for mediation analysis for a dichotomous outcome. Am J Epidemiol. 2010;172:1339–48.
30. Seaman SR, White IR. Review of inverse probability weighting for dealing with missing data. Stat Methods Med Res. 2013;22:278–95.
31. Crane CA, Hawes SW, Weinberger AH. Intimate partner violence victimization and cigarette smoking: a meta-analytic review. Trauma Violence Abuse. 2013;14:305–15.
32. Cook BL, Wayne GF, Kafali EN, Liu Z, Shu C, Flores M. Trends in smoking among adults with mental illness and association between mental health treatment and smoking cessation. JAMA. 2014;311:172–82.

33. Stene LE, Jacobsen GW, Dyb G, Tverdal A, Schei B. Intimate partner violence and cardiovascular risk in women: a population-based cohort study. J Women's Health (Larchmt). 2013;22:250–8.
34. Allsworth JE, Zierler S, Lapane KL, Krieger N, Hogan JW, Harlow BL. Longitudinal study of the inception of perimenopause in relation to lifetime history of sexual or physical violence. J Epidemiol Community Health. 2004; 58:938–43.
35. Allsworth JE, Zierler S, Krieger N, Harlow BL. Ovarian function in late reproductive years in relation to lifetime experiences of abuse. Epidemiology. 2001;12:676–81.

9

Prophylactic salpingo-oophorectomy & surgical menopause for inherited risks of cancer: the need to identify biomarkers to assess the theoretical risk of premature coronary artery disease

Zarah Batulan[1], Nadia Maarouf[1], Vipul Shrivastava[1] and Edward O'Brien[1,2*]

Abstract

Background: Some women with genetic risk of breast and/or ovarian cancer (e.g., BRCA1/2) opt to undergo prophylactic salpingo-oophorectomy (PSO, or surgical removal of the ovaries & fallopian tubes) in order to reduce their risk of cancer. As a consequence, these women experience "surgical menopause" – accompanied by more severe climacteric symptoms that occur in a much shorter time frame. While the risk of coronary artery disease (CAD) rises with menopause, little is known about how the sudden loss of ovarian function from PSO alters the whole-body physiology, and whether it predisposes women to premature CAD.

Methods/Design: To manage CAD risk there is a prerequisite for reliable biomarkers that can help guide risk assessment and therapeutic interventions. To address these needs, this prospective, observational cohort study will evaluate surrogate markers reflective of CAD health in women experiencing surgical menopause after PSO. Twenty women representing each of the following groups will be enrolled over 3 years (total participants = 240): (i) pre-menopausal PSO, (ii) post-menopausal PSO, (iii) pre-menopausal women undergoing other pelvic surgery, and (iv) pre-menopausal controls (no surgery). All participants will provide blood plasma samples pre- and 1, 3, 6, & 12 months post-operatively, with serial samples collectively assessed for measurements of the study's primary endpoints of interest. These include a hormone profile (estradiol, follicle stimulating hormone (FSH), luteinizing hormone (LH), and progesterone) and both conventional (lipid profile) and novel biomarkers (Heat Shock Protein 27 (HSP27), HSP27-antibodies (HSP27 Ab), proprotein convertase subtilisin/kexin 9 (PCSK9), inflammatory cytokines) of CAD. Another aspect of this study is the measurement and analysis of retinal vessel diameters – an emerging physiological parameter reflective of CAD risk. Finally, a patient engagement exercise will result in the drafting of patient-generated questionnaires that address the well-being and health concerns of these women as they transition through premature menopause and work with our research team to identify and discuss their health priorities.

(Continued on next page)

* Correspondence: ermobrie@ucalgary.ca
[1]Department of Cardiac Sciences, Libin Cardiovascular Institute of Alberta, University of Calgary, Health Research Innovation Centre, GB42, 3280 Hospital Dr NW, Calgary, AB T2N 4Z6, Canada
[2]Department of Cardiac Sciences, Libin Cardiovascular Institute of Alberta, Health Research Innovation Centre, Room GAA16, 3280 Hospital Drive NW, Calgary, AB T2N 4Z6, Canada

(Continued from previous page)

Discussion: The protocol of our planned study investigating the effects of PSO on CAD is described herein. Characterization of novel CAD markers in women experiencing surgical menopause will yield new insights into the role of the functional ovary in modulating lipid parameters and other CAD risk factors such as HSP27 and HSP27 Ab.

Keywords: Atherosclerosis, Cardiovascular disease, Cardiovascular risk factors, Coronary artery disease, Estrogen, Heat shock protein 27, HSP27, Inflammatory cytokines, Menopause, PCSK9, Prophylactic salpingo-oophorectomy, Retinal vessel analysis, Surgical menopause

Background

It is widely recognized that pre-menopausal women are relatively protected from cardiovascular disease (CVD), including the manifestations of (*i*) coronary artery diseases (CAD, e.g., angina & heart attacks), and (*ii*) stroke. However, this advantage is lost after menopause [1–3]. In fact, one-third of all deaths in post-menopausal women are due to CAD [4], with a higher risk and overall mortality in women who experience premature or early-onset menopause [5]. As more women worldwide with hereditary breast and ovarian cancer mutations consider surgical removal of their ovaries and fallopian tubes ("prophylactic salpingo-oophorectomy", PSO) to reduce their cancer risk, it is increasingly important to highlight the potential cardiovascular risks that accompany such an intervention and the ensuing premature, "surgical" menopause. The aim of this study will thus be to investigate whether PSO leads to increased cardiovascular risk as assessed by the measurement of conventional and novel surrogate markers for CAD. The rationale and methodology is thereby presented herein as a *study protocol* manuscript.

Menopause

Menopause is a complex physiological process that results from reduced secretion of ovarian hormones, estrogen and progesterone. Clinical manifestations of this physiological transition include vasomotor symptoms e.g. 'hot flashes', urogenital problems, sexual dysfunction, sleep disturbances, depression and osteoporosis [6]. Another common clinical presentation post-menopause is accelerated changes in CAD risk factors, as first reported in the Healthy Women Study (HWS) [7, 8], and later supported by various other studies, including the Study of Women Across the Nation (SWAN) [9]. These observations led to the assumption that estrogens are cardio-protective, a theory which was initially supported by retrospective observational studies in women [1, 10, 11], and later by in vivo animal studies demonstrating that estrogen exerts beneficial physiological effects on: i) the vascular endothelium; and ii) plasma lipoprotein profiles (e.g., by increasing levels of "good" cholesterol – high density lipoprotein (HDL) – while reducing insulin resistance biomarkers [12, 13]).

Evidence accumulated at that time indicated that increased CAD risk post-menopause most likely occurs because of a loss of ovarian hormones. Therefore, several subsequent clinical trials tested the therapeutic potential of post-menopausal hormone therapy (MHT). However, the cardio-protective hypothesis of MHT was refuted by several major randomized clinical trials assessing both primary and secondary CAD prevention (these included the Women's Health Initiative (WHI) and the Heart Estrogen/Progestin Replacement Study (HERS) [14, 15]). In fact, the early termination of the WHI study occurred when the safety monitoring board concluded that the risks of using MHT to prevent / treat CAD exceeded the benefits. This trial brought into sharper focus the conclusion that MHT is associated with adverse cardiovascular outcomes and increased risk of stroke, thromboembolism and breast cancer, most likely through changes in the blood coagulation index favoring the direction of enhanced clotting and increased inflammation [16]. Consequently, there was a marked decline in MHT use worldwide. More recently, this discordance between the theoretical benefit of MHT and the clinical outcomes of the randomized clinical trials has undergone critical reappraisal and new experimental data strongly argued for a second look at MHT [17, 18]. An important fact which may help explain the incongruity between the expected athero-protective effects of MHT and the lack of cardiovascular benefits in patients is the 'timing hypothesis'. Based on the premise that MHT affects CAD outcomes more favorably in younger, compared to older women [19], this hypothesis has drawn attention to the fact that in the WHI study the introduction of MHT was, on average, 7 years post-menopause and probably too late to generate athero-protective benefits. Moreover, there is the theoretical argument that compared to arteries free of atherosclerosis, estrogen receptor responsiveness in CAD may be diminished [20]. Thus, exogenous estrogens (i.e., MHT) may be ineffective late after the onset of menopause if CAD is already present or progressing. Unfortunately, there are currently few (if any) robust therapeutic options to lower cardiovascular risk for post-menopausal women – and to a large degree, this reflects the lack of enrollment and study of women in cardiovascular prevention trials. While this neglectful in-attention to the plight of coronary artery disease in women has a history that spans decades [21], even the most important cardiovascular trials reported in 2017 have woefully low percentages of women enrolled in them (e.g., 16–26%) [22].

"Surgical" menopause

In the first half of the twentieth century, there were already reports of European women undergoing surgical removal of the ovaries and fallopian tubes (or prophylactic salpingo-oophorectomy, PSO) to prevent the onset and/or progression of breast cancer. Hence, more than 100 years ago, female hormones, particularly estrogens, were already being implicated in tumorigenesis. Unfortunately, the negative impact of removing the source of estrogens (via surgical intervention) on a woman's cardiovascular (and cognitive) health was not considered nor deemed important – most likely because it seemed to be the lesser of two evils (i.e., risk of cancer outweighing cardiovascular disease). Historically, community-based studies for CAD did not focus on women; however, epidemiological studies in the mid-1900s began to indicate that women have a lower tendency of developing cardiovascular disease compared to men – a situation that reverses after menopause. Indeed, concerns surfaced regarding the cardiovascular health of women who underwent PSO and the ensuing "surgical" menopause. An illustrative example is a study of Scottish women (≤ 35 yrs. old) who underwent PSO between 1934 and 1938 and then followed for 20 years post-surgery, showing higher CAD events in PSO patients compared to controls [23]. These findings were independently observed by other research groups during that time [23–29].

Advances in genetic diagnostic testing within the past decade have led to the early identification and detection of women with hereditary cancer-causing mutations [30, 31]. The popular actress and human rights advocate, Angelina Jolie, was one such woman diagnosed with a breast cancer-causing BRCA1/2 genetic mutation, who opted to undergo PSO to reduce her risk of developing cancer. Her personal health saga was widely covered by the mass media, and consequently, the number of women diagnosed with BRCA-related mutations, as well as instances of PSO intervention, rose significantly [32, 33]. Less highlighted, however, was the possible negative impact on cardiovascular health. The need to balance the cancer-sparing benefit of PSO with its theoretical risk of premature CAD is thus starting to emerge. Now is the time for women who are considering surgical removal of their ovaries and fallopian tubes (to lower their hereditary cancer risk) to be aware of the cardiac health risks they may face in the future.

PSO as clinical intervention to reduce cancer risk

Historically, it appears that removal of the ovaries and fallopian tubes delayed and/or reduced the severity of breast and ovarian cancers, despite the lack of a clear understanding of how precisely estrogens (and other female hormones) instigate and/or regulate cancer onset and progression. Nowadays, there is a better mechanistic understanding of how estrogen, which is essentially a proliferative factor, can promote the dysregulated growth of tumor cells (Fig. 1a) [34–36]. Women with genetic predispositions to ovarian cancer may thus opt to ablate/eliminate/remove their ovaries – their main source of estrogen [37]. As well, since there is growing concern that the fallopian tubes may also be a source of malignant cells, they are also removed. Currently, the following genes are the most commonly linked to hereditary breast & ovarian cancers:

BRCA1/2

It is estimated that ~ 15% of women with epithelial ovarian cancer have mutations in BRCA1 or 2 [38]. Both genes were first implicated as causative factors for hereditary breast and ovarian cancers in the mid-1990s [39, 40] and have since been characterized extensively as multifunctional proteins that play key roles in DNA repair, replication, chromatin stability, and cell cycle control [41]. Given its importance in promoting genomic stability, its high disease penetrance (30–70% lifetime risk for cancer) is not surprising. To date, 61 missense mutations (70.5% in BRCA1 & 29.5% in BRCA2) have been documented [42]; however, it is not yet clear if patients have higher cancer risk depending on the type of BRCA mutation. Regardless of the actual cancer risk inherent in a particular mutation, an increasingly common clinical recommendation for BRCA1/2 gene mutation carriers is PSO, as it has been shown by several groups to lower risk of ovarian, fallopian tube, and epithelial cancer by 80%, and reduce mortality risk by 77% [37, 43–45].

Lynch syndrome-associated genes

Women with Lynch syndrome, caused by mutations in DNA mismatch repair genes (MSH2, MLH1, MSH6, PMS2, EPCAM), usually develop colorectal cancer but may also be at high risk for ovarian and endometrial cancers [46]. These women may also be advised to undergo PSO to lower their risk of ovarian cancer [47].

PSO, surgical menopause, and increased cardiovascular risk

Although PSO may lower cancer risk, the effect of surgical menopause leads not only to more severe menopausal symptoms [48], but also elevated risks in cardiovascular disease particularly in younger pre-menopausal women (< 45 years of age at surgery) [23, 49]. The abrupt drop of serum sex hormones (i.e., estrogen), is associated with a doubled risk of myocardial infarction, an increase in the relative risk for fatal & nonfatal coronary heart disease, stroke, as well as higher incidence of

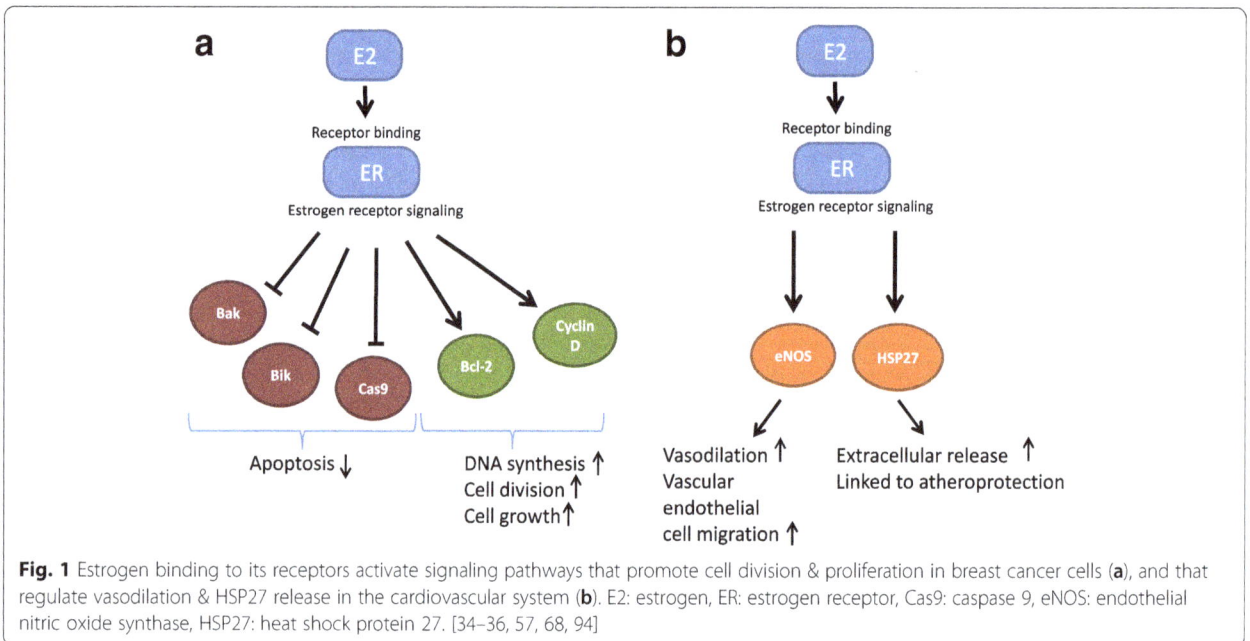

Fig. 1 Estrogen binding to its receptors activate signaling pathways that promote cell division & proliferation in breast cancer cells (**a**), and that regulate vasodilation & HSP27 release in the cardiovascular system (**b**). E2: estrogen, ER: estrogen receptor, Cas9: caspase 9, eNOS: endothelial nitric oxide synthase, HSP27: heat shock protein 27. [34–36, 57, 68, 94]

metabolic syndrome [50, 51]. There are also increased concerns regarding an accelerated risk of dementia in women who have undergone PSO at young, pre-menopausal ages [52, 53]. Post-menopausal dementia may be a form of vascular cognitive impairment, possibly attributable to inflammatory cytokines [54]. Recent epidemiological studies have associated bilateral oophorectomy to increased rates of multimorbidity (as defined by the assessment of chronic conditions associated with aging, including indices of cardiovascular and mental health) [49, 55] suggesting that PSO can accelerate the aging process.

How does the sudden drop in estrogen post-PSO worsen women's cardiovascular risk profile? Athero-sclerosis is driven by both inflammation and cholesterol accumulation, and since estrogen's multitude of physiological effects include the attenuation of both of these processes, its abrupt loss after PSO can thus aggravate atherogenesis. Estrogen has both direct and indirect effects on the endothelium of the vasculature, acting as a vasodilator and helping to repair damaged endothelium via recruitment of new endothelial cells and its action on immune cells (Fig. 1b) [56–58]. Related to lipid regulation, estrogen is inversely correlated with serum levels of low density lipoprotein (LDL) and PCSK9 [59, 60], a recently characterized negative mediator of cholesterol metabolism.

Surrogate markers of cardiovascular risk
HSP27

Over the past 15 years, our group has also focused on HSP27, a molecular chaperone protein that associates with estrogen receptor-beta. It was rather fortuitous that we made a key clinical observation that HSP27 protein expression in human coronary arteries diminishes as the stage of coronary atherosclerosis advances [61]. Interestingly, four other groups using objective (proteomic discovery) approaches, also demonstrated that expression of HSP27 diminishes with the development and progression of atherosclerosis. [62–65] Of clinical importance, we found that HSP27 is a novel cardiovascular biomarker, as elevated serum levels are associated with a lower 5-year risk of having a myocardial infarction, stroke or cardiovascular death [66]. HSP27 is more than a conventional intracellular chaperone protein as it has an extracellular signaling function that is instrumental in protecting against the development of atherosclerosis [67]. For example, we showed in atherosclerosis-prone apolipoprotein E null (ApoE$^{-/-}$) mice that augmentation of extracellular HSP27 levels reduces both serum and plaque cholesterol content, as well as promotes the formation of plaques with histological features of enhanced plaque stability [66, 68, 69]. The mechanisms by which HSP27 reduces atherogenesis appear to be distinct from its chaperone function. From our initial studies we suggested that this atheroprotection occurred because HSP27 promoted the release of the anti-inflammatory chemokine IL-10 [68, 70] and attenuated foam cell formation by binding to and/or reducing the expression of scavenger receptor AI (SR-AI) [68, 71]. We now believe that the cholesterol lowering effect of HSP27 is due to its modulation of a key mediator of cholesterol metabolism, PCSK9, and that estrogens may play an important role in this process.

HSP27 Ab
Recent findings in the O'Brien Laboratory suggest that HSP27 Ab are significantly lower in coronary artery disease patients compared to controls (unpublished data). Others have shown variable HSP27 Ab levels in the context of heart disease, with elevations first noted during acute coronary events followed by a rapid drop [72] and both increases and decreases observed in cardiovascular disease patients (unpublished data) [73, 74]. The functional role of circulating HSP27 Ab is unclear and currently is the subject of much study in our laboratory.

PCSK9
Interest in PCSK9 arose in 2003 when a gain-of-function *PCSK9* mutation was linked with autosomal dominant hypercholesterolemia [75]. This was subsequently confirmed when loss-of-function mutations in PCSK9 were shown to lower LDL [76]. Later experiments indicated that PCSK9 interferes with clearance of LDL from the circulation by binding to LDL-receptor (LDL-R) and facilitating its degradation [77]. Higher circulating plasma levels of PCSK9 has been shown to positively correlate with plasma levels of LDL and susceptibility to CAD; individuals with a PCSK9 loss of function display reduced LDL levels and lower risk of CAD [78]. Findings from the Dallas Heart Study suggest that PCSK9 levels are higher in post- menopausal compared to pre-menopausal women [79]. Of note, our laboratory obtained promising in vitro and in vivo results supporting the role of recombinant HSP27 in reducing PCSK9 levels in both liver cells / tissue and serum (unpublished data).

Retinal vessel analysis
With advances in technology, relatively low cost, excellent reproducibility and radiation free testing, assessment of retinal arterioles is an attractive screening modality for assessing CAD risk [80–84]. Recently, changes in retinal microvessels were reported to correlate with cardiovascular outcomes [85]. Narrower retinal arterioles and wider retinal venules were associated with increased long-term risk of cardiovascular mortality and ischemic stroke both in male and female patients. Measurements of the central retinal arteriolar equivalent (CRAE) and the central retinal venular equivalent (CRVE) were also linked to cardiovascular disease, and in women were predictive of stroke [85]. Hence, retinal arteriolar narrowing is an early marker of systemic microvascular dysfunction with a higher sex-specific risk predictability for atherosclerotic disease in women [85]. Studies are ongoing to determine if retinal vessel parameters are static or can improve with cardiovascular risk factor modification (e.g., ClinicalTrials.gov identifiers: NCT02853747 and NCT02796976) [86]. Therefore, we are using retinal vessel analysis as a

surrogate CAD endpoint as it has previously been indicated to be predictive of atherosclerotic events (i.e., small arteriole: large venule diameter ratio) [85].

This study will address the hypothesis that PSO intervention in pre-menopausal women, which causes an abrupt drop in estrogen and premature menopause, leads to physiological changes that increase cardiovascular risk. Surrogate markers for CAD (conventional and novel biomarkers, as well as measurement of an emerging physiological parameter reflective of CAD – retinal vessel analysis) will be used as tools to evaluate cardiovascular risk, with the long-term goal of potentially using these markers as predictive determinants of cardiovascular health in other at-risk populations.

Methods / design
Study design
This is a single-center, prospective, cross-sectional study which addresses whether women undergoing PSO develop features of cardiovascular disease as assessed by conventional (e.g., cholesterol) and novel biomarkers, including HSP27. Candidates for surgery will be introduced to the study by medical genetics counselors and gynecologists specializing in minimally invasive PSO (University of Calgary's affiliated hospitals, Calgary, Alberta). Patients who decide to undergo surgery and are interested in participating in this study are then scheduled for a cardiac consultation with EOB (University of Calgary). To determine if the sudden drop in estrogen following PSO leads to increases in cardiovascular disease markers, the study population will involve women representing the following four different treatment groups:

1) *Pre-menopausal women undergoing PSO*. This patient group is predicted to develop the most obvious changes in cardiovascular disease markers, as previously indicated by increases in total cholesterol and LDL levels [59, 60] – this is most likely attributed to the abrupt loss in estrogen after surgical removal of functional ovaries.

2) *Post-menopausal women undergoing PSO*. Comparison with this group of women will address whether the surgical removal of ovaries alone (which are non-cycling), and not the sudden drop in estrogen per se, contributes to increases in cardiovascular disease markers.

3) *Pre-menopausal women experiencing other pelvic surgeries* that spare both ovaries and fallopian tubes (e.g., hysterectomy, salpingectomy). This "surgical control" group is included to eliminate the possibility that surgical interventions in the pelvic region affect levels of cardiovascular disease markers over time.

4) *Pre-menopausal women, no surgery.* It is expected that women in this non-surgical, pre-menopausal control group will not exhibit remarkable changes in cardiovascular disease markers during the study's time frame, and as such, will be used to compare with both groups of pre-menopausal women having undergone surgery (PSO or other pelvic surgery).

Patients with pre-existing malignancy or who have experienced a myocardial infarction event in the year prior to their surgery will be excluded from the study since these populations exhibit elevated HSP27 serum levels [63, 87–90]. Once patients decide to enroll in the study and provide signed informed consent, they will undergo a standardized cardiac consultation that includes a detailed personal health history (e.g., medication use, incidence of hypertension, diabetes mellitus, and prior cardiovascular events), cardiovascular physical examination and an ECG. Patients will then be asked to give blood and urine samples before and at various times after surgery (University of Calgary). Retinal images will also be captured before and after surgery (Calgary Retina Consultants). The time commitment required for participation in this study is 1 year (following surgery), with an option to extend participation for an additional year.

Participant recruitment
Depending on family history and outcome of genetic testing, women that are positive for mutations in BRCA1/2 or Lynch syndrome associated-genes (e.g., HNPCC) may be referred by the University of Calgary's team of genetic counselors for an information sharing consultation with gynecologists who specialize in minimally invasive PSO. During the medical genetics consultation, patients will be given a cursory introduction to this study via dissemination of an information pamphlet. After discussing with their gynecologist, who will further elaborate on the details of this study, patients who decide to undergo PSO and are interested in participating will then be scheduled for an appointment with a cardiologist (EOB). Post-menopausal women considering PSO and pre-menopausal women undergoing other pelvic surgeries will be introduced to the study by the same team of medical genetics counsellors and gynecologists, while non-surgical control participants will be enrolled through the use of recruitment flyers posted at the University of Calgary and its affiliated hospitals. Active patient enrollment for this study will take place over 3 years. Recruitment targets for each of the four patient treatment groups are 20 per year, totalling 240 participants for the duration of the study.

Data collection
Cardiac consultations will take place before and at 6- and 12-months after surgery, during which patients will be given an ECG and monitored for incident hypertension, diabetes mellitus, and cardiovascular events (e.g., myocardial infarction, stroke). Fasting blood and urine samples will be collected before surgery (PSO or other pelvic) and at 1, 3, 6, and 12 months after surgery. In addition to routine blood tests (glucose, hemoglobin A1c), Calgary Lab Services will conduct the following analyses: lipid profile (total cholesterol, HDL, LDL, triglycerides) and a female endocrine panel (estradiol, progesterone, FSH, LH). Our research laboratory will separately analyze blood samples at these time points for assessment of novel cardiovascular biomarkers. Plasma will be extracted from blood samples, aliquoted, and stored at -80 °C for future testing (e.g., enzyme-linked immunosorbent assays for HSP27, HSP27 antibodies, PCSK9, as well as inflammatory cytokine arrays [performed by EVE Technologies on campus]). Urine samples will also be stored at -80 °C for future isolation of microparticles and exosomes (ultracentrifugation) and detection of HSP27 and PCSK9 (Western blot and mass spectrometry). Retinal images will be captured by digital photography before and at 6 and 12 months after surgery by a high-volume retinal referral clinic (Calgary Retina Consultants) and images will be securely transferred to the University of Wisconsin Retina Core lab for analysis (Drs. Ron and Barbara Klein). In addition to the above data collection time points, patients will be given the option of extending their participation for an additional year, which will involve cardiac consultations, blood draws, and retinal imaging at 18- and 24-months post-surgery.

To complement this work, our collaborator, Dr. Denise Nebgen (MD Anderson, Houston; **W**omen choos**I**ng **S**urgical **P**revention "**WISP**" trial [ClinicalTrials.gov Identifier: NCT02760849] researcher) will also provide plasma samples before and after PSO in their cohorts diagnosed with BRCA- or Lynch syndrome-associated mutations (~ 35 WISP participants).

Outcomes
The primary outcome is a change in levels of HSP27 following PSO. Plasma HSP27 will be measured using ELISA methods before and 1, 3, 6, and 12 months following surgery. Since previous findings have shown that higher HSP27 serum levels correlate with cardiovascular health [66], it is likely that women experiencing premature menopause after PSO will experience a worsening of their cardiovascular health (as measured by total cholesterol and LDL) and consequently, lower levels of HSP27. HSP27 localized to microparticles isolated from plasma and urine will also be measured using Western blotting and mass spectrometry. Additional primary outcomes assessed at the same time points and analyzed by ELISA are: HSP27 natural antibodies, which appear to be elevated in healthy controls compared to coronary artery

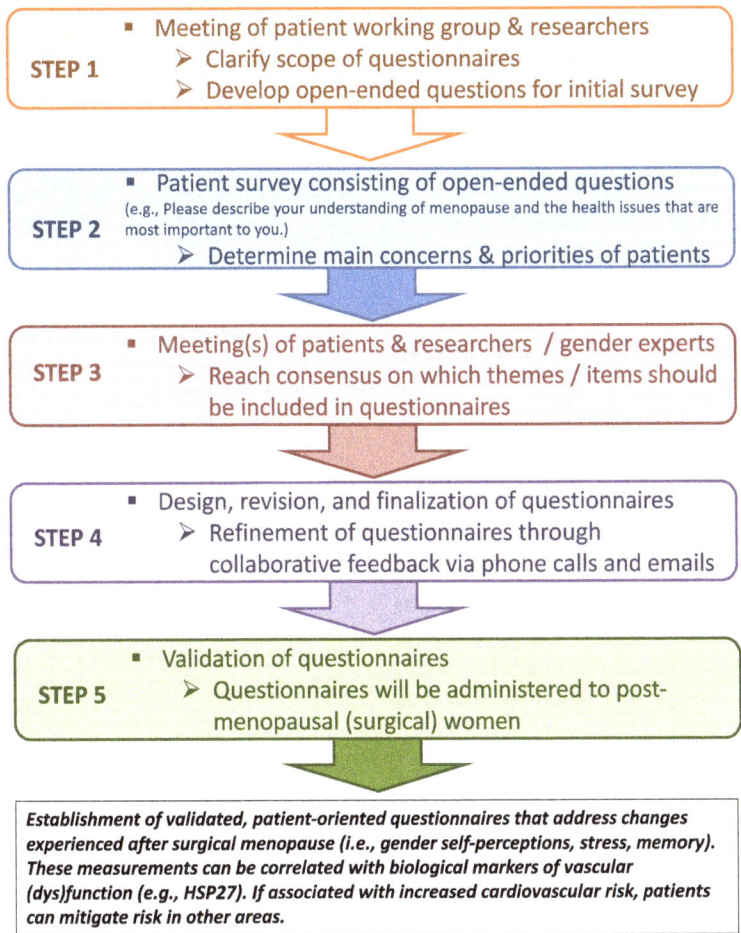

STEP 1
- Meeting of patient working group & researchers
  - ➢ Clarify scope of questionnaires
  - ➢ Develop open-ended questions for initial survey

STEP 2
- Patient survey consisting of open-ended questions
  (e.g., Please describe your understanding of menopause and the health issues that are most important to you.)
  - ➢ Determine main concerns & priorities of patients

STEP 3
- Meeting(s) of patients & researchers / gender experts
  - ➢ Reach consensus on which themes / items should be included in questionnaires

STEP 4
- Design, revision, and finalization of questionnaires
  - ➢ Refinement of questionnaires through collaborative feedback via phone calls and emails

STEP 5
- Validation of questionnaires
  - ➢ Questionnaires will be administered to post-menopausal (surgical) women

Establishment of validated, patient-oriented questionnaires that address changes experienced after surgical menopause (i.e., gender self-perceptions, stress, memory). These measurements can be correlated with biological markers of vascular (dys)function (e.g., HSP27). If associated with increased cardiovascular risk, patients can mitigate risk in other areas.

Fig. 2 Workflow of development of questionnaires that reflect patient priorities

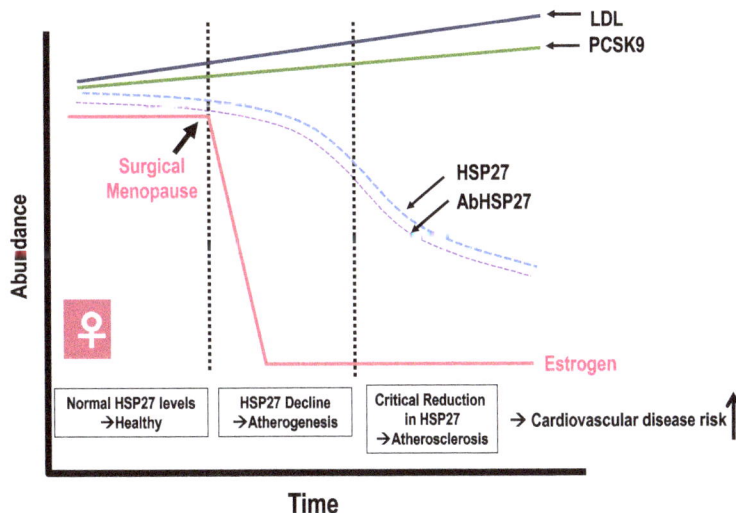

Fig. 3 Proposed interplay of HSP27 & estrogens

disease patients, and PCSK9, which itself may be regulated by HSP27 (unpublished data). Secondary outcome variables are lipids (total cholesterol, triglycerides, HDL, LDL), ovarian hormones (estradiol, FSH, LH, progesterone), cytokines, and retinal vessel (arteriole and venule) diameters. Abnormally high lipid levels and/or severe post-menopausal symptoms following PSO may necessitate alterations in management and treatment by attending physicians.

Sample size calculation
To date, there are no prospective studies investigating HSP27, HSP27 Ab, and PCSK9 levels in women following PSO and the ensuing premature, surgical menopause. To estimate the necessary sample size, we assumed an effect size of 0.3, Type 1 error rate $\alpha = 0.05$, and desired power = 0.90. Based on our conservative assumptions, a minimal sample size of at least 160 participants (40 per group) is needed for the study. Assuming 10% attrition rate over the course of the study, a minimum of 178 participants will be required (which is well below our recruitment target of 240). Once there is sufficient enrollment ($n = 6$ / group), effect size will be recalculated based on pilot data (again presuming $\alpha = 0.05$ and power = 0.90) and the sample size adjusted accordingly as the study continues.

Statistical analyses
Data analysis will be performed using Statistical Analysis System (SAS) software. Probability (p) of less than 0.05 will be considered significant. Experimental outcomes for continuous variables will be expressed as means ± standard deviation for each time point and the variance between the groups will be analyzed using ANOVA. Categorical variables will be compared with a chi-square test. In order to examine the relationship between variables, regression analysis will be performed. If more than one predictor variable is found to affect the outcome, multivariate regression will be employed to identify significant associations.

Patient engagement activities
In addition to identifying biological markers associated with cardiovascular dysfunction in women experiencing surgical menopause, we are also interested in understanding how shifts in gender perception (which includes subjective measurements of stressful experiences) can heighten CAD risk. The idea that gender (a construct distinct from "sex" that encompasses social perceptions and expectations regarding the roles of men and women) can shape the clinical outcome of CVD patients is illustrated by a recent study using the GENESYS Gender Index [91, 92], suggesting that a feminine gender score, but not female sex, was associated with heart disease risk factors. We thus hope to identify how surgical menopause

influences the subjective health perceptions, feelings, and lifestyle changes of women after PSO, and if these can affect their vascular health. Together with a focus group of women in Calgary that have undergone PSO, we will co-create questionnaires exploring changes in perceptions of the patient experience (Fig. 2). We will also plan a research forum open to the general public that will address the health concerns most relevant to PSO patients.

Study limitations
We recognize the importance of incorporating a Quality of Life (QOL) assessment that collects data on diet, exercise, and other lifestyle measures. Although there is no formal component in the pilot phase of this study, we plan to include this in the future. Additionally, one of the patient engagement working group's goals is to generate questionnaires together with our research team that directly reflect the patient experience following PSO – these will contain questions on self-reports of lifestyle changes. We also acknowledge that sample size in this study is small; however, it can provide the basis for future, larger studies involving multiple centres.

Discussion
Women with hereditary cancer mutations increasingly elect to undergo PSO as a risk-reducing treatment option, but it is important to be aware of potential ensuing cardiovascular health consequences. As the association of cancer risk with a particular mutation is not fully characterized, the advantages and disadvantages of PSO must be carefully weighed. Besides increased risks of cardiovascular disease and cognitive dysfunction, there are also other associated morbidities that are elevated after PSO, and adjustments to changes in lifestyle (e.g., sexual performance [93]) and in gender self-perceptions are additional issues that should not be ignored.

The "biological arm" of this study will determine how the abrupt loss of estrogen after PSO influences levels of established (e.g., lipids) and novel biomarkers (e.g., HSP27, retinal vessel diameters) in pre-menopausal women. We predict that after surgery, the sudden drop in estrogen will lead to gradual increases in LDL and PCSK9, with concomitant decreases in HSP27 and HSP27 Ab, making these women more susceptible to cardiovascular disease risk (Fig. 3). Results from this pilot work will inform future studies involving larger patient populations, with the long-term goal of using these markers as predictors of cardiovascular health in susceptible populations. Ongoing in vivo studies in our laboratory using an atheroprone murine model suggest that ovariectomy leads to an exacerbation of atherogenesis and that HSP25 (the murine orthologue of HSP27) can substantially reduce the development of aortic atherosclerosis. Hence, HSP27 may serve not only as a marker for cardiovascular disease but possibly as a novel therapeutic in post-menopausal women.

Abbreviations

BRCA1/2: Breast cancer susceptibility gene 1/2; CAD: Coronary artery disease; CVD: Cardiovascular disease; HSP27 Ab: HSP27 antibodies; HSP27: Heat shock protein 27; MHT: Post-menopausal hormone therapy; NO: Nitric oxide; PCSK9: Proprotein convertase subtilisin/kexin type 9; PSO: Prophylactic salpingo-oophorectomy; WISP: Women choosing surgical prevention trial

Acknowledgements

We are indebted to our many collaborators who have provided critical comments and helped with the design of these studies. We would also like to thank Ms. Zhiying (Jane) Liang (Mozell Family Analysis Core Laboratory, University of Calgary) for invaluable biostatistics support, and Mr. Matthew Clarkson, Dr. Jingti Deng, and Ms. Catherine Diao (O'Brien Lab, University of Calgary) for helpful discussions and technical support.

Funding

This research is supported by a Canadian Institutes of Health Research (CIHR) bridge funding grant (PJT-149015), a CIHR-sponsored Strategy for Patient-Oriented Research (SPOR) Collaboration grant (PEG-151774), and seed funding from CIHR's Canadian Vascular Network (CVN).

Authors' contributions

All authors contributed to literature review, writing, and figure presentation of the manuscript. EOB and ZB were involved in the design of the study. All authors edited and approved the manuscript.

Competing interests

The authors declare that they have no competing interests.

References

1. Grodstein F, Manson JE, Colditz GA, Willett WC, Speizer FE, Stampfer MJ. A prospective, observational study of postmenopausal hormone therapy and primary prevention of cardiovascular disease. Ann Intern Med. 2000;133(12):933–41.
2. Barrett-Connor E. Menopause, atherosclerosis, and coronary artery disease. Curr Opin Pharmacol. 2013;13(2):186–91
3. Witteman JC, Grobbee DE, Kok FJ, Hofman A, Valkenburg HA. Increased risk of atherosclerosis in women after the menopause. BMJ. 1989; 298(6674):642–4.
4. Wenger NK. Coronary heart disease: an older woman's major health risk. BMJ. 1997;315(7115):1085–90.
5. Muka T, Oliver-Williams C, Kunutsor S, Laven JSE, Fauser BCJM, Chowdhury R. Association of age at onset of menopause and time since onset of menopause with cardiovascular outcomes, intermediate vascular traits, and all-cause mortality. JAMA Cardiol. 2016;1(7):767–76.
6. Nelson HD. Menopause. Lancet. 2008;371(9614):760–70.
7. Matthews KA, Kuller LH, Chang Y, Edmundowicz D. Premenopausal risk factors for coronary and aortic calcification: a 20-year follow-up in the healthy women study. Prev Med. 2007;45(4):302–8.
8. Kuller LH, Matthews KA, Sutton-Tyrrell K, Edmundowicz D, Bunker CH. Coronary and aortic calcification among women 8 years after menopause and their premenopausal risk factors : the healthy women study. Arterioscler Thromb Vasc Biol. 1999;19(9):2189–98.
9. Chae CU, Derby CA. The menopausal transition and cardiovascular risk. Obstet Gynecol Clin N Am. 2011;38(3):477–88.
10. Stampfer MJ, Colditz GA, Willett WC, Manson JE, Rosner B, Speizer FE, Hennekens CH. Postmenopausal estrogen therapy and cardiovascular disease. Ten-year follow-up from the nurses' health study. N Engl J Med. 1991;325(11):756–62.
11. Henderson BE, Paganini-Hill A, Ross RK. Decreased mortality in users of estrogen replacement therapy. Arch Intern Med. 1991;151(1):75–8.
12. Sobrino A, Oviedo PJ, Novella S, Laguna-Fernandez A, Bueno C, Garcia-Perez MA, Tarin JJ, Cano A, Hermenegildo C. Estradiol selectively stimulates endothelial prostacyclin production through estrogen receptor-{alpha}. J Mol Endocrinol. 2010;44(4):237–46.
13. Tostes RC, Nigro D, Fortes ZB, Carvalho MH. Effects of estrogen on the vascular system. Braz J Med Biol Res. 2003;36(9):1143–58.
14. Rossouw JE, Writing Group for the Women's Health Initiative Investigators. Risks and benefits of estrogen plus progestin in healthy postmenopausal women: principal results from the Women's Health Initiative randomized controlled trial. JAMA. 2002;288:321–33.
15. Hulley S, Grady D, Bush T, Furberg C, Herrington D, Riggs B, Vittinghoff E. For the H, estrogen/progestin replacement study research G: randomized trial of estrogen plus progestin for secondary prevention of coronary heart disease in postmenopausal women. JAMA. 1998;280(7):605–13.
16. Riggs BL, Hartmann LC. Selective estrogen-receptor modulators – mechanisms of action and application to clinical practice. N Engl J Med. 2003;348(7): 618–29.
17. Harman SM, Black DM, Naftolin F, Brinton EA, Budoff MJ, Cedars MI, Hopkins PN, Lobo RA, Manson JE, Merriam GR, et al. Arterial imaging outcomes and cardiovascular risk factors in recently menopausal women: a randomized trial. Ann Intern Med. 2014;161(4):249–60.
18. Hodis HN, Mack WJ, Shoupe D, Azen SP, Stanczyk FZ, Hwang-Levine J, Budoff MJ, Henderson VW. Methods and baseline cardiovascular data from the early versus late intervention trial with estradiol testing the menopausal hormone timing hypothesis. Menopause. 2015;22(4):391–401.
19. Clarkson TB, Melendez GC, Appt SE. Timing hypothesis for postmenopausal hormone therapy: its origin, current status, and future. Menopause. 2013;20(3):342–53.
20. Losordo DW, Kearney M, Kim EA, Jekanowski J, Isner JM. Variable expression of the estrogen receptor in normal and atherosclerotic coronary arteries of premenopausal women. Circulation. 1994;89(4):1501–10.
21. Cassidy M. Coronary disease; the Harveian oration of 1946. Lancet. 1946; 2(6426):587–90.
22. Roeters van Lennep JE. Why women are not small men. Maturitas. 2017;107:A3–4.
23. Oliver MF, Boyd GS. Effect of bilateral ovariectomy on coronary-artery disease and serum-lipid levels. Lancet. 1959;274(7105):690–4.
24. Wuest JH Jr, Dry TJ, Edwards JE. The degree of coronary atherosclerosis in bilaterally oophorectomized women. Circulation. 1953;7(6):801–9.
25. Rivin AU, Dimitroff SP. The incidence and severity of atherosclerosis in estrogen-treated males, and in females with a hypoestrogenic or a hyperestrogenic state. Circulation. 1954;9(4):533–9.
26. Robinson RW, Higano N, Cohen WD. Increased incidence of coronary heart disease in women castrated prior to the menopause. Arch Intern Med. 1959;104:908–13.
27. Cochran R, Gwinup G. Coronary artery disease in young females. Possibility of oophorectomy as an etiologic agent. Arch Intern Med. 1962;110:162–5.
28. Sznajderman M, Oliver MF. Spontaneous premature menopause, ischemic heart-disease and serum-lipids. Lancet. 1963;281(7288):962–5.
29. Johansson BW, Kaij L, Kullander S, Lenner HC, Svanberg L, Astedt B. On some late effects of bilateral oophorectomy in the age range 15-30 years. Acta Obstet Gynecol Scand. 1975;54(5):449–61.
30. Neff RT, Senter L, Salani R. BRCA mutation in ovarian cancer: testing, implications and treatment considerations. Therapeutic advances in medical oncology. 2017;9(8):519–31.
31. Lancaster JM, Powell CB, Chen LM, Richardson DL, Committee SGOCP. Society of Gynecologic Oncology statement on risk assessment for inherited gynecologic cancer predispositions. Gynecol Oncol. 2015;136(1):3–7.
32. Jolie A: My medical journey. New York Times 2013:A25.
33. Jolie A: Diary of a surgery. New York Times 2015:A23.

34. Tyson JJ, Baumann WT, Chen C, Verdugo A, Tavassoly I, Wang Y, Weiner LM, Clarke R. Dynamic modelling of oestrogen signalling and cell fate in breast cancer cells. Nat Rev Cancer. 2011;11(7):523–32.

35. Frasor J, Barnett DH, Danes JM, Hess R, Parlow AF, Katzenellenbogen BS. Response-specific and ligand dose-dependent modulation of estrogen receptor (ER) alpha activity by ERbeta in the uterus. Endocrinology. 2003;144(7):3159–66.

36. Perillo B, Sasso A, Abbondanza C, Palumbo G. 17beta-estradiol inhibits apoptosis in MCF-7 cells, inducing bcl-2 expression via two estrogen-responsive elements present in the coding sequence. Mol Cell Biol. 2000;20(8):2890–901.

37. Hartmann LC, Lindor NM. The role of risk-reducing surgery in hereditary breast and ovarian Cancer. N Engl J Med. 2016;374(5):454–68.

38. Walsh T, Casadei S, Lee MK, Pennil CC, Nord AS, Thornton AM, Roeb W, Agnew KJ, Stray SM, Wickramanayake A, et al. Mutations in 12 genes for inherited ovarian, fallopian tube, and peritoneal carcinoma identified by massively parallel sequencing. Proc Natl Acad Sci U S A. 2011; 108(44):18032–7.

39. Miki Y, Swensen J, Shattuck-Eidens D, Futreal PA, Harshman K, Tavtigian S, Liu Q, Cochran C, Bennett LM, Ding W, et al. A strong candidate for the breast and ovarian cancer susceptibility gene BRCA1. Science. 1994; 266(5182):66–71.

40. Wooster R, Neuhausen SL, Mangion J, Quirk Y, Ford D, Collins N, Nguyen K, Seal S, Tran T, Averill D, et al. Localization of a breast cancer susceptibility gene, BRCA2, to chromosome 13q12-13. Science. 1994;265(5181):2088–90.

41. Takaoka M, Miki Y. BRCA1 gene: function and deficiency. Int J Clin Oncol. 2018; 23(1):36–44.

42. Corso G, Feroce I, Intra M, Toesca A, Magnoni F, Sargenti M, Naninato P, Caldarella P, Pagani G, Vento A, et al. BRCA1/2 germline missense mutations: a systematic review. Eur J Cancer Prev. 2018;27(3):279–86.

43. Finch A, Bacopulos S, Rosen B, Fan I, Bradley L, Risch H, McLaughlin JR, Lerner-Ellis J, Narod SA. Preventing ovarian cancer through genetic testing: a population-based study. Clin Genet. 2014;86(5):496–9.

44. Finch AP, Lubinski J, Moller P, Singer CF, Karlan B, Senter L, Rosen B, Maehle L, Ghadirian P, Cybulski C, et al. Impact of oophorectomy on cancer incidence and mortality in women with a BRCA1 or BRCA2 mutation. J Clin Oncol. 2014;32(15):1547–53.

45. Finch A, Beiner M, Lubinski J, Lynch HT, Moller P, Rosen B, Murphy J, Ghadirian P, Friedman E, Foulkes WD, et al. Salpingo-oophorectomy and the risk of ovarian, fallopian tube, and peritoneal cancers in women with a BRCA1 or BRCA2 mutation. JAMA. 2006;296(2):185–92.

46. Carethers JM, Stoffel EM. Lynch syndrome and lynch syndrome mimics: the growing complex landscape of hereditary colon cancer. World J Gastroenterol. 2015;21(31):9253–61.

47. Schmeler KM, Lynch HT, Chen LM, Munsell MF, Soliman PT, Clark MB, Daniels MS, White KG, Boyd-Rogers SG, Conrad PG, et al. Prophylactic surgery to reduce the risk of gynecologic cancers in the lynch syndrome. N Engl J Med. 2006;354(3):261–9.

48. Benshushan A, Rojansky N, Chaviv M, Arbel-Alon S, Benmeir A, Imbar T, Brzezinski A. Climacteric symptoms in women undergoing risk-reducing bilateral salpingo-oophorectomy. Climacteric. 2009;12(5):404–9.

49. Rocca WA, Gazzuola-Rocca L, Smith CY, Grossardt BR, Faubion SS, Shuster LT, Kirkland JL, Stewart EA, Miller VM. Accelerated accumulation of multimorbidity after bilateral oophorectomy: a population-based cohort study. Mayo Clin Proc. 2016;91(11):1577–89.

50. Parker WH, Broder MS, Chang E, Feskanich D, Farquhar C, Liu Z, Shoupe D, Berek JS, Hankinson S, Manson JE. Ovarian conservation at the time of hysterectomy and long-term health outcomes in the nurses' health study. Obstet Gynecol. 2009;113(5):1027–37.

51. Kallen AN, Pal L. Cardiovascular disease and ovarian function. Curr Opin Obstet Gynecol. 2011;23(4):258–67.

52. Rocca WA, Bower JH, Maraganore DM, Ahlskog JE, Grossardt BR, de Andrade M, Melton LJ 3rd. Increased risk of cognitive impairment or dementia in women who underwent oophorectomy before menopause. Neurology. 2007;69(11):1074–83.

53. Phung TK, Waltoft BL, Laursen TM, Settnes A, Kessing LV, Mortensen PB, Waldemar G. Hysterectomy, oophorectomy and risk of dementia: a nationwide historical cohort study. Dement Geriatr Cogn Disord. 2010; 30(1):43–50.

54. Au A, Feher A, McPhee L, Jessa A, Oh S, Einstein G. Estrogens, inflammation and cognition. Front Neuroendocrinol. 2016;40:87–100.

55. Rocca WA, Gazzuola Rocca L, Smith CY, Grossardt BR, Faubion SS, Shuster LT, Kirkland JL, Stewart EA, Miller VM. Bilateral oophorectomy and accelerated aging: cause or effect? J Gerontol A Biol Sci Med Sci. 2017;72(9):1213–7.

56. Billon-Gales A, Krust A, Fontaine C, Abot A, Flouriot G, Toutain C, Berges H, Gadeau AP, Lenfant F, Gourdy P, et al. Activation function 2 (AF2) of estrogen receptor-alpha is required for the atheroprotective action of estradiol but not to accelerate endothelial healing. Proc Natl Acad Sci U S A. 2011;108(32): 13311–6.

57. Menazza S, Murphy E. The expanding complexity of estrogen receptor signaling in the cardiovascular system. Circ Res. 2016;118(6):994–1007.

58. Mendelsohn ME, Karas RH. The protective effects of estrogen on the cardiovasclar system. N Engl J Med. 1999;340(23):1801–11.

59. Persson L, Henriksson P, Westerlund E, Hovatta O, Angelin B, Rudling M. Endogenous estrogens lower plasma PCSK9 and LDL cholesterol but not Lp(a) or bile acid synthesis in women. Arterioscler Thromb Vasc Biol. 2012;32(3):810–4.

60. Ghosh M, Galman C, Rudling M, Angelin B. Influence of physiological changes in endogenous estrogen on circulating PCSK9 and LDL cholesterol. J Lipid Res. 2015;56(2):463–9.

61. Miller H, Poon S, Hibbert B, Rayner K, Chen YX, O'Brien ER. Modulation of estrogen signaling by the novel interaction of heat shock protein 27, a biomarker for atherosclerosis, and estrogen receptor beta - mechanistic insight into the vascular effects of estrogens. Arteriosclerosis Thrombosis and Vascular Biology. 2005;25(3):E10–4.

62. Martin-Ventura JL, Duran MC, Blanco-Colio LM, Meilhac O, Leclercq A, Michel JB, Jensen ON, Hernandez-Merida S, Tunon J, Vivanco F, et al. Identification by a differential proteomic approach of heat shock protein 27 as a potential marker of atherosclerosis. Circulation. 2004;110:2216–9.

63. Park HK, Park EC, Bae SW, Park MY, Kim SW, Yoo HS, Tudev M, Ko YH, Choi YH, Kim S, et al. Expression of heat shock protein 27 in human atherosclerotic plaques and increased plasma level of heat shock protein 27 in patients with acute coronary syndrome. Circulation. 2006;114(9):886–93.

64. Lepedda AJ, Cigliano A, Cherchi GM, Spirito R, Maggioni M, Carta F, Turrini F, Edelstein C, Scanu AM, Formato M. A proteomic approach to differentiate histologically classified stable and unstable plaques from human carotid arteries. Atherosclerosis. 2009;203(1):112–8.

65. Liang W, Ward LJ, Karlsson H, Ljunggren SA, Li W, Lindahl M, Yuan XM. Distinctive proteomic profiles among different regions of human carotid plaques in men and women. Sci Rep. 2016;6:26231.

66. Seibert TA, Hibbert B, Chen Y-X, Rayner K, Simard T, Hu T, Cuerrier CM, Zhao X, de Belleroche J, Chow BJ. Serum heat shock protein 27 levels represent a potential therapeutic target for atherosclerosis: observations from a human cohort and treatment of female mice. J Am Coll Cardiol. 2013;62(16):1446–54.

67. Batulan Z, Pulakazhi Venu VK, Li Y, Koumbadinga G, Alvarez-Olmedo DG, Shi C, O'Brien ER. Extracellular release and signaling by heat shock protein 27: role in modifying vascular inflammation. Front Immunol. 2016;7:285.

68. Rayner K, Chen Y-X, McNulty M, Simard T, Zhao X, Wells DJ, de Belleroche J, O'Brien ER. Extracellular release of the atheroprotective heat shock protein 27 is mediated by estrogen and competitively inhibits acLDL binding to scavenger receptor-a. Circ Res. 2008;103(2):133–41.

69. Cuerrier CM, Chen YX, Tremblay D, Rayner K, McNulty M, Zhao X, Kennedy CR, de BJ PAE, O'Brien ER. Chronic over-expression of heat shock protein 27 attenuates atherogenesis and enhances plaque remodeling: a combined histological and mechanical assessment of aortic lesions. PLoS One. 2013;8(2):e55867.

70. De AK KKM, Yeh BS, Miller-Graziano C. Exaggerated human monocyte IL-10 concomitant to minimal TNF-alpha induction by heat-shock protein 27 (Hsp27) suggests Hsp 27 is primarily an antiinflamatory stimulus. J Immunol. 2000;165(7):3951–8.

71. Raizman JE, Chen YX, Seibert T, Hibbert B, Cuerrier CM, Salari S, Zhao X, Hu T, Shi C, Ma X, et al. Heat shock protein-27 attenuates foam cell formation and atherogenesis by down-regulating scavenger receptor-a expression via NF-kappaB signaling. Biochim Biophys Acta. 2013;1831(12):1721–8.

72. Ghayour-Mobarhan M, Saber H, Ferns GA. The potential role of heat shock protein 27 in cardiovascular disease. ClinChimActa. 2012;413(1–2):15–24.

73. Pourghadamyari H, Moohebati M, Parizadeh SM, Falsoleiman H, Dehghani M, Fazlinezhad A, Akhlaghi S, Tavallaie S, Sahebkar A, Paydar R, et al. Serum antibody titers against heat shock protein 27 are associated with the severity of coronary artery disease. Cell Stress Chaperones. 2011;16(3):309–16.

74. Shi C, Chen Y, Li Y, O'Brien ER. When auto-antibodies potentiate: the paradoxical Signalling role of anti-HSP27 auto-antibody immune complexes improves Athero-protection. Circulation. 2014;130(Suppl 2):A12771.

75. Abifadel M, Varret M, Rabes JP, Allard D, Ouguerram K, Devillers M, Cruaud C, Benjannet S, Wickham L, Erlich D, et al. Mutations in PCSK9 cause autosomal dominant hypercholesterolemia. Nat Genet. 2003;34(2):154–6.

76. Cohen J, Pertsemlidis A, Kotowski IK, Graham R, Garcia CK, Hobbs HH. Low LDL cholesterol in individuals of African descent resulting from frequent nonsense mutations in PCSK9. Nat Genet. 2005;37(2):161–5.

77. Yan H, Ma YL, Gui YZ, Wang SM, Wang XB, Gao F, Wang YP. MG132, a proteasome inhibitor, enhances LDL uptake in HepG2 cells in vitro by regulating LDLR and PCSK9 expression. Acta Pharmacol Sin. 2014;35(8):994–1004.

78. Zhang Y, Xu RX, Li S, Zhu CG, Guo YL, Sun J, Li JJ. Association of plasma small dense LDL cholesterol with PCSK9 levels in patients with angiographically proven coronary artery disease. Nutr Metab Cardiovasc Dis. 2015;25(4):426–33.

79. Lakoski SG, Lagace TA, Cohen JC, Horton JD, Hobbs HH. Genetic and metabolic determinants of plasma PCSK9 levels. J Clin Endocrinol Metab. 2009;94(7):2537–43.

80. Sharrett AR, Hubbard LD, Cooper LS, Sorlie PD, Brothers RJ, Nieto FJ, Pinsky JL, Klein R. Retinal arteriolar diameters and elevated blood pressure: the atherosclerosis risk in communities study. Am J Epidemiol. 1999;150(3):263–70.

81. Klein R, Clegg L, Cooper LS, Hubbard LD, Klein BE, King WN, Folsom AR. Prevalence of age-related maculopathy in the atherosclerosis risk in communities study. Arch Ophthalmol. 1999;117(9):1203–10.

82. Ikram MK, de Jong FJ, Bos MJ, Vingerling JR, Hofman A, Koudstaal PJ, de Jong PT, Breteler MM. Retinal vessel diameters and risk of stroke: the Rotterdam study. Neurology. 2006;66(9):1339–43.

83. McGeechan K, Liew G, Macaskill P, Irwig L, Klein R, Klein BE, Wang JJ, Mitchell P, Vingerling JR, de Jong PT, et al. Prediction of incident stroke events based on retinal vessel caliber: a systematic review and individual-participant meta-analysis. Am J Epidemiol. 2009;170(11):1323–32.

84. Couper DJ, Klein R, Hubbard LD, Wong TY, Sorlie PD, Cooper LS, Brothers RJ, Nieto FJ. Reliability of retinal photography in the assessment of retinal microvascular characteristics: the atherosclerosis risk in communities study. Am J Ophthalmol. 2002;133(1):78–88.

85. Seidelmann SB, Claggett B, Bravo PE, Gupta A, Farhad H, Klein BE, Klein R, Di Carli M, Solomon SD. Retinal vessel calibers in predicting long-term cardiovascular outcomes: the atherosclerosis risk in communities study. Circulation. 2016;134(18):1328–38.

86. Hanssen H, Nickel T, Drexel V, Hertel G, Emslander I, Sisic Z, Lorang D, Schuster T, Kotliar KE, Pressler A, et al. Exercise-induced alterations of retinal vessel diameters and cardiovascular risk reduction in obesity. Atherosclerosis. 2011;216(2):433–9.

87. Zhao M, Ding JX, Zeng K, Zhao J, Shen F, Yin YX, Chen Q. Heat shock protein 27: a potential biomarker of peritoneal metastasis in epithelial ovarian cancer? Tumour Biol. 2014;35(2):1051–6.

88. Gruden G, Carucci P, Lolli V, Cosso L, Dellavalle E, Rolle E, Cantamessa A, Pinach S, Abate ML, Campra D, et al. Serum heat shock protein 27 levels in patients with hepatocellular carcinoma. Cell Stress Chaperones. 2013;18(2):235–41.

89. Zimmermann M, Nickl S, Lambers C, Hacker S, Mitterbauer A, Hoetzenecker K, Rozsas A, Ostoros G, Laszlo V, Hofbauer H, et al. Discrimination of clinical stages in non-small cell lung cancer patients by serum HSP27 and HSP70: a multi-institutional case-control study. Clin Chim Acta. 2012;413(13–14):1115–20.

90. Jin C, Phillips VL, Williams MJ, van Rij AM, Jones GT. Plasma heat shock protein 27 is associated with coronary artery disease, abdominal aortic aneurysm and peripheral artery disease. Spring. 2014;3:635.

91. Pelletier R, Khan NA, Cox J, Daskalopoulou SS, Eisenberg MJ, Bacon SL, Lavoie KL, Daskupta K, Rabi D, Humphries KH, et al. Sex versus gender-related characteristics: which predicts outcome after acute coronary syndrome in the young? J Am Coll Cardiol. 2016;67(2):127–35.

92. Pelletier R, Ditto B, Pilote L. A composite measure of gender and its association with risk factors in patients with premature acute coronary syndrome. Psychosom Med. 2015;77(5):517–26.

93. Tucker KL. Nutrient intake, nutritional status, and cognitive function with aging. Ann N Y Acad Sci. 2016;1367(1):38–49.

94. Rayner K, Sun J, Chen Y-X, McNulty M, Simard T, Zhao X, Wells DJ, de Belleroche J, O'Brien ER. Heat shock protein 27 protects against Atherogenesis via an estrogen-dependent mechanism role of selective estrogen receptor Beta modulation. Arterioscler Thromb Vasc Biol. 2009; 29(11):1751–6.

10

Unintended pregnancy: a framework for prevention and options for midlife women in the US

Versie Johnson-Mallard[1]*, Elizabeth A. Kostas-Polston[2], Nancy Fugate Woods[3], Katherine E. Simmonds[4], Ivy M. Alexander[5] and Diana Taylor[6]

Abstract

Recently unintended pregnancies have been described as "a new kind of mid-life crisis." Given the high prevalence of unwanted or mistimed pregnancy in the US, we examined the sexual and reproductive health patterns of sexually active midlife women. An examination of the prevalence of unintended pregnancy among midlife women revealed a gap in data indicating unmet sexual and reproductive health needs of midlife women. The application of a framework for primary, secondary and tertiary prevention for unintended pregnancy may assist with guiding care for women and identifying implications for reproductive health policy and potential political interference as they relate to sexual and reproductive health in midlife women.

Keywords: Reproductive health, Menopause, Contraception, Pregnancy, Abortion, Transition, Framework, Age, Women, Sex

Background

An unintended pregnancy is one that was mistimed or unwanted. Mistimed pregnancies are those that occur among women who do not want to become pregnant at the time the pregnancy occurred, but who want to become pregnant at some time in the future. Unwanted pregnancies are those that women experience when they do not want to become pregnant then or at any time in the future. An intended pregnancy is one that is desired at the time it occurred or sooner [1]. Although one might imagine that adult women, in particular midlife women, would be experienced in fertility control and family planning, even older women do not seem to be immune to the experience of unintended pregnancy [2].

James [3] conducted a systematic review of studies of multiple unintended pregnancies spanning the period from 1979 to the present. She found 8 studies that provided incidence rates on multiple unintended pregnancies ranging from 7.4 to 30.9 per 100 person-years and

prevalence rates ranging from 17% to 31.6%. In addition, she examined factors associated with multiple unintended pregnancies: increasing age, identifying as Black or Hispanic, having an income below the poverty level, experiencing a non-voluntary first sexual intercourse and especially at a very young age, participating in sex trade, experiencing stressful life events, and having had a previous abortion. Factors associated with reduced risk of multiple unintended pregnancies were use of IUDs or combined oral contraceptives. Some of these risk factors are modifiable, for example, contraceptive type and use. Others reflect pervasive effects of poverty and other social determinants of health disparities.

In addition to the above reasons for unintended pregnancy among midlife women, sexual health of midlife women is often over-looked by both primary care providers and researchers, with most effort focused on younger women. Nonetheless, midlife women are at greater risk of new sexually transmitted infections and unintended pregnancy than previously imagined [4]. In addition to recent changes in relationships that make many women single again, a limited knowledge of safer sexual practices, less predictable menstrual cycles, and health care providers who may not evaluate sexual

* Correspondence: Vjmallard@ufl.edu
[1]Department of Family, Community, and Health System Science, Robert Wood Johnson Nurse Faculty Scholar Alum, University of Florida, College of Nursing, Gainesville, FL, USA
Full list of author information is available at the end of the article

health risks among this population of women may contribute to the incidence of unintended pregnancy [4].

The U. S. has the highest rates of unintended pregnancy among the most developed nations of the world, with nearly half of pregnancies being unintended [1]. Despite efforts to improve access to evidence-based and culturally sensitive reproductive health care, outcomes of unintended pregnancy prevention efforts in the United States lag behind those in many other countries. Some progress in reducing the risk of unintended pregnancy can be attributed to the implementation of the Affordable Care Act (ACA) from 2009 to 2016 [5]. The ACA improved coverage for contraceptive services for adolescents and young adult reproductive age women up to 26 years of age. In addition, provisions required insurance plans to cover contraceptives for all women, regardless of their age, with no out of pocket cost required [5].

Given the high prevalence of unintended pregnancy in the US, the purposes of this paper are to:

- describe sexual and reproductive health (SRH) patterns of sexually active midlife women;
- examine the prevalence of unintended pregnancy among midlife women;
- apply a framework for primary, secondary and tertiary prevention for unintended pregnancy grounded in a primary health care perspective to midlife women; and
- explore reproductive health policy and potential political interference as they relate to sexual and reproductive health in midlife women.
Sexual and Reproductive Health Patterns of Midlife Women.

Why is sexual and reproductive health important for midlife women?

Women remain sexually active well into their postmenopausal years and many sexually active midlife women not using an effective family planning method are at risk for pregnancy. Evidence supports pregnancy in sexually active women can occur over the age of 50 years, with women remaining potentially fertile. Sexually active couples are at risk for pregnancy until women reach approximately 54 years, at which age menopause has occurred in 95% [6]. Indeed, women are often advised to continue using birth control/family planning methods until they have not had a menstrual period for one calendar year.

The menopausal transition challenges women to manage their fertility and complicates their family planning efforts. As they begin the menopausal transition, women's menstrual cycles become irregular, with some experiencing long periods (months) of amenorrhea during the latter part of the menopausal transition prior to their final menstrual period [7]. In general, this period of amenorrhea of variable duration has stimulated guidelines that one year of amenorrhea be observed prior to confirming a women's cycle pattern as consistent with post-menopause. Despite this conservative definition, there are rare occurrences of another menses following a year of amenorrhea.

Mercer and colleagues surveyed midlife women in the United Kingdom, finding that those 35–44 years reported an average of 4 episodes of sexual intercourse over the past month and those 45–54 reported 3.5 episodes [8]. Similar data from women in the U.S. by Finer and Philibin reported 75% of women aged 40 to 44 years were sexually active, a small percentage 4% of the 75% reported not using contraception and actively trying to conceive [9].

In Great Britain, 25% of women 40–44 years of age reporting using no contraception, compared with 28% of women 45–49 years of age [8]. In a similar study conducted with a cohort of sexually active women 40–44 years in the USA, 31% of women reported not using any form of contraception [10]. As seen in the data in Table 1, use of hormonal contraceptives was low in both the UK and the US. In both countries, women 40–44 years of age relied on female and partner sterilization and male condoms, with the latter being used by a greater proportion of those in the UK [10]. In the US 13% reported relying on vasectomy/partner sterilization, 35% relied on female sterilization compared to 25% of UK participants relying on partner sterilization and 15% on female sterilization [8, 11]. Thus US and UK data indicate a majority of midlife women are using condoms, male and female sterilization [8–10]. The U. S. data on contraceptive use collected by National Survey of Family Growth (NSFG) included women aged 15–44 years. These data did not provide information about the latter midlife years. Only recently (2015) has data collection

Table 1 Contraceptive Method of Women 40–44 years in Great Britain and U.S

Age 40–44 years	Great Britain %	United States
Male condom	21%	8%
Pill	13%	8%
IUD	8%	<1%
Hormonal IUS	7%	<1%
Injection	3%	1%
Implant	1%	<1%
Patch	<1%	1%
Female Sterilization	15%	35%
Partner Sterilization	25%	13%

Adapter from: Finer, L. B., & Philbin, J. M. (2014). Trends in ages at key reproductive transitions in the United States, 1951–2010. Women's Health Issues, 24(3), e271-e279; Hardman, S. M., & Gebbie, A. E. (2014). The contraception needs of the perimenopausal woman. *Best Practice & Research Clinical Obstetrics & Gynaecology*, 28(6), 903–915 expanded to include upper bound of age range 44 to 49 years.

One might also ask whether women are confused about using hormone therapy (HT) to manage symptoms related to menopause and hormones used in contraceptive methods. Although hormone therapy does not provide effective contraceptive effects, both hormone therapy and hormonal contraceptives can mask the onset of menopause by stimulating regular withdrawal bleeding. Use of hormonal contraception and hormone therapy (HT) for menopause-related symptoms in combination is not recommended. Once ovulation inhibition is no longer a concern, lower dosed menopause-specific methods can be considered for managing symptoms such as hot flashes that are not well-controlled by other means. Risks for adverse clinical outcomes exist for women continuing hormonal contraceptive use after menopause [11].

Prevention of unintended pregnancy
What are the risks of unintended pregnancy in midlife women?
Data on unintended pregnancy rates in U.S. among women older than 45 years does not appear to be intentionally collected by the NSFG at the time of writing this paper. Estimates are that for women 40–44 years of age, 48% of pregnancies are unintended [12–15]. However, Europe has reported unplanned pregnancy estimates as high as 30% among women 45–49 years of age [12, 13].

In the United States, birth rates for women up to age 44 years have been trending upward since the 1990s with 0.3 births per 1000 to 0.7 births per 1000 in 2012 to 0.8 births /1000 in 2013 [15, 16]. The increase in live births among some midlife women in the U.S. is reportedly due to planned births and increasing use of assisted reproductive technology [17]. Unintended pregnancy rates for nearly half of U.S. women 40–44 years old and the international data from Europe reporting unplanned pregnancy rates as high as 30% in women 45–49 years of age are concerning. Framing and addressing unintended pregnancy at a global level is imperative for the health of women and children.

Prevention and Management of Unintended Pregnancy for midlife women: A framework
What is a framework for prevention and management of unintended pregnancy in midlife women?
Taylor and colleagues proposed using a comprehensive, culturally appropriate public health framework in which primary, secondary, and tertiary measures are integrated into nationally supported clinical guidelines and incorporated into primary care competencies for health professionals [13]. The proposed framework for prevention

and management of unintended pregnancy rests on foundational work by the World Health Organization on Primary Health Care that is grounded in public health and primary medical care. Such a framework is used widely in national health services outside the U.S., e.g. Canada, UK. In this framework, public health care models include primary, secondary, and tertiary prevention strategies. (In the US primary, secondary, and tertiary care refers to both settings and type of clinical care and is not systematically linked to a public health framework).

In the public health model proposed in this paper, primary prevention includes services designed to promote intended, healthy pregnancies with healthy mothers and infants and reduction of personal perinatal, neonatal, and family adverse events. Primary prevention services incorporate preconception care, reproductive life plan development and evaluation and contraception and emergency contraception dispensing or prescribing. Secondary prevention services are focused on identification of unintended pregnancies early in order to improve reproductive health outcomes. Secondary prevention services incorporate pregnancy diagnosis, pregnancy options counseling and management, referral and counseling for pregnancy care, adoption or early abortion referral and care. Tertiary prevention is focused on preventing complications associated with a later unintended pregnancy and support for women and their families who experience later unintended pregnancy [13]. Tertiary prevention for midlife women may incorporate prevention efforts specific to women who have experienced multiple unintended pregnancies [13].

Primary prevention of unintended pregnancy
Why primary prevention of unintended pregnancy?
The concept of preconception health is important for girls and women from birth to death, with the goal being optimal health which may involve getting healthy, staying healthy, and managing health problems. Preconception health is not age-specific but based on individual health, and not only for those planning a pregnancy, since about half of pregnancies are unplanned. The concept of preconception health is important for midlife women. Embedded within the concept of preconception health are the notions of the *Well Woman Visit*, an opportunity to promote health by addressing health concerns and educating women about pregnancy risks. Women experience aging differently and their care should be individualized. Aging into midlife should not be a barrier to addressing sexual health topics. Midlife women have sexual concerns and sometimes may want their healthcare provider to breach the subject first, thereby opening the door to two way and trusting conversation.

Nurses, physicians and other providers of primary prevention services for midlife women during transition to menopause should incorporate counseling and education in regard to fluctuating fertility and methods to prevent unplanned pregnancies. The incorporation of reproductive life plan development and topics of discussion should include safe and effective contraceptive methods, diagnosis and management of common age-related medical conditions such as hypertension, diabetes and breast cancer, transition to menopause and hormone therapy to manage menopause-related symptoms. The American College of Obstetricians and Gynecologists guidelines recommend family planning counseling and contraceptive protection for women at risk for pregnancy until they are 55 years old [14]. Safe and effective contraceptive methods for midlife women exist in many forms and delivery methods (see Table 2).

Midlife women at risk for pregnancy may have a twofold benefit from use of certain contraceptive methods. Hormonal contraceptives can help alleviate irregular menstrual bleeding, hot flashes, night sweats and vaginal dryness while simultaneously lowering pregnancy risk. Contraceptive methods should be individualized based on the women's health history: for example, contraceptives containing estrogen may not be ideal for women with hypertension, diabetes, cancer or other chronic medical conditions. Newer combined oral contraceptive (COC) preparations contain low dose estrogen and progestogen and are safe, and monophasic pill with 30 mcg or less of estrogen are considered an appropriate first line choice, safe and effective for women with chronic medical conditions [10, 11, 18]. (see Table 2). Women using contraceptive methods can be advised to stop

Table 2 Contraceptives methods: Type, details and route of delivery

Type	Progestin Only Contraceptive			
Descriptive	• alleviates bleeding irregularities		• not effective with alleviated vasomotor symptoms or vaginal dryness • women ≥ 45 years at time insertion can rely on IUS for 7yrs or until menopause	
Routes of delivery	pill	subdermal implant	injectable	Intra Uterine System (IUS)
Type	Combined Hormonal Methods			
Descriptive	• reduces vasomotor symptoms • relieves irregular bleeding • methods with ≤ 30 mcg of ethinylestradiol are considered appropriate first line choice,		• Risk of medical morbidity must balance the risk	
Route of delivery	pills		transdermal patch	vaginal
Type	Barrier Methods			
Descriptive	• None hormonal • User dependent		• Requires use of spermicide	
Route of delivery	Condoms (Male and female)		Diaphragm	
Type	Natural Family Planning			
Descriptive	Low effectiveness • Menstrual cycle is unpredictable in perimenopausal women which makes these method problematic			
Route of delivery	Basal body temperature		Calendar/rhythm	
Type	Sterilization (mechanical occlusion, electrocoagulation, vasectomy)			
Descriptive	Female sterility •Natural sterility is pending in perimenopausal women making surgical/invasive method potentially less cost effective		Male sterility • Male controlled fertility method popular, • permanent, safe	
Route of delivery	Surgical tubal ligation or blockage		Surgical vas deferens occlusion	

Adapted from Finer, L. B., & Philbin, J. M. (2014). Trends in ages at key reproductive transitions in the United States, 1951–2010. Women's Health Issues, 24(3), e271-e279
10. Hardman, S. M., & Gebbie, A. E. (2014). The contraception needs of the perimenopausal woman. Best Practice & Research Clinical Obstetrics & Gynaecology, 28(6), 903–915

contraception at age 55 providing they have stopped menses for at least one year.

What does pregnancy risk look like at midlife?

Godfrey et al.' estimated that over three-quarters of women aged 45–50 were at risk for an unintended pregnancy due to their low use of contraception [14]. Many midlife women believe they are no longer able to conceive and may choose not to use contraception. For others, the use of hormonal contraception becomes riskier if the woman has a medical conditions that increase the risks associated with a particular method (e.g., combined estrogen-progestogen contraceptives) [15]. Healthcare providers, too, fail to educate midlife women about important non-contraceptive benefits of hormonal contraception, including reduction of vasomotor symptoms, treatment of abnormal uterine bleeding, decreased risk of ovarian and endometrial cancer, and maintenance of bone mineral density. For example, the levonorgestrel (LNG) intrauterine system (IUS) (a long-acting reversible contraceptive method), is a first-line therapy for heavy menstrual bleeding which is commonly experienced during midlife [15]. Perhaps more importantly, the LNG-IUS is not only an alternative to uterine ablation and hysterectomy, but also provides superior contraceptive effectiveness (equivalent to sterilization) [16].

As fertility declines in midlife, recognition of pregnancy may become more problematic. Changes in a midlife woman's body, such as changing bleeding patterns or prolonged periods of amenorrhea, may be mistaken as normal, instead of as signs of an unintended pregnancy [17]. Vasomotor symptoms (e.g., hot flashes), changes in menstrual patterns, body weight, vaginal discharge, and mood may be interpreted by the midlife woman as indicating menopause [17]. With advancing age, midlife women with chronic gynecological issues (e.g., uterine fibroids, endometriosis) also experience decreased fertility. It would be reasonable, then, for a midlife woman not to think about the risk of unintended pregnancy when her understanding of her changing body is related to *the change of life* or to her gynecological issue.

Secondary prevention of unintended pregnancy

Secondary prevention of unintended pregnancy optimizes early diagnosis of a pregnancy. Clinical care for women who suspect unintended pregnancy begins with a health history and physical exam, as well as engagement with women to support their decision process.

Why a health history? Obtaining a health history is the first step during a pregnancy testing encounter. Open-ended questions are used to gather information about a midlife woman's physical, psychological, social, and sexual history. Because it is common for midlife women to experience unpredictable menstrual bleeding, such as skipping a month or having multiple bleeding episodes in a month, they may experience difficulty with estimating gestational age. Therefore, a woman's sexual and other health history will serve as a database on which to date gestational age, as well as to provide insight as to how a woman feels about the possibility of a pregnancy or termination.

Why a physical examination?

In addition to obtaining a health history, a physical examination may be helpful when attempting to diagnose a pregnancy. If too early in a pregnancy, physical changes of the vagina, cervix, and uterus may not be evident. Inconsistencies among and between a woman's health history, physical examination, and pregnancy test results may warrant a quantitative (serum) pregnancy test and/or transvaginal ultrasound.

What is emergency contraception?

If desired, within 5 days of unprotected sexual intercourse, a midlife woman should be offered emergency contraception (EC). EC consists of methods that can be used to prevent pregnancy. Effectiveness of EC methods vary depending on the method and most importantly, timing of administration. In the United States (US), four options are available (the Cu-IUD [intrauterine copper contraceptive] and three types of emergency contraceptive pills [ECPs]). See Table 3, for EC types, timing of initiation, and evidence summary. It is critically important to note that not all midlife women are eligible to use all forms of EC. Healthcare providers should refer to the *U.S. Medical Eligibility Criteria for Contraceptive Use, 2016* [18] for guidance as to whether women with particular medical conditions or lifestyle behaviors can use specific EC methods.

Why pregnancy confirmation?

A woman may suspect pregnancy and seek confirmation, or be unaware of the possibility of pregnancy due to increasingly sporadic menstrual periods during midlife. She may choose to either perform an over-the-counter pregnancy test in the privacy of her home, or visit her healthcare provider to appraise the cause of her amenorrhea. During visit with the healthcare provider, a pregnancy test and ultrasound may be performed. The pregnancy test results and ultra sound gestational age assessment are shared with the woman. Simmonds and Likis [19] have identified four steps for delivering options counseling after a confirmed pregnancy: 1) exploring feelings about the pregnancy, 2) identifying support systems and assessing risks, 3) assisting with decision making, and 4) providing desired service or referral.

Table 3 Types of Emergency Contraception

Intrauterine Device (IUD)		
IUD	Initiation of EC	Evidence Summary
Cu-IUD (intrauterine copper contraceptive)	• Can be inserted within 5 days of 1st act of unprotected sexual intercourse as an EC. • Additionally, when can estimate the day of ovulation, can be inserted beyond 5 days after sexual intercourse (as long as insertion does not occur >5 days after ovulation).	• Highly effective. • Can be continued as regular contraception (Cleland et al., 2012).
Emergency Contraceptive Pills (ECPs)		
ECPs	Initiation of EC	Evidence Summary
Ulipristal acetate (UPA) • Single dose (30 mg)	• Take as soon as possible within 5 days of unprotected sexual intercourse.	• Similar effectiveness to Cu-IUD when taken within 3 days after unprotected sexual intercourse. • Shown to be more effective than LNG formulation 3–5 days after unprotected sexual intercourse (Glasier et al., 2010).
Levonorgestrel (LNG) • Single dose (1.5 mg) or • Split dose (1 dose of 0.75 mg of levonorgestrel, followed by a 2nd dose of 0.75 mg of levonorgestrel 12 h later	• Take as soon as possible within 5 days of unprotected sexual intercourse.	• Similar effectiveness to Cu-IUD when taken within 3 days after unprotected sexual intercourse (Glasier et al., 2010). • LNG may be less effective than UPA in obese women (Jatlaoui, 2016).
Combined estrogen and progestin in 2 doses (Yuzpe regimen) • 1 dose of 100 µg of ethinyl estradiol plus 0.50 mg of levonorgestrel followed, by a 2nd dose of 100 µg of ethinyl estradiol plus0.50 mg of levonorgestrel 12 h later	• Take as soon as possible within 5 days of unprotected sexual intercourse.	• Less effective than UPA or LNG. • Associated with more frequent occurrence of side effects (nausea and vomiting) (Raymond et al., 2004).

Adapted from Curtis et al. (2016). U.S. Selected Practice Recommendations for Contraceptive Use, 2016. MMWR Recomm Rep 2016;65(No. RR-4): [1–66]

How to explore feelings about the pregnancy?

When exploring a woman's feelings, healthcare providers should use open-ended questions which will allow the woman to freely express her thoughts or concerns. A starting point may include, "How do you feel about this pregnancy?" Such a question will create a safe space for the woman, as well as allow the healthcare provider to appraise whether she has made any decisions about the pregnancy and provide insight into her understanding of available options (Table 4).

Why identify support systems and assess risks?

Identifying support systems and social risk of violence, abuse, and/or sexual and reproductive coercion are important for the physical and mental well-being of a woman. Pregnancy resulting from non-consensual sexual intercourse may require involving a Social Worker, Psychologist, and/or Psychiatrist in the care of the pregnant woman. What is more, such situations necessitate careful contemplation and collaboration, on behalf of the pregnant woman, as mandated reporting may further compromise a woman's health and well-being.

There appears to be no link between abortion and adverse mental health outcomes like depression [20, 21]. However women with pre-existing mental health problems and those with a history of sexual abuse and/or intimate partner violence are at risk for mental health issues. Robinson, Stotland, and Russo determined the best predictor of serious mental health issues after abortion was emotional health prior to abortion [22]. Obtaining an accurate and thorough woman's physical, psychological, social, and sexual health history will help the healthcare provider identify and treat pre-existing psychiatric problems and psychosocial stressors.

Table 4 Open-ended Questions to Facilitate Communication When Exploring Pregnancy Options

Exploring Feelings
• "How do you feel about this pregnancy?" • "I want to be sure that you know what all of your options are, and I will help you get good care no matter what you decide to do about this pregnancy." • "Tell me what you have heard about adoption?" • "Tell me what you have heard about abortion?" • "Do you have any questions about what it would be like to be a parent?" • "Do you have any questions about what it would be like to place a child for adoption?" • "Do you have any questions about what it would be like to have an abortion?"

Adapted from Simmonds, K. & Likis, F. E. (2011). Caring for women with unintended pregnancies. *Journal of Obstetric, Gynecologic, and Neonatal Nursing*, 40(6), pp. 794–807; and Simmonds, K. & Stern, L. (2017). The challenge of unintended pregnancies. In Alexander, I., Johnson-Mallard, V., Kostas-Polston, E. A., Fogel, C. I., & Woods, N. F. (Eds.), *Women's Health Care in Advanced Practice Nursing*. New York: Springer Publishing Company, LLC

Why assist with decision-making?

Prior to presenting for a healthcare encounter a woman who suspects pregnancy may have already made her decision about the pregnancy. She may have decided to continue with the pregnancy and keep the baby, to continue with the pregnancy and relinquish the baby for adoption, or to have an abortion. Once a decision has been made a referral for appropriate services can help provide a seamless transition.

Are coordination of services and referral important for midlife women?

Providing or referring for appreciate services is essential for transition of care for the midlife woman experiencing an unintended pregnancy. Helping her to make appointments and navigate the system is an essential component of reproductive health care services, particularly when women must seek pregnancy termination outside of the care system, county, or state. Should she decide to continue the pregnancy, a woman should establish obstetrical care and begin prenatal care. If she decides to relinquish the baby for adoption a referral to an adoption agency will be needed. If she decides to terminate the pregnancy, referral for safe, competent abortion care is also essential transition care. Although referral patterns are often clear for other health problems midlife women encounters, these arrangements are often left to the women to navigate alone.

Why pregnancy options counseling?

Regardless of whether intended, unwanted, mistimed, or ambivalent, pregnancy is a life-changing event. Providing counseling and information regarding pregnancy options will be guided by a woman's circumstance and desires. Regardless of circumstance, the possibility of an unintended pregnancy becomes a woman's private health matter—oftentimes, a burden for her to bear. Each woman's situation, presentation, and timing for appraisal of pregnancy exposure or pregnancy confirmation, lend themselves to individual but related healthcare encounters: pregnancy confirmation and counseling on options (i.e. maintaining the pregnancy, relinquishing the baby for adoption, or abortion). A woman should be allowed to self-identify what she perceives are viable options. Parenting, adoption, and abortion are options. Many factors may influence women's decision making. It is important that healthcare providers establish a climate of trust and deliver non-judgmental active listening.

Is maintaining pregnancy an option?

Recent studies suggest that women who carry unwanted pregnancies to term are likely to be in poverty, have depressive symptoms, and have reason to worry about the negative impact of an unintended birth on that child as well as on their existing children [20, 23, 24].

Choosing to continue with an unwanted pregnancy can be emotionally painful and negatively impact a woman's mental health. Herd, Higgins, Sicinski, and Merkurieva[25] examined the association between unwanted and mistimed pregnancies and mental health in women whose pregnancies occurred prior to the legalizaton of abortion [25, 26]. Experiencing unwanted pregnancies, especially after a woman or couple has reached a desired number of children, appears to be strongly associated with poor mental health effects for women later in life. Although not statistically significant, the authors reported more depressive symptoms and a greater likelihood of having a significant episode of depression in the now midlife women who carried an unwanted pregnancy to term and raised the infant. Caretaking stressors; social and economic burdens; changes in educational, career, and health trajectories; and poorer quality relationships between the parent/s and child were posited as causative.

A study to assess differences in child health and development outcomes for women who were denied an abortion and carried an unwanted pregnancy to term compared with women who obtained an abortion found lower scores on child development for the children of women denied abortions [20, 24]. Evidence suggests that unintended births may lead to poorer quality relationships between parents and children thereby negatively influencing parental well-being [21]. Therefore, when midlife women seek out a healthcare provider, the provider has a window of opportunity for detection and intervention. In such cases, a multidisciplinary approach to prenatal care will be in the best interest of both the pregnant woman and her future child.

Is adoption an option?

It is estimated that approximately 14,000 women choose adoption annually [27, 28]. Most unintended pregnancies result in a woman choosing to keep the infant or have an abortion. In fact, only 3% of US White unmarried women and fewer than 2% of Black unmarried women are estimated to place an infant for adoption during their reproductive lifetime [27, 28]. Data regarding the number of infants relinquished each year, and the demographics of women who relinquish their parental rights to infants (birth mothers) is limited; largely due to the low number of infants put up for adoption (Child Welfare Information Gateway, 2011) [27]. The small proportion of women who choose relinquishment of parental rights makes it difficult to collect and generalize data concerning this population [27]. In the US, federal legislation ensures that all pregnant women are offered the opportunity to receive impartial information regarding prenatal care and delivery; infant care, foster care, or adoption; and pregnancy termination (Title X of Public Law 91–572, Section 1008, 1970) [29].

Further, adoption laws differ by state, therefore it is important that healthcare providers are able to: 1) counsel women and provide state-specific information regarding the different options of adoptions, including the different manners in which adoptions can be processed (e.g., public or private agency, adoption lawyer), 2) discuss with the woman, her rights as a birth mother, and 3) refer the woman to an impartial adoption professionals such as social worker [19, 30]. Women considering adoption should establish prenatal care as well as be provided information reinforcing prenatal care and education. The healthcare provider should also review hospital policies regarding adoption with the woman well in advance of her delivery [19, 30].

Is abortion an option?

Women come to a decision to terminate a pregnancy for many different reasons: the most commonly reported include concerns or responsibilities to care for others, inability to afford a child, and the belief that having a baby would interfere with other work and life commitments [31]. For midlife women, concerns related to their age, such as the increased risk of a fetal genetic anomaly or the belief that their family is complete, may also be a factor in their decision. Currently, 19% of all pregnancies in the US end in abortion; most (90%) take place in early pregnancy (before 13 weeks' gestation) [32], and are performed or initiated in ambulatory clinic [33, 34].

What is abortion counseling?

Women who decide to have an abortion should be informed about the estimated gestational age of the pregnancy and encouraged to seek care as early as possible, as the risks of abortion increase in more advanced gestations, and it is also more expensive and can be harder to obtain. It is important that women understand that delayed decision making may be problematic as advanced gestational age abortions are associated with poorer maternal health outcomes, may be difficult to obtain, and/or may be illegal in some states. Recent evidence suggests that carrying an unintended pregnancy to term or being denied an abortion raises an important policy issues affecting women's health. When women do not have freedom to make a decision or cannot act on their decision to end a pregnancy, they may experience long-term psychological sequelae. A recent study of women's mental health and well-being five years after receiving or being denied an abortion (The Turn-away Study) revealed that women denied abortion reported more anxiety symptoms, lower self-esteem, lower life satisfaction, and similar levels of depression [24, 35]. Being denied an abortion [and continuing an unwanted pregnancy] was associated with greater risk of initial experience of adverse psychological outcomes. Over time, psychological well-being improved with both groups of women having similar levels of well-being [24].

Often the decision to have an abortion, as compared to other health decisions can be a subject of conflict. To explore this belief, researchers used the *Decisional Conflict Scale* (DCS), an instrument widely used in many health specialties and considered the gold standard for measuring decisional conflict, as well as the Taft-Baker Scale (TBS), a valid and reliable instrument for use to measure decisional certainty in women seeking abortion and to predict a decision to continue a pregnancy [23, 36]. The majority of women (ages 15 and older), reported that they were certain of their decision when presenting for abortion care. Similar to other studies, women reported that although the decision to have an abortion was not an easy one, they were confident that they had made the right decision [23, 36].

What are the current abortion demographics? Nationally, the abortion rate has fallen in recent years, from a historic high of 29.3/1000 women in 1980–81 to 14.6/1000 in 2014 [1, 33]. This trend has been attributed to the combined effects of increases in the use of highly effective contraceptive methods, as well as the widespread passage of restrictive abortion legislation that makes it more difficult for some women to access services [33]. Though the overall rate has declined, on closer examination, disparities in utilization and inequities in access to services are evident. Women who are poor and low-income, Black, and young are disproportionately represented among abortion patients [33]. Disproportionate patterns exist that mirror those previously discussed with unintended pregnancy (See Table 5), and which are inextricably linked to the broader contexts of unequal access to health care, economic resources and education, and other social determinants of health [37, 38].

With regard to age, in 2014 women age 40 and older had low rates of abortion (3.1/1000) compared to all other age groups [38]. While a table demonstrating the specific demographics among midlife women who experience unintended pregnancy and undergo abortion would likely be very illuminating, such data are not readily available [39]. Data on unintended pregnancies and abortion are published in the aggregate. More often specific demographics are available for younger women. Perhaps this dearth of data is a reflection of the common misperception that midlife women are not sexually active, and therefore may not be at risk for unintended pregnancy. Furthermore, midlife women, even those who are known to be sexually active, are infrequently counseled about contraception.

Table 5 Demographics of Women Obtaining Abortions in 2014: Age, Race/Ethnicity, Relationship Status and Sexual Orientation

AGE	PERCENT	RACE/ETHNICITY	PERCENT
Younger than 20	11.9	White	38.7
20–29	60.0	Black	27.6
30–34	15.9	Hispanic	24.8
35–39	9.1	Asian/Pacific Islander	5.5
Older than 40	3.1	Other	3.4
RELATIONSHIP STATUS	PERCENT	SEXUAL ORIENTATION	PERCENT
Married	14.3	Heterosexual	94.4
Living together not married	31.0	Homosexual	0.3
Single/never married/not living together	45.9	Bisexual	4.2
History of being married, not living together	8.8	Something else	1.1

Adapted from Jones RK, Finer LB, Singh S. Characteristics of US abortion patients, 2008. New York: Guttmacher Institute, 2010, 20,101–8

Between 2008 and 2014, however, this older group experienced a modest increase (6.2%) in abortion utilization, which contrasts with the dramatic declines (25.2–44%) observed among women between 15 and 20 years old during the same period. This decrease in rates among adolescents has been linked to broader declines in teenage pregnancy, which are not attributable to changes in patterns of sexual activity or contraceptive use, but rather are theorized to be a result of greater educational opportunities, and media and economic influences [38, 40].

Are there different abortion methods and providers?

The Centers for Disease Control and Prevention (CDC) defines "legal induced abortion" as an intervention performed by a licensed clinician (e.g. a physician, nurse-midwife, nurse practitioner or physician assistant) that is "intended to terminate an ongoing pregnancy" [41]. In surveillance reporting, most states and systems distinguish between two major categories of abortion, "surgical" and "medical," however the alternative terms "aspiration" and "medication" have been advanced, as the former "obfuscates the differences in the procedures and the training requirements for provision, as well as evokes scary imagery that contributes to wider misunderstanding" ([42], p78).

Regardless of the terminology, procedural abortion involves the removal of pregnancy and supporting endometrial tissue from the uterus via electric or manual vacuum aspiration [42]. In gestations of greater than 14–15 weeks, the procedure typically requires the use of additional instrumentation, a method referred to as "dilation and evacuation" (or D & E). Alternatively, abortion can be provoked by the administration of medication. A combination of the drugs mifepristone and misoprostol is the most common regimen used for early abortions in the US [42]. These medications interrupt pregnancy development and stimulate its expulsion from the uterus. Medication can also be administered later in pregnancy to stimulate uterine contractions that lead to the passage of a fetus. This approach – commonly referred to as "labor induction abortion" – is an uncommon method of abortion in the US at this time (<1.0%) [43].

Uterine aspiration is currently the most common method of abortion in the US, comprising approximately 77% of all abortions [43]. Due to outdated state laws, only physicians are legally permitted to perform this procedure in most states [43]. In abortions beyond 14–15 weeks' gestation, abortion is restricted to physicians with advanced clinical training and skill. In 2016, the Food and Drug Administration (FDA) revised the label for mifepristone to expand the type of licensed healthcare providers, however, as of this writing, 37 states still require a physician to prescribe the medication, even though advanced practice nurses and physician assistants in many states have prescriptive authority. Though laws and regulations in the majority of states require a physician to provide or be involved in the delivery of abortion services, in most settings care is provided by multi-disciplinary teams that include a range of health care workers such as medical assistants, nurses, counselors, social workers, physician assistants, and others. See Table 6 for a comparative overview of medication and aspiration abortion, the two most common methods in the US.

Does disparity in abortion access exist?

Bommaraju, Kavanaugh, Hou and Bessett assert that abortion is often more difficult to access than other types of reproductive health services in the US as a result of the convergence of "three major mutually-reinforcing factors: lack of public financing for abortion services, legislative efforts to restrict access, and stigma associated with the procedure" ([44] p. 62). Women who are members of "vulnerable" populations, including racial or ethnic minorities, youth, socioeconomically disadvantaged, underinsured, or those with certain medical conditions are known to be at greater risk of disparate health care access [45], and may have particular difficulty accessing abortion services. Such vulnerabilities have been associated with delays in care, and in some cases, the continuation of unwanted pregnancies [46, 47].

Rural-residing women generally have less access to health care compared to those who live in urban areas [33, 38], and this pattern is also found with abortion services. In 2014, 90% of US counties - where 39% of all US

Table 6 Early Abortion methods

	Medication abortion	Aspiration abortion
Efficacy	95–98%	99%
Gestational age eligibility	Can use up to 10 weeks' gestation	Up to 14–15 weeks' gestation
Typical number of visits to abortion provider	2 (one to initiate process; one to confirm completion of abortion)	Typically 1–2; one for procedure; follow up can be with abortion provider or primary care provider
Advantages	• Does not require invasive procedure • Some women feel it is more "natural" • Offers more privacy as abortion occurs at home (or other chosen place) • May be accessible in remote/less-densely populated areas	• Complete within a short, defined period of time (several minutes) • Trained health personnel are present throughout procedure • Bleeding is typically light after the procedure
Disadvantages	• Process can take hours to complete • Failure of method requires aspiration of uterus • Cramping can be strong, and last longer than with aspiration abortion • Heavy bleeding is common	• Requires instrumentation of uterus • Providers generally located in areas with higher density populations • Pain medication and anesthesia can cause side effects

Adapted from the Reproductive Health Access Project. (2016). Early Abortion Options, Retrieved from http://www.reproductiveaccess.org/wp-content/uploads/2014/12/early_abortion_options.pdf;
University of California at San Francisco Medical Center. (2016). Medical versus Surgical Abortion, Retrieved from https://www.ucsfhealth.org/education/medical_versus_surgical_abortion/
And the Center for Reproductive Health in Family Medicine. (n.d.) Comparison of early abortion options. Retrieved from http://www.earlypregnancylossresources.org/resources/clinical-resources/

women lived – had no abortion provider [47] legislation specifically aimed at regulating abortion providers (referred to as Targeted Regulation of Abortion Providers or "TRAP" laws) has led some to stop providing services altogether [47, 48] resulting in increases in average travel distances for women in some states [48]. Overall, TRAP laws have been associated with delays in obtaining or forgoing abortion care altogether, as well as increasing attempts at self-abortion by women [47–49]. Decreased access to abortion limits women's ability to make the best decisions about childbearing for themselves and their families.

Women of lower socioeconomic status and women of color in the United States have higher rates of abortion than women of higher socioeconomic status and White women. These disparities are related to systemic hardships experienced by disadvantaged communities, including decreased access to health care, higher levels of stress, exposure to racial discrimination, and poorer living and working conditions [50, 51]. Disparities in abortion rates are related to disparities in unintended pregnancy, and associated disparities in contraceptive use. Structural factors, including economic disadvantage, neighborhood characteristics, lack of access to family planning services, and mistrust in the medical system underlay these disparities in abortion. Reduced access to abortion will result in more women experiencing later abortions or having an unintended childbirth which will worsen health disparities [52].

Are abortions safe?
Overall, abortion is very safe; a first-trimester abortion is one of the safest medical procedures and carries minimal

risk—less than 0.05%—of major complications that might need hospital care [53–55]. Mortality is extremely rare when abortion is performed by qualified, competent licensed healthcare providers and occurs early in pregnancy [56]. The risk of death associated with abortion increases with gestational age, from 0.3 per 100,000 abortions at or before eight weeks to 6.7 per 100,000 at 18 weeks or greater [56]. These rare deaths are usually the result of such things as adverse reactions to anesthesia, embolism, infection, or uncontrollable bleeding. In comparison, a woman's risk of death during pregnancy and childbirth is ten times greater [56]. The abortion mortality rate was at least as low as the mortality rate associated with plastic surgery at licensed or accredited ambulatory surgical centers in the same decade, approximately equivalent to the proportion of marathon runners who died during races in the same time period [52, 57].

When compared against the risk of morbidity and mortality that occur during pregnancy for women over 35 years of age, abortion is a far safer option. Morbidity and adverse events during hospital delivery and postpartum maternal hospitalization increased 75% and 114%, respectively from 1998 to 1999 to 2008–2009 [58]. The risk of morbidity increases with maternal age, ranging, for example, from 6.6% for preeclampsia to 18.6% for obesity [59]. The risk for negative infant outcomes, such as stillbirth, disability, and prenatal demise, increases as well [59]. The most common types of morbidity associated with pregnancy for midlife women are hypertensive disorders of pregnancy [59]. Among almost 55,000 women, morbidity identified across service settings were experienced by 2.1% who had a medication abortion, and by 1.3% in the first trimester and 1.5% in the second trimester or later among those who had an abortion procedure [34].

Serious abortion related adverse events (clinical errors) or morbidity (conditions due to pregnancy or abortion process) are rare and are defined as those resulting in intervention (surgical repair for uterine perforation, transfusion for hemorrhage) occur less than 0.1%) and hospitalization for pelvic infection/sepsis or hemorrhage occur less than 0.5%. [34]. The most common non-serious (minor) adverse event (incomplete abortion) or morbidity (continued uterine bleeding) often requires re-aspiration or repeat abortion in an outpatient setting [60]. Other potential adverse events or morbidity diagnoses following abortion or with midlife pregnancy are provided in Table 7.

Tertiary prevention of unintended pregnancy
What is tertiary prevention of unintended pregnancy?
Tertiary prevention of unintended pregnancy emphasizes prevention of adverse events associated with a later term unintended pregnancy, supporting women and their families who experience later term unwanted pregnancy and may include prevention efforts for women who have had multiple unintended pregnancies. Women who are at high risk, including those who carry an unwanted pregnancy to term or experience a later term abortion will require more professional attention and care coordination than women having an unintended pregnancy that is diagnosed very early in gestation. Although public financing for prenatal care has been expanded, there continue to be documented disparities in receipt of unplanned pregnancy care and disparities in maternal and infant outcomes by race and SES [61]. Improving the accessibility and quality of unintended pregnancy care can further ensure that all women who continue their unplanned pregnancies have the best

possible pregnancy and parenting outcomes. A tertiary approach to preventing unintended pregnancy should be combined with multifaceted public health interventions addressing health disparities in reproductive health services, toxic stress, and economic supports [13].

What might the future hold for reproductive Health Research, rights, and justice?
What are the future issues for research related to unintended pregnancy prevention and midlife women?
At this writing and without a crystal ball, we can only guess at the future of unintended pregnancy prevention and care as it relates to all women and specifically midlife women. What we do know is that in the current political climate there are likely to be fewer resources for research and increasing political interference and disparities with access to quality sexual and reproductive health care.

The consequences of political interference for women's reproductive health and justice not only limit care options, but also impose restrictions on research [61]. Harris investigated the consequences of antiabortion politics trumping science by questioning the legitimacy of abortion research and stigmatizing the status of the work. Moreover, in addition to deterring investigators from studying abortion through limiting federal funding for the research, in vitro fertilization (IVF) research and research on human embryonic stem cell lines has also been limited by policies affecting what the National Institutes of Health is empowered to fund. Consequences of these policies has been limitation of access for women and families to knowledge that would inform a wide range of reproductive health issues spanning a range from establishing a pregnancy to ending one [39, 61]. Harris has pointed out the threat to reproductive justice that has been imposed by limiting research on topics

Table 7 Adverse Events/Morbidities Associated with Abortion and Pregnancy

Adverse Events/ Associated with Abortion	* Maternal Morbidities Associated with Pregnancy in Women over 35 Years of Age
Anesthesia side-effects	Acute Renal Failure
Incomplete abortion (retained products of conception)	Cesarean section delivery
Continuing pregnancy/Missed Ectopic Pregnancy	Gestational Diabetes/Diabetes
Pelvic Infection	Hemorrhage
Hemorrhage (> 500 cm^3 uterine bleeding) resulting from uterine perforation	Hypertension disorders of pregnancy
Uterine/cervical perforation	GU Infections
Bleeding/Disseminated intravascular coagulation (DIC)	Hematometra
Bowel or bladder injury	Hemorrhage (> 500 cm^3 uterine bleeding) Myocardial Infarction
Cervical shock	Obesity and Weight Gain
	Placenta Previa
	Preeclampsia
	Preterm Labor
	Pulmonary Embolism
	Respiratory Distress Syndrome
	Shock

Callaghan, Creanga, & Kuklina, 2012; Franz & Husslein, 2010; Grossman, Anderson, et al., 2015; Hand, 2014; Lim & Singh, 2014; Raymond, Grimes, 2012; Raymond, Grossmam, & Weaver, 2014; Taylor, et al., 2017
*Maternal complications only

such as IVF to private funding sources and the consequent access to IVF to a subset of women with financial resources to obtain IVF services and thus contribute to IVF research efforts. Balancing research needs for contraception, all unintended pregnancy prevention interventions, and fertility enhancement during midlife in federal research portfolios would serve the goal of reproductive justice.

At this time, we have identified many important questions for research pertaining to midlife women and unplanned pregnancy. Contemporary research on the menopausal transition and early postmenopausal has provided novel research findings, positioning scientists to understand more fully the optimal approaches to prevention of unplanned pregnancy for midlife women. Appreciation of the influence of chronic illness, in particular multiple chronic illnesses on midlife women's health could contribute to refinement of prevention strategies to help women avoid unintended pregnancy while minimizing their risk of adverse outcomes related to the use of some types of contraceptives or decisions to have sterilization procedures. At the same time, expanded research about contemporary midlife women's sexual behavior patterns could enrich the evidence on which primary prevention of unplanned pregnancy is based, by providing data about US women comparable to that available in Europe. In addition, understanding the consequences for midlife women of carrying an unintended pregnancy to term and parenting an infant would benefit from additional research on which to base approaches to care, such as tertiary prevention of unintended pregnancy. In particular, advancing understanding of repeated unintended pregnancy and factors that interfere with women's ability to manage their fertility warrant attention in national data gathering efforts that would drive research agendas [3]. Finally, recent research findings from an evaluation of abortion services point to the need for further research to improve services offered to women. Pain management challenges for

over 5000 women having early aspiration abortions was a common theme in women's descriptions of their experiences, as was the need to address the stigma and shame many of these women felt about their need for abortion [62].

What concerns are there about Reproductive Health? Rights, Justice, and Politics.

Republican majorities in the federal government and in most states are putting at risk existing protections for abortion, parenting, and birth control rights. Midlife women have an opportunity to help shape policy that affects not only their portion of the population, but all women.

Before abortion became legal through the Supreme Court case Roe v. Wade, an estimated 1.2 million women per year sought illegal abortions. Today, while legal abortion is safe, there has been increasing political interference (legislation, regulations) that threatens reproductive health access. Within the past decade alone, US women have experienced both increased and reduced options related to sexual and reproductive health care. With the passage of the Affordable Care Act in 2010, women were assured that contraceptive methods would be available to them as an insurance benefit without co-payment and that insurers would be obligated to provide coverage/ benefits to women instead of viewing them as having a pre-existing condition – being a woman [5]. With the weakening of policy insuring contraceptive access as a result of a Supreme Court Case (Burwell vs Hobby Lobby) which allowed employers to limit contraceptive benefits in health insurance based on the employers' religious beliefs, women's access to contraceptives as envisioned in the original ACA was limited. In addition, increasing restrictions on access to abortion in state legislation and regulation, such as those limiting the types of facilities in which abortions could be performed, further threatens women's reproductive choice. Indeed, in some states, politicians have pushed for laws and regulations restricting ethical standards of

Table 8 Reproductive Health Policy Resources

Resource	Location of Resource
Reproductive Health Policy Resources	http://www.womenshealthpolicyreport.org/articles/daily.html?referrer=http://go.nationalpartnership.org/site/PageServer?pagename=report_daily http://www.nationalpartnership.org/our-impact/
Policy advocacy/action	http://www.reprohealthwatch.org/?referrer=http://www.womenshealthpolicyreport.org/articles/monthly/#5
Contraception policy	http://www.nationalpartnership.org/issues/repro/birth-control.html
Abortion policy	http://www.nationalpartnership.org/issues/repro/abortion.html
Impact of abortion restrictions	http://www.scholarsstrategynetwork.org/scholar-spotlight/what-trump-means-abortion-access
What if Roe fell? Impact at state level (Center for Reproductive Rights)	https://www.reproductiverights.org/sites/default/files/documents/Roe_PublicationPF4a.pdf
Organizations working toward reproductive justice like the	National Network of Abortion Funds, ACCESS Reproductive Justice, Sister Song, and Sister Reach.

care for women and are imposing politics and ideology on evidence-based clinical care as outlined by the recent policy report "Politics in the Exam Room" led by a coalition of 24 nursing, medical, health and advocacy organizations, the Coalition to Protect the Patient-Provider Relationship (http://www.coalitiontoprotect.org). For more detailed information about policy resources related to reproductive health, see Table 8.

In addition, politics has trumped evidence supporting who may provide abortion services [63]. A strategy to reduce access to abortion has been state regulation limiting the type of health care provider who may provide medication and aspiration abortion. A recent study evaluating the outcomes of over 11,000 early aspiration abortions completed by physicians, and newly trained nurse practitioner, certified nurse midwives, and physician assistants in California revealed that abortion adverse effects were clinically equivalent among these groups of health professionals, supporting policies to allow these providers to perform early aspirations [60]. Moreover, updated findings from this study based on over 16,000 women having early aspiration underscore the very low rate of adverse complications/effects associated with this procedure [64].. Changing state regulations to improve access to early aspiration abortion for women by expanding the types of health professionals allowed to provide the service would seem a logical next step.

As a consequence of increasing threat to women's reproductive health rights, future options for midlife women's management of unintended pregnancy may be constrained. With political threats to defund Planned Parenthood, one of the primary resources for women's reproductive health care is at risk and with it a resource providing US women with the full range of approaches to preventing unintended pregnancy. Protecting reproductive rights and promoting reproductive justice for women demands activism at all levels of the society. The political becomes personal as midlife and younger women may find themselves unable to access a broad range of unintended pregnancy prevention services. Limitations on women's access to these services intersect with social determinants of their health, ultimately affecting women who are most vulnerable and who already suffer from marginalization and discrimination in the larger society. Using strategies to socially construct fertile women as "welfare queens" and "teen moms" has reinforced the political disenfranchisement of the population of all fertile women, contributing to our national failure to create effective reproductive health policy [65].

There is an urgent need to expand and protect policies that insure access to care to help women prevent unintended pregnancy. Moreover, there is an urgent need to protect the patient-provider relationship, insuring that health care professionals are not limited in providing the care to midlife women that they need and desire. Research and policy that recognizes the importance of all aspects of women's reproductive health—including pregnancy prevention, abortion care, pregnancy services, and economic supports—are essential to meeting the sexual and reproductive health care needs of low-SES women and women of color [39].

In the current political maelstrom, US women will continue to experience unintended pregnancies, in some parts of the country without access to the option of pregnancy termination. In addition, many women who have benefitted from the access to coverage of contraception by health insurance policy changes provided by the Affordable Care Act may find themselves with more limited access, if not inability to obtain affordable contraception. Likely consequences are that unintended pregnancy will continue to be a problem for many women in one of the world's most developed nations. In addition, public and private insurance coverage for abortions especially for low income women and women of color remains in jeopardy depending on contemporary political targets.

Acknowledgements
Not applicable.

Funding
No funding to disclose by any author, all authors free of conflict.

Human subjects
Not applicable.

Authors' contributions
VJM made substantial contributions to the conception of the manuscript, led the literature review and had primary responsibility for final editing of the manuscript. She developed content on sexual and reproductive care and services. DT, KS, and IA contributed content related to pregnancy termination. DT contributed to policy issues and the prevention of unintended pregnancy framework. EKP contributed to the current clinical practice in sexual and reproductive health care of women during midlife and menopause. NFW contributed to revision of the manuscript for important intellectual content. All authors have read and approved the final manuscript.

Author's information
Elizabeth A. Kostas-Polston, PhD, APRN, WHNP-BC, FAANP, FAAN*.
*The contents of this publication are the sole responsibility of the author and do not necessarily reflect the views, assertions, opinions or policies of the Uniformed Services University of the Health Sciences or the Department of Defense. Mention of trade names, commercial products, or organizations does not imply endorsement by the U.S. Government.

Competing interests
The authors declare that they have no competing interests.

Author details

[1]Department of Family, Community, and Health System Science, Robert Wood Johnson Nurse Faculty Scholar Alum, University of Florida, College of Nursing, Gainesville, FL, USA. [2]Daniel K. Inouye Graduate School of Nursing, Uniformed Services University of the Health Sciences, Bethesda, MD, USA. [3]Biobehavioral Nursing and Health Informatics, Interim Associate Dean for Diversity, Equity, and Inclusion, University of Washington School of Nursing, Seattle, WA, USA. [4]MGH Institute of Health Professions, Boston, MA, USA. [5]Director of Advance Practice Programs, Storrs, CT, USA. [6]UCSF School of Nursing, Research Faculty, Advancing New Standards in Reproductive Health Program (ANSIRH), UCSF Bixby Center for Global Reproductive Health, University of California, San Francisco, CA, USA.

References

1. Guttmacher Institute. Fact Sheet. Unintended Pregnancy in the United States. September 2016, Guttmacher institute (2016). Data center. https://www.guttmacher.org/united-states/abortion. Accessed 28 Feb 2017.
2. Swartz LH, Sherman CA, Harvey SM, Blanchard J, Vawter F, Gau J. Midlife women online: evaluation of an internet-based program to prevent unintended pregnancy & STIs. Journal of women & aging. 2011, 23, 4. 342–59.
3. Aztlan-James EA, McLemore M, Taylor D. Multiple unintended pregnancies in US women: a systematic review. Womens Health Issues. 2017;
4. Taylor D, James EA. Risks of being sexual in midlife: what we don't know can hurt us. The Female Patient. 2012;37:17–20.
5. Hall KS, Fendrick AM, Zochowski M, Dalton VK. Women's Health and the affordable care act: high hopes versus harsh realities? Am J Public Health. 2014;104:e10–3. https://doi.org/10.2015/AJPH,2014.302045.
6. Harlow SD, Crawford S, Dennerstein L, Burger HG, Mitchell ES, Sowers MF, ReSTAGE Collaboration. Recommendations from a multi-study evaluation of proposed criteria for staging reproductive aging. Climacteric. 2007;10:112–9.
7. Harlow SD, Gass M, Hall JE, Lobo R, Maki P, Rebar RW, Sherman S, Sluss PM, de Villiers TJ. Executive summary of STRAW+10: addressing the unfinished agenda of staging reproductive aging. Climacteric. 2012;15:105–14.
8. Mercer CH, Tanton C, Prah P, Erens B, Sonnenberg P, Clifton S, Macdowall W, Lewis R, Field N, Datta J, Copas AJ, Phelps A, Welllings K, Johnson AM. Changes in sexual attitudes and lifestyles in Britain through the life course and over time: findings from the National Surveys of Sexual Attitudes and Lifestyles (Natsal). Lancet, 2013; 382: 9907, 1781-1794.
9. Finer L B, Philbin J M. Trends in ages at key reproductive transitions in the United States, 1951–2010. Women's Health Issues, 2014; 24:3, e271-e279.
10. Hardman SM, Gebbie, AE. The contraception needs of the perimenopausal woman. Best Practice & Research Clinical Obstetrics & Gynaecology, 2014; 28:6, 903–915.
11. Ruan X, Alfred OM. "Oral contraception for women of middle age." Maturitas, 2015 82:3 (2015): 266–270.
12. Finer, LB, Mia RZ. "Declines in unintended pregnancy in the United States, 2008–2011." New England Journal of Medicine, 2016; 374:9, 843–852
13. Taylor D, James EA. An evidence-based guideline for unintended pregnancy prevention. Journal of Gynecologic, Obstetric, and Neonatal Nursing. 2011;4:782–93.
14. Godfrey EM, Zapata LB, Cox CM, Curtis KM, Marchbanks PA. Unintended pregnancy risk and contraceptive use among women 45-50 years old: Massachusetts, 2006, 2008, and 2010. Am J Obstet Gynecol. 2016;214(6):712–e1.
15. Long ME, Faubion SS, MacLaughlin KL, Pruthi S, Casey PM. Contraception and hormonal management in the perimenopause. Journal of Women's Health, 2015; 24:1, 3–10.
16. Linton, A, Golobof, A, Shulman, LP. Contraception for the perimenopausal woman. Climacteric, 2016; 19:60, 526–534.
17. Sunderam, S. "Assisted reproductive technology surveillance—United States, 2014." MMWR. Surveillance.
18. Curtis KM, Jatlaoui TC, Tepper N K, Zapata LB, Horton LG, Jamieson DJ, Whiteman MK. U.S. Selected Practice Recommendations for Contraceptive Use, 2016. MMWR Recomm Rep 2016; 65(No. RR-4):[1–66].
19. Simmonds K, Likis FE. Caring for women with unintended pregnancies. Journal of Obstetric, Gynecologic, and Neonatal Nursing, 2011; 40:6, 794–807.
20. Biggs MA, Upadhyay UD, McCulloch C, Foster DG. Women's Mental health and well-being 5 years after receiving or being denied an abortion: a prospective, longitudinal cohort study. JAMA psychiatry. 2016;
21. Barber JS, Axinn WG, Thornton A. Unwanted childbearing, health, and mother-child relationships. J Health Social Behavior. 1999;40(3):231–57.
22. Robinson GE, Stotland NL, Russo NE. Is there an "abortion trauma syndrome"? Critiquing the evidence. Harvard Review of Psychiatry. 2009;17:268–90.
23. Rocca CH, Kimport K, Gould H, Foster DG. Women's Emotions one week after receiving or being denied an abortion in the United States. Perspectives Sexual Reproductive Heatlh. 2013;45:122–31.
24. Drey EA, Foster DG, Jackson RA, Lee SJ, Cardenas LH, Darney PD. Risk factors associated with presenting for abortion in the second trimester. Obstet Gynecol. 2006;107(1):128–35.
25. Herd P, et al. "The implications of unintended pregnancies for mental health in later life." American journal of public health, 2016 106:3, 421–429.
26. Roev. Wade, 410 U.S. 113 [1973].
27. Gateway CWI. How many children were adopted in 2007 and 2008? Washington, DC: U.S. Department of Health and Human Services, Children's Bureau; 2011.
28. Coleman PK, Debbie G. From birth mothers to first mothers: toward a compassionate understanding of the life-long act of adoption placement. Issues L & Med. 2016;31:139.
29. Title X of Public Law 91–572, Section 1008, 1970.
30. Moss DA, Snyder MJ, Lu L. Options for women with unintended pregnancy. Am Fam Physician. 2015;91:544–9.
31. Finer LB, et al. Reasons U.S. women have abortions: quantitative and qualitative perspectivesPerspect Sex Reprod Health. 2005;37:3,110–8.
32. Jatlaoui TC, Curtis KM. Safety and effectiveness data for emergency contraceptive pills among women with obesity: a systematic review. Contraception. 2016;94:605–11. doi:10.1016/j.contraception.2016.05.002.
33. Jones RK, Jerman J. How far did US women travel for abortion services in 2008? J Women's Health. 2013;22:8,706–13.
34. Upadhyay UD, Tracy AW, Rachel KJ, Rana EB, Diana GF. "Denial of abortion because of provider gestational age limits in the United States." American Journal of Public Health, 2014; 104:9, 1687-1694.
35. Roberts SC, Biggs MA, Chibber KS, Gould H, Rocca CH, Foster DG. Risk of violence from the man involved in the pregnancy after receiving or being denied an abortion. BMC Med. 2014;12:1,144.
36. Sereno S, Leal I, Maroco J. The role of psychological adjustment in the decision-making process for voluntary termination of pregnancy. Journal of reproduction & infertility. 2013;14:3,143.
37. Ralph LJ, Foster DG, Kimport K, Turok D. Roberts SC. Contraception: Measuring decisional certainty among women seeking abortion, 2016.
38. Jones RK, Finer LB, Singh S. Characteristics of US abortion patients. New York: Guttmacher Institute. 2008;2010:20101–8.
39. Taylor DL, Upadhyay UD, Fjerstad M, Battistelli MB, Weitz TA, Paul ME. Standardizing the classification of abortion incidents: the procedural abortion incident reporting and surveillance (PAIRS) framework, Contraception, 2017, 96 (1). 1 13. ISSN 0010-7824, https://doi.org/10.1016/j.contraception.2017.05.004. Available at http://www.sciencedirect.com/science/article/pii/S0010782417301361
40. Jerman J, Jones RK, Onda T. Characteristics of U.S. abortion patients in 2014 and changes since 2008. New York: Guttmacher Institute; 2016.
41. Pazol K, Andreea AC, Denise JJ. Abortion surveillance United States, 2012. MMWR Surveill Summ. 2015;64(10):1–40.
42. Weitz TA, Foster A, Ellertson C, Grossman D, Stewart FH. Medical and surgical abortion: rethinking the modifiers. Contraception. 2004;69(1):77–8.
43. Jatlaoui TC. Abortion surveillance—United States, 2013. MMWR Surveill Summ. 2016;65
44. Bommaraju A, Kavanaugh ML, Hou MY, Bessett D. Situating stigma in stratified reproduction: abortion stigma and miscarriage stigma as barriers to reproductive healthcare. Sexual & Reproductive Healthcare. 2016;10:62–9.

45. Waisel DB. Vulnerable populations in healthcare. Current Opinion in Anesthesiology. 2013;26:2,186–92.

46. Roberts SCM, Heather G, Katrina K, Tracy AW, Diana GF. Out-of-pocket costs and insurance coverage for abortion in the United States. Women's Health Issues. 2014 24:2, e211-e218.

47. Jones RK, Jerman J. Abortion incidence and service availability in the United States, 2011. Perspectives on sexual and reproductive health. 2014, 46:1, 3–14.

48. Fessenden-Raden J, Fitchen JM, Heath JS. Providing risk information in communities: Factors influencing what is heard and accepted. Science, Technology, & Human Values. 1987, 12:3/4, 94–101.

49. Mercier RJ, Buchbinder M, Bryant A. TRAP laws and the invisible labor of US abortion providers. Critical public health. 2016;26:1,77–87.

50. Roberts D. Killing the Black Body: Race reproduction, and the meaning of liberty. NY, NY: Pantheon Books,1997, Vintage.

51. Dominguez TP, Dunkel-Schetter C, Glyn LM, Hobel C, Sandman CA. Racial differences in birth outcomes: the role of general, pregnancy, and racism stress. Health Psychol. 2008;27:2,194–2003.

52. Dehlendorf C, Harris LH, Weitz TA. Disparities in abortion rates: a public health approach, AJPH, 2013; 103:10; 1772–1779. Doi:10.2105/AJPH.2013.301339.

53. Hand L, Abortion C, Raymond EG, Grimes DA. The comparative safety of legal induced abortion and childbirth in the United States. Obstetrics & Gynecology, 2014. 2012;119(2 Pt 1):215–9.

54. Raymond EG, Grossman D, Weaver MA, Toti S, Winikoff B. Mortality of induced abortion, other outpatient surgical procedures and common activities in the United States. Contraception, 2014, 90:5, 476–9.

55. Upadhyay UD, Desai S, Zlidar V, Weitz TA, Grossman D, Anderson P, et al. Incidence of emergency department visits and complications after abortion. Obstetrics & Gynecology, 2015, 125:1, 175–183.

56. Zane S, Creanga AA, Berg CJ, Pazol K, Suchdev DB, Jamieson DJ, Callaghan WM. Abortion-related mortality in the United States: 1998-2010. Obstet Gynecol. 2015;26(2):258–65.

57. Raymond EG, Grimes DA. The comparative safety of legal induced abortion and childbirth in the United States. Obstetrics & Gynecology. 2012; 119(2, Part 1):215–9.

58. Callaghan WM, Creanga AA, Kuklina EV. Severe maternal morbidity among delivery and postpartum hospitalizations in the United States. Obstetrics & Gynecology, 2012; 120:5, 1029–1036.

59. Franz MB, Husslein P. Obstetrical management of the older gravida. Women's Health, 2010; 6:3, 463–468.

60. Weitz TA, Taylor D, Desai S, Uphadyay UD, Waldman J, Battistelli MF, Drey EA. Safety of aspiration abortion performed by nurse practitioners. Certified Nurse Midwives, and Physician Assistants under a California legal waiver American Journal of Public Health. 2013:e1–8. doi:10.2105/AJPH.2012. 301159.

61. Harris LH. Abortion politics and the production of knowledge. Contraception. 2013;88:200–3.

62. McLemore M, Desai S, Freedman L, James EA, Taylor D. Women' know best – findings from the thematic analysis of 5,214 surveys of abortion care experience. Womens Health Issues. 2014;24:594–9.

63. Taylor D, Safriet B, Weitz T. When politics trumps evidence: legislative or regulatory exclusion of abortion from advanced practice clinician scope of practice. Journal of Midwifery and Women's Health. 2009;54:4–7.

64. Weitz, TA, Taylor, D, Upadhyay, UD, Desai, S, Battistelli, M. Research informs abortion care policy change in California. American Journal of Public Health 2014, 104:10:e3-e4.

65. James EA, Rashid M. "Welfare queens" and "teen moms": how the social construction of fertile women impacts unintended pregnancy prevention policy in the United States. Policy, Politics, and Nursing Practice. 2013;14: 125–32.

11

Methods in a longitudinal cohort study of late reproductive age women: the Penn Ovarian Aging Study (POAS)

Ellen W. Freeman[1][*] and Mary D. Sammel[2]

Abstract

Background: This report describes the methods utilized in the Penn Ovarian Aging Study (POAS), which is a longitudinal cohort study of hormone dynamics and menopausal symptoms of women in the menopause transition.

Methods/Design: The cohort is a community-based sample of generally healthy women enrolled in the late reproductive years. The study population is a stratified random sample of African-American and Caucasian women, identified by random digit dialing.

Of the 1427 women who were identified as potentially eligible, 578 women were eligible after full screening; 75 % of the eligible women enrolled in the study (436/578). At Period 14 (14 years after study enrollment), 67 % remained active and were fully evaluated (293/436). Attrition was non-differential with respect to the sample characteristics.

The aims of the project overall are to 1) identify within-woman trends of reproductive hormones (estradiol, follicle stimulating hormone, hormone, lutinizing hormone, inhibin B, dehydroepiandrosterone, testosterone, and anti-mullerian hormone), cofactors such as race, body mass index (BMI), age, physical and behavioral symptoms, and their predictions of menopausal symptoms, and patterns around the final menstrual period; 2) identify associations of hormone dynamics with physical and behavioral symptoms that occur with ovarian aging and identify racial differences in these factors; 3) identify associations of genetic polymorphisms with levels and longitudinal trends in menopausal symptoms. The cohort consists of 436 late reproductive-age women at enrollment, and now has 18 years of approximately annual follow-up assessments. Menopausal stage based on concurrent menstrual dates is identified at each follow-up period.

Discussion: Studies of the cohort have shown that hot flashes can occur well before menopause and extend 10 or more years beyond menopause for sizeable numbers of women; provide evidence for new-onset depressed mood in the menopause transition and show that the final menstrual period is pivotal in the increases in depressive symptoms prior to menopause and decreases postmenopausal; suggest that poor sleep is common in the late reproductive years but increases in relation to the final menstrual period in only a small proportion of women; and show effects of obesity on reproductive hormones in the menopause transition. To date, more than 50 studies of the cohort are published in medical journals, demonstrating the relevance of these data to the clinical care of mid-life women.

Keywords: Menopause, Menopause transition, Menopausal symptoms, Reproductive hormones, Midlife cohort

* Correspondence: freemane@mail.med.upenn.edu
[1]Department of Obstetrics/Gynecology and Department of Psychiatry, 3701 Market Street, Suite 820 (Mudd Suite), Philadelphia, PA 19104, USA
Full list of author information is available at the end of the article

Background

More than 80 % of U.S. women experience physical or behavioral symptoms around menopause, most commonly hot flashes and night sweats, depressive symptoms, and sleep disturbances [1]. Although the severity of these symptoms varies widely, many women seek medical relief for distressing symptoms that disrupt their functioning. However, whether these symptoms are associated with the biological changes of ovarian senescence or with age-related changes and other behavioral and psychosocial conditions of mid-life has only recently been a target of scientific investigation, and knowledge of the efficacy of therapeutic treatments is limited.

Calls for research have aimed to increase understanding of biological and behavioral changes associated with ovarian aging, and to identify whether there are racial differences in these changes. Recent cohort studies of mid-life or late reproductive age women are elucidating associations between symptoms and reproductive aging and providing new information that can lead to better preventive and therapeutic strategies and reduce the short- and long-term morbidity of women's mid-life and postmenopausal years.

The purpose of this report is to describe the methods in the Epidemiologic Study of the Late Reproductive Years, which is also termed the Penn Ovarian Aging Study (POAS), supported by the National Institute of Aging (RO1-AG12745). The POAS cohort consists of healthy, mid-life women in their late reproductive years, who were randomly identified through random digit dialing in Philadelphia County, Pennsylvania, with stratification to obtain equal numbers of African American and Caucasian women. The cohort has continued for 18 years with approximately annual follow-up evaluations.

POAS studies focus on hormone dynamics and associated symptoms of menopause. The participants were premenopausal at enrollment and then entered and moved through stages of the menopause transition. The overall aims of the project are to 1) identify how within-woman trends of reproductive hormones (estradiol, follicle stimulating hormone, luteinizing hormone, inhibin B, dehydroepiandrosterone, testosterone, and anti-mullerian hormone) and cofactors such as race, body mass index (BMI), age, physical and behavioral symptoms predict the progression through the menopause transition; 2) identify associations of hormone dynamics with physical and behavioral symptoms that occur with ovarian aging and identify racial differences in these factors; 3) compare hormone levels and longitudinal trends between African American and Caucasian women; 4) identify associations of genetic polymorphisms with levels and longitudinal trends and with menopausal symptoms.

Methods

Overview of study design

This longitudinal study has 14 complete assessment periods followed by 4 partial assessment periods for a total of 18 assessment periods. In each full assessment period, data were collected at 2 visits scheduled between days 2 and 6 of 2 consecutive menstrual cycles (or 1 month apart in non-cycling women). In the first five years of the project (Phase 1), the follow-up assessment periods were approximately 9 months apart. In Phase 2 (years 6–10) and Phase 3 (years 11–15), follow-up assessments were conducted annually. There were 14 complete assessment periods due to a one-year delay in funding in year 11. Limited follow-up was conducted annually by telephone interview for follow-up periods 15–17. Full follow-up with home visits was resumed in year 18.

Study visits were conducted at participants' homes. At each visit, a trained research interviewer administered a structured interview questionnaire and obtained anthropometric measures and blood samples for the hormone assays. Participants also completed standard self-report questionnaires to assess physical, behavioral and mood factors and completed a daily symptom report for 1 menstrual cycle at each assessment period.

Sample selection and recruitment

A sample of 436 healthy women (218 African American, 218 Caucasian) was recruited in Philadelphia County over a 16-month period in 1996–1997. Recruitment was stratified by race to obtain equal numbers of African American and Caucasian participants. In a two-phase recruitment process, potentially eligible women were first identified through random-digit dialing, using a modified Mitoksky-Waksberg method [2]. The women who were identified through random digit dialing were then contacted by a research interviewer, who explained the details of the study and screened for study eligibility.

Women were eligible for study participation if they were between 35 and 47 years of age, experienced regular menstrual cycles in normal range (22–35 days) in the past 3 months, and had at least one ovary and a uterus. Women were excluded from enrollment if they were pregnant, taking hormone therapy or using hormonal contraception, taking psychotropic medications, had a history of illness that could affect hormonal function (e.g., diabetes, liver disease, breast or endometrial cancer, et al.), had a history of drug or alcohol abuse or a major psychiatric disorder in the previous 12 months, or were non-English speaking.

The age range was carefully considered when the cohort was recruited in order to evaluate ovarian aging *prior to observable menstrual cycle changes*. The lower age limit of 35 years was selected as an age when follicular depletion accelerates, resulting in subtle increases in follicle-stimulating hormone (FSH) and decreases in inhibin [3], and is consistent with standard age groupings as in U.S. census data (e.g., ages 35–39 years). The upper age limit of 47 years was selected as an accepted median age for women entering the perimenopause, as shown in the estimates of Treloar [4] and McKinlay [5]. This provided a unique baseline of premenopausal women for the subsequent follow-up through the menopause transition.

A cohort size of $N = 300$ women (150 in each racial group) was predetermined using a 2-sided alpha error of 0.05 and 80 % power to detect clinically relevant differences in hormones and symptoms. The enrollment number was increased to 436 women to account for estimated dropout in the first 4 years of the study. However, it is noteworthy that retention far exceeded the initial estimate (see below), and the powered estimate of 300 participants remained at Year 12. Further post-hoc calculations of statistical power for hypothesis testing have remained strong throughout the years of the study.

To obtain the cohort of 436 women, 1427 potentially eligible women were identified through random digit dialing. Of these, 129 (9 %) could not be contacted further by the research staff, 308 (22 %) declined to participate without providing eligibility information, and 412 (29 %) were ineligible. Reasons for ineligibility included hysterectomy ($n = 111$), use of hormonal contraception ($n = 87$), menstrual irregularities or no menses ($n = 92$), known to be leaving the area during the study period ($n = 31$), medical contraindications ($n = 30$), pregnant, breast feeding or attempting pregnancy ($n = 24$), alcohol or drug abuse ($n = 6$). Of the 578 women eligible after full screen, 436 (75 %) enrolled, and 142 (25 %) declined. Neither eligibility nor participation differed significantly by race.

Informed consent for study participation and follow-up contact was approved by the Institutional Review Board of the University of Pennsylvania, signed and witnessed at the first study visit and repeated thereafter when there were protocol changes (e.g., the addition of another hormone assay). Verbal consent was given for telephone contacts in the screen period and at later follow-up telephone contacts.

Sample characteristics at enrollment

Four- hundred-thirty- six women enrolled in the cohort (218 African American, 218 Caucasian). All participants were premenopausal with regular menstrual cycles in normal range (22–35 days) at enrollment. The mean age was 41.4 (SD 3.5) years (range 35–47 years). The mean cycle day of the blood draw was 4.0 (SD 1.0). Mean (SD) hormone levels were FSH: 8.3 (5.2) mIu/mL; inhibin b: 78.0 (77.0) pg/mL; LH: 3.4 (2.6) mIU/mL; estradiol: 44.1 (38.8) pg/mL. [6]. The mean BMI was 29.1; 38 % (166/436) were current smokers; 81 % were employed; 33 % were

high school graduates, 11 % had less than high school education, 56 % had college or technical training beyond high school; 57 % were married, 43 % were single, divorced, separated or widowed.

Data collection

a. *Interview questionnaire.* A structured interview questionnaire was constructed and tested for the study and administered by a trained research interviewer at the first visit of every assessment period. Primary components of the interview included standard demographic information; menstrual cycle characteristics (most importantly, the dates of the current and previous two menstrual periods); menopausal symptoms (using a validated menstrual symptom questionnaire [7], which were reported for the past month and the past year and included frequency and severity of each symptom; general and gynecological health (current, history and contraceptive use), all current medications; health practices and behaviors (including smoking and alcohol consumption); physical activity (adapted from the validated College Alumni Health Study questionnaire [8] with additional questions such as number of city blocks walked daily, etc., that are shown to be a major source of physical activity among African American women [9]; sleep disturbance (using the validated St Mary's Hospital Sleep Questionnaire [10, 11]; decreased functioning due to symptoms (using the Sheehan Disability Scale [12]).

b. *The Menopausal Symptom List (MSL)* [7]. This validated symptom list included 12 common menopausal symptoms: hot flashes/night sweats; aches/joint pain/stiffness; depressed mood; poor sleep; decreased libido; vaginal dryness; urine leaks; headache; irritability; mood swings; anxiety; and concentration difficulties. The symptom list was embedded in the structured Interview Questionnaire and administered by the research interviewer at each assessment period (periods 1–18). For each symptom, the interviewer asked whether the symptom occurred in the past month, whether the symptom occurred in the past year, and asked the participant to rate the frequency (number per day, week or month) and severity (none, mild, moderate, severe) of each symptom. The MSL was validated for the study [7], and several reports of associations between the symptoms and menopausal stages are published [13, 14].

c. *Mood and anxiety diagnosis.* Current mood disorders were screened for all women at enrollment using the Symptom-Driven Diagnostic System (SDDS-PC) [15], which was developed from the Structured Clinical Interview for DSM III R Diagnosis (SCID) [16]. The SDDS is a validated screening measure for DSM diagnoses of major mood disorders, its symptom checklist is rapid and easily used by the participants, it provides symptom information collected systematically from all participants, and the screening information can be obtained in the telephone interview followed by in-person evaluation of screen positives at the next study visit.

Clinical diagnosis was made using the Primary Care Evaluation of Mental Disorders (PRIME-MD) [17] to obtain DSM diagnoses of depression and anxiety disorders at each assessment period through Period 6. The Prime-MD is a 2-stage system where the participant first completes a 26-item self-administered questionnaire that screens for 5 of the most common groups of disorders in primary care: depressive, anxiety, alcohol, somatoform and eating disorders. Algorithms are provided, and when the checklist scores indicate a defined severity level, trained interviewers administer a brief set of questions to determine a DSM diagnosis. The Prime-MD is validated and highly correlated with full SCID interviews for DSM diagnosis.

The Patient Health Questionnaire (PHQ) [18] was administered in Periods 7 through 14. The PHQ is a self-administered version of the Prime-MD to provide DSM diagnosis of major depressive disorder, other depressive syndromes, panic disorder, other anxiety syndromes, eating disorder and alcohol abuse. It also queries bothersome problems, current medications and reproductive events. The PHQ is extensively validated and has a sensitivity of 0.88 and specificity of 0.88 for the diagnosis of MDD [19].

d. *Behavioral symptom measures.* Six self-report questionnaires were completed by the participants at each assessment period. All measures are validated and published in the literature.

Depressive symptoms were evaluated at each assessment period using the Center for Epidemiologic Studies Depression Scale (CES-D) [20]. The CES-D is a 20-item self-report inventory that was developed for epidemiologic research, is widely used and validated. The standard CES-D cutoff score of 16 or greater indicates high depressive symptoms. A higher CES-D score of 25 or greater can be examined as a closer approximation of a clinical diagnosis of depression [17, 21].

Anxiety symptoms were evaluated at every assessment period using the Zung Anxiety Index, a validated, 20-item self-report measure that is sensitive to the frequency of both affective and somatic symptoms of anxiety [22]. Zung established score ranges to classify normal anxiety [20–35], mild to moderate anxiety [36–47], and high anxiety (48–60).

Perceived stress was evaluated using the Perceived Stress Scale (PSS) [23] at each assessment period. The PSS is a 14-item widely validated self-report measure of the degree to which situations are appraised as stressful.

Quality of life was evaluated with the Quality of Life Enjoyment and Satisfaction Questionnaire (Q-les-Q) [24], which assesses various aspects of quality of life. The 16-item summary scale was used in this project. The Q-les-Q has high reliability and validity, addresses

general functioning rather than disease-specific issues, and has considerable normative data available. The Utian Quality of Life Scale (UQOL) [25] was added in Periods 11–14. This validated instrument is specific to a perimenopausal population and quantifies "sense of well-being".

General health. The SF-12 Health Survey [26] was administered at each assessment period to monitor health outcomes. The SF-12 is a 12-item short form developed from the SF-36 Health Survey. There are two summary scales, which have demonstrated equivalence to the SF-36 and yield reliable summary scales for physical and mental health.

e. *Sleep disturbance.* The St. Mary's Hospital Sleep Questionnaire (SMHSQ) [11], a standard, self-administered questionnaire, was administered to assess sleep disturbances at each assessment period through Period 8. We adapted the SMHSQ by adding items to assess the etiology of nocturnal awakenings, the frequency of sleep medication use, and whether the previous night of sleep was comparable to usual sleep and deleting items about bedtime, fall-asleep time, wake time, time out of bed, and the "depth" of sleep, resulting in a total of 20 items.

We subsequently conducted a factor analysis of the SMHSQ, using all data from the first assessment period [27]. The factor analysis identified 3 factors: sleep quality, sleep complaints, and sleep latency. The sleep quality factor explained the largest proportion of variability in responses (37 %) and was used as a primary outcome variable for sleep studies in the cohort [27, 28].

"Poor sleep" (frequency and severity) was included as a symptom in the validated menopausal symptom questionnaire, administered at each assessment period through 18 years of follow-up [7]. This sleep item had a high correlation with the sleep quality factor score derived from the SMHSQ (r = 0.83) [27] and has been used as a primary outcome measure in sleep studies in this cohort [28, 29].

The Women's Health Initiative Insomnia Rating Scale (WHIIRS) [30] was collected in assessment periods 10–14. The WHIIRS is a 5-item self-report questionnaire that is sensitive to sleep disturbances over time and validated in a perimenopausal population. The Multivariable Apnea Prediction Index (MAP) [31] was administered in Periods 10–14).

f. *The Female Sexual Functioning Index (FSFI)* [32] was collected in each assessment period 8–14. The FSFI is a 19-item, multi-dimensional, self-report instrument for assessing the key dimensions of sexual function in women. Domains include desire, arousal, lubrication, orgasm, satisfaction, and pain. The instrument has been validated and scaled on a sample of women with clinically diagnosed female sexual dysfunction.

Symptoms of decreased libido and vaginal dryness were included in the validated Menopausal Symptom

Questionnaire, administered by interview at each assessment period. The items were "Please tell me if you have experienced a decreased libido or interest in sex in the past month" and "Have you experienced vaginal dryness or discomfort in the past month."

A 30-day and a 1-year time period were queried; participants rated the severity (none, mild, moderate, severe) and the frequency of the items.

g. *The Social Adjustment Scale (SAS)* [33] was completed by participants at assessment Periods 1–3, 6–8, and 11–13. The scale provides domain scores that evaluate the participant's role performance, interpersonal relationships, friction, feelings and satisfaction in work, and social and leisure activities

h. *Cognition.* Brief tests of cognitive memory were completed at each assessment period. These included the Buschke-Fuld Selective Reminding Test [34], which provided scores for total recall, short-term recall and long-term storage; the Digit Symbol Substitution test (Weschler Adult Intelligence Test-III) [35], a sensitive measure of cognitive processing speed [36]; and the Digit Symbol Copy test (WAIS-III) [35] to assess sensorimotor processing speed. These are widely used, brief cognitive tests, with extensive data published in the literature.

i. *Daily Symptom Reports (DSR)* were completed by participants for one menstrual cycle (or one month if not cycling) at each assessment period to determine prospectively the occurrence and severity of symptoms in relation to the menstrual cycle. The DSR lists 20 symptoms specific to reproductive aging as described in the menopause literature. Participants rated the symptoms daily on a 5-point scale of severity according to written descriptors (0 = not present to 4 = very severe). The symptoms included on the DSR were also included in the Menopausal Symptom List (above), which was administered by interview at each assessment period.

j. *Anthropometric measures.* Measures of height, weight, waist and hip circumferences were made at each assessment period 1–14. Height (without shoes) was measured to the nearest 0.5 cm with a vertical ruler. Body weight (light clothing only) was measure to the nearest 0.2 kg. Waist circumference was measured at the maximum abdominal girth, in duplicate, to the nearest 0.5 cm. Hip circumference was measured at the maximal protrusion of the hips at the level of the symphysis pubis, in duplicate, to the nearest 0.5 cm. The average of duplicate measures was calculated for analysis.

Body mass index (BMI) was calculated by computer algorithm from the measures of height and weight at each assessment period, using the average of the duplicate measures of height and weight at each assessment period (weight (kg) divided by the square of height (cm)).

k. *Hormone measures.* Blood samples were obtained at each study visit (2 visits per assessment period). Visits were scheduled throughout the day in days 2–6 of the menstrual cycle or approximately one month apart in the assessment period for non-cycling women. Standardizing the collection of blood samples to the first 6 days of the menstrual cycle was maintained for cycling women throughout the project. Less than 1 % of the blood samples from cycling women were outside the 6-day window.

Blood samples (2 ½ ounces, non-fasting) were drawn from the non-dominant arm into vacutainer serum separator (tiger top) tubes containing separator gel and clot activator. The tubes were kept on ice, centrifuged for 20 min and frozen in aliquots (−80 C.) using polypropylene tubes.

Hormone values were measured by radioimmunoassay in the Clinical and Translational Research Center (CTRC) of the University of Pennsylvania. Assays were conducted in batched samples of 20 participants, with 4 samples at 4 time points per participant, to reduce the within-subject variability due to assay conditions. Estradiol, follicle stimulating hormone (FSH), luteinizing hormone (LH), dehydroepiandrosterone (DHEAS), testosterone, and sex hormone binding globulin (SHBG) were assayed using commercial kits (Coat-a-Count, Diagnostic Products Corp). Anti-mullerian hormone (AMH) assays were conducted using ELISA commercial kits (GEN 2, Beckman Coulter). Assays of Inhibin b were initially conducted in the laboratory of Dr. Patrick Sluss (Massachusetts General Hospital, Boston, MA) (assessment periods 1–10), and then conducted in the CTRC (assessment periods 11–14) using a commercial kit (Diagnostic Systems). Assays were performed in duplicate for all hormones and repeated if values differed by more than 15 %. Inter- and intra-assay coefficients of variation were calculated for the study samples in each study phase and were consistently less than 5 %.

l. *Genomic DNA and genetic polymorphisms.* Genomic DNA was obtained from 95 % of the cohort (413/436). Extraction of genomic DNA was performed using the QIAamp 96 DNA Buccal Swab Biorobot Kit and performed on a 9604 Biorobot (Qiagen, Inc., Valencia, CA). We identified seven genes involved in the downstream metabolism of estrogen and chose functionally relevant SNPs with a sufficiently high allele frequency to provide adequate power for testing first order interactions in the cohort. These SNPs were: *COMT* Val158Met (rs4680), *CYP19* Arg 264Cys, (re700519), *CYP1A2*1 F (rs762551), *CYP1B1*4 (Asn452Ser, rs1800440), *CYP1B1*3 (Leu432-Val, rs1056836), *CYP3A4*1B (rs2740574), *SULT1A1* Arg213His (*2; rs9282861), *SULT1A1*3 (Met223Val, rs1801030), *SULT1E1* (−64G > A Promoter Variant; rs3736599), and *SULT1E1* A220G 3'UTR Variant (rs3786599). Genotypes were determined using previously described methods [37, 38].

m. *Other behavioral measures.* Additional validated behavioral measures were included at selected assessment periods to assess variables for pre-specified studies. The validated Kaiser Physical Activity Survey (KPAS) [39] was included in Periods 13–14. The Bristol Female Lower Urinary Tract Symptoms Scored Form (BFLUTS-SF) [40] was administered at Periods 11–14. A 61-item Dietary Assessment Questionnaire (DAQ) from the Nurses' Health Study [41] was completed by participants at Periods 2, 5, 6, 7, and 9. Table 1 presents a summary of the outcome measures by study visits.

Definition of menopausal status

We defined 5 stages of the menopause transition based on menstrual bleeding patterns and adapted from the initial Stages of Reproductive Aging Workshop (STRAW) [42] in order to capture the early changes in the menopausal transition [43]. The following 5 categories were defined in the cohort: 1) Premenopausal: regular menstrual cycles in the 22–35 day range. (Note: all participants were premenopausal at cohort enrollment). 2) Late premenopausal: a change in cycle length of 7 days or more in either direction from the participant's personal baseline at enrollment in the cohort and observed for at least one cycle in the study. 3). Early transition: changes in cycle length of 7 days or more in either direction from the participant's personal baseline at enrollment in the cohort and observed for at least 2 consecutive cycles in the study or 60 days amenorrhea. 4). Late transition: more than 60 days to 11 months amenorrhea. 5). Postmenopausal: 12 months or more amenorrhea, excluding hysterectomy. As participants progressed beyond menopause, the number of years since the final menstrual period were identified for analysis of the postmenopausal stage. Analyses have been conducted comparing early and later postmenopause as follows: <2 versus > =2 years [44]; 0–3 versus >3–11 years [45]; 0–5 versus 6–14 years [46].

Menopausal stage was identified at each assessment period, using the menstrual dates recorded at each study visit. This included the date of the current menstrual cycle (visits were conducted within 6 days of bleeding) and the dates for the 2 previous menstrual cycles, which were recorded at each visit. The 6 dates recorded at 2 visits provided consecutive menstrual dates for approximately 4 months in each assessment period. Additional confirmatory data were obtained from the daily symptoms diaries that participants recorded for one menstrual cycle at each assessment period (the diary date was used in cases of disagreement). Other confirmatory data included the reported number of menstrual periods between assessments, cycle length and the number of bleeding days, which were obtained in the structured interviews and the daily diaries.

Hormonal contraception, hysterectomy, pregnancy and breast feeding were exclusions at study enrollment. When these events occurred during the study, the information was coded and menopausal stage for these subjects was classified separately in categories of "hysterectomy", "hormone use", and "pregnancy/breast feeding" in the relevant assessment periods.

Identification of final menstrual period (FMP)

The final menstrual period was identified retrospectively after 12 or more months of no menstrual bleeding. The FMP marked entry into the postmenopausal stage. The small number of participants with surgical menopause were categorized separately.

Study adherence and attrition

Attrition occurred primarily in the early years of the study (Table 2). Nineteen percent (83/436) discontinued in the first 6 years. Half of these discontinued in the first year of the study, when they refused further participation or could not be located for the first follow-up evaluation. Only 10 % (42/436) discontinued in Phase 2 (years 7–10), and 4 % (18/436) discontinued in Phase 3 (years 11–14), for a total of 33 % attrition (143/436) over 14 years. Attrition through Period 14 was classified as lost to follow-up ($n = 51$), no reason given ($n = 40$), withdrew consent ($n = 22$), personal constraints or problems ($n = 16$), and deceased ($n = 14$).

We conducted a systematic analysis of study participation in the first 4 years, as reported in Nelson et al. [47]. Nelson examined demographic, behavioral, psychosocial and hormonal variables of the study that included age, race (African-American and Caucasian), education, marital status, body mass index, depressive symptoms, menopausal symptoms, perceived stress, anxiety, and reproductive hormone levels. There were no racial differences in study participation. Reproductive hormone levels at baseline did not differ between active and dropout groups. Only 2 variables marginally differed between active participants and dropouts: the dropout group was less likely to have high school education and less likely to report menopausal symptoms. Attrition to date has not significantly differed by race.

Effect of attrition on power

The pre-enrollment estimates for sample size indicated that a cohort of 300 women would detect clinically relevant differences in hormones and symptoms, using a 2-sided alpha error of 0.05 and 80 % power. We enrolled 436 women based on estimates of attrition in the first 4 years of the study. At the 12-year follow-up, 300 participants remained active and 293 participants remained active at Year 14.

We consider the home visits to be the key element in maintaining the high completion rate, which has far exceeded the original estimates. All data and blood samples were collected at home visits from enrollment through Period 14, resulting in minimal missing data

Table 1 Outcome measures by study visits

Domain	Measure	Study visits[1]
Demographic	Interview questionnaire	1,3,5,7,9,11,13
Menstrual cycle:	Interview questionnaire	1,3,5,7,9,11,13
menstrual dates, cycle characteristics ovulation test		2,4,6,8,10,12
Menopausal symptoms	Symptom questionnaire[5]	all odd visits 1-27
	Daily symptom reports	all odd visits 1-27
Health: gynecologic, reproductive, medications, health practices/behaviors	Interview questionnaire	all odd visits 1-27
General	SF-12 Health Survey[24]	all odd visits 1-27
Physical activity	Questionnaire[6]	4,12,16,20,22,24,25,27
	Kaiser Physical Activity Survey[37]	25,27
Sleep	SMH Sleep Questionnaire[8,9]	1,3,5,7,11,13,15,19
	WHI Insomnia Rating Scale[28]	19,21,23,25,27
	Apnea Prediction Index[29]	19,21,23,25,27
Mood and anxiety	PRIME-MD[15]	2,4,6,8,10,12
	Patient Health Questionnaire[16,17]	14,16,18,20,21,23,25 27
	CES-Depression Scale[18,19]	all odd visits 1-27
	Zung Anxiety Scale[20]	all odd visits 1-27
	Perceived Stress (PSS)[21]	2,4,6,8,10,12,3–27 (odd visits)
Quality of Life	Q-les-Q[22]	all odd visits
	Utian QOL Scale[23]	21,25,27
Sexual function	Female Sexual Function Index[30]	15,17,19,22,24,26,28
	Interview Questionnaire:	
	Abuse	11,17,19,23
	Interest	17,19,21,23,25,27
	Libido	all odd visits 1-27
Vaginal	Urinary Tract Rating (BFLUTS-SF)[38]	21,24,26,28
	Interview Questionnaire	
	Dryness	odd visits 3-27
	Urine leaks	odd visits 3-27
Social support	Interview Questionnaire	1, 9, 15, 19
	Social Adjustment Scale[31]	1,3,5,11,13,15,22
	Life Events	9,11,13,17,21,24,25,27
Cognition	Cognitive memory tests Buschke-Fuld Selective Reminding Test[32] Digit Symbol Substitution[33] Digit Symbol Copy[33]	all even visits 2-28
Diet	Dietary Assessment Questionnaire[39]	4, 10, 12, 14, 18
	Interview Questionnaire	3,5,7,11,15,19-17 (odd)

Table 1 Outcome measures by study visits *(Continued)*

Anthropomorphic	Measurement:	
	Height, weight, waist, hip	all odd visits 1-27
	Wrist	23,25,27
Hormones	Estradiol, follicle stimulating hormone, Luteinizing hormone, DHEAS, Testosterone, inhibin b	all visits 1-28
	Sex hormone binding globulin	all visits 13-28
	Anti-mullerian hormone	V1 to variousendpoints
Genotypes		413 participants

throughout the study. Incentives were provided to the participants, such as a small payment and a gift (e.g., mugs, magnets, throws, etc.) at the completion of each visit. In the intervals between the annual follow-up assessments, study staff maintained contact with participants by sending birthday cards and holiday cards each year. Participants were closely monitored via mailings and telephone calls around the dates of estimated menses in order to schedule visits on days 2–6 of the menstrual cycle. If a participant could not be located by mail or telephone, an interviewer went to the most recent home address to make contact and/or to query neighbors for information to locate the participant.

Data management

Two separate but related database management systems were established. The first Management Information System (MIS) addressed the internal study procedures. This included a database of all eligible women with the phone numbers, addresses, and persons who could be contacted on their behalf if the participant could not be located. The database also included a full register of the menstrual cycle dates reported by each participant at each visit and a record of the blood collections as they were stored in freezers or sent for assay. This database was used by the study coordinator to track and schedule the study visits, to identify the freezer location of blood samples, and to select and batch blood samples for laboratory assays.

Table 2 Study continuation and attrition by assessment period

PERIOD	CONTINUING, N (%)	DROPPED, N (%)
1	436	—
2	394 (90)	42 (10)
3-4	366 (84)	28 (6)
5-6	353 (84)	13 (3)
7-8	320 (73)	33 (8)
9-10	311 (71)	9 (2)
11-12	301 (69)	10 (2)
13-14	293 (67)	8 (2)
TOTAL	293 (67)	143 (33)

The second MIS contained all interview and questionnaire data collected for the study. These data were coded as they were collected and entered into computer files. A computer technician performed range checks and other organizing procedures to prepare the data for statistical analysis.

Potential bias and quality control

Menopausal symptom assessment is inherently based on subjective perception. In order to limit expectancy effects of menopause, the participants were told that the study was a women's health study. Specific questions about menopause were embedded in questionnaires with many other health questions. The menopause symptom questionnaire was validated and administered within the much longer structured Interview Questionnaire that assessed many aspects of women's health. We assessed the major symptoms of interest with *both* structured interview questions and more detailed validated self-report measures.

To reduce recall bias, the reference time frame for symptoms information was current, the data were collected concurrently with the blood draws, and participants additionally rated symptoms prospectively in daily symptom reports for one menstrual cycle (or month) at each assessment period.

To control for menstrual cycle effects in the hormone measures, all data were collected in the first 6 days of the menstrual cycle in cycling women. Neither the interviewers nor the participants had information from the study on the participants' hormone levels, making it unlikely that the women reported their symptoms based on hormone information.

To assure systematic data collection, we used structured interviews, and the interviewers were trained in the use of standard probes. Review sessions were conducted with the interviewers on an ongoing basis as part of the quality control process to address problems, develop consistent probes and promote systematic data collection. All interviewers were trained for SCID interviews via taped SCID interviews and training sessions with an experienced SCID interviewer. Interviewers checked that data for completion at each home visit. In addition, the study coordinator further reviewed all collected data when the data were returned to the research site. In the event of missing data, interviewers re-contacted participants to complete the missing items.

Representativeness of the cohort

The cohort participants were randomly identified by random digit dialing in a large metropolitan area of the U.S., with stratification to obtain equal numbers of African American and Caucasian women. The exclusion criteria limited the cohort to healthy women with a uterus and ovary at enrollment. Consequently the data are generalizable to generally healthy African American and Caucasian women in large urban areas of the U.S. who experience natural menopause. Findings may not be generalized to other racial groups or to women with surgical menopause, hormone users, serious illnesses or chronic disease without further studies.

Discussion

The POAS cohort was established to address the limited scientific understanding of menopausal hormone changes and symptoms and their relationships to health and morbidity of mid-life women. The cohort followed the large epidemiologic Study of Women's Health Across the Nation (SWAN), with specific aims to evaluate an earlier baseline of symptoms and hormones in late reproductive age women before they entered the transition to menopause. Annual evaluations followed the participants as they traversed the menopause transition. After 18 years of follow-up, the cohort remains viable with adequate statistical power for studies of the natural menopause transition and early postmenopausal years.

Strengths of the cohort addressed several limitations of earlier studies. The longitudinal data identified menopausal stages as they were observed rather than by long-term recall. Menopausal stages were based on the initial STRAW [42], utilizing bleeding patterns to classify premenopausal, transition and postmenopausal stages. Hormone levels and symptoms were measured concurrently. To control for menstrual cycle effects, all data, including the blood samples, were collected within days 2–6 of the menstrual cycle in cycling women. Menopausal stage was determined annually and, together with calendar age, can be analyzed to identify the independent effects of these key markers of menopausal status. Longitudinal assessments from a premenopausal baseline allowed *new-onset* symptoms to be identified in the menopause transition. Extensive symptom assessments included identifying psychiatric diagnoses to more clearly interpret menopausal symptoms. The cohort was population-based, participants were randomly-identified and in general good health for this study of behavioral and hormonal factors in relation to natural menopause.

Limitations to consider include the following: the cohort includes only Caucasian and African American women, who were enrolled in equal numbers, and does not include other racial or ethnic groups. Blood samples were collected in the early follicular phase of the menstrual cycle (days 2–6) to control for menstrual cycle effects, but do not include luteal phase measures and cannot describe across-cycle hormone effects. Hysterectomy and hormone use were exclusions at enrollment and in subsequent follow-up did not occur in sufficient numbers to analyze these factors. Attrition naturally occurred over the 18 years of follow up (described above), but the cohort remains viable with adequate statistical power.

More than 50 studies based on this cohort are published in medical journals at this time, demonstrating the relevance of these data to the clinical care of mid-life women. (See Additional file 1: Appendix 1). Several examples of the POAS data as they elucidate clinical issues are the following: studies of the timing and duration of hot flashes show that hot flashes can occur well before menopause and extend 10 or more years beyond menopause for sizeable numbers of women [48, 49]; data provide evidence for new-onset depressed mood in the menopause transition and show that the final menstrual period is pivotal in the premenopausal increase and postmenopausal decrease in depressive symptoms [44, 50, 51]; data show that poor sleep is common in the late reproductive years but suggest that only a small proportion of women experience increases in poor sleep in relation to the final menstrual period [28]; studies provide evidence of effects of obesity on reproductive hormones in the menopause transition [45, 52]; show the relationship between smoking and hot flashes as a function of genetic variation in sex-steroid metabolizing enzymes [46, 53]; indicate decreased libido in the menopause transition [54, 55]; menopause effects on verbal memory [56]; and anti-mullerian hormone as a predictor of time to menopause [57, 58].

In conclusion, longitudinal data are critical for the understanding of hormone changes and symptoms that are experienced by mid-life women and influence other physical conditions of aging. The POAS cohort and other recent cohorts of mid-life women exist to address questions about these menopausal changes. Increasing scientific information about the biological and behavioral changes associated with menopause contributes to improving the health care of women,

Abbreviations
AMH: anti-mullerian hormone (AMH).; BMI: body mass index; DHEAS: dehydroepiandrosterone; FSH: follicle stimulating hormone; LH: luteinizing hormone; POAS: Penn Ovarian Aging Study; SHGB: sex hormone binding globulin; STRAW: Stages of Reproductive Aging Workshop; SWAN: Study of Women's Health Across the Nation; T: testosterone.

Competing interests
The authors report no competing interests for this study.

Authors' contributions
EF drafted and wrote the manuscript. MS participated in the design (aims) of the review and helped draft the manuscript. Both authors read and approved the final manuscript.

Acknowledgements
This cohort and its studies were funded by the National Institute of Aging, RO1 AG12745, Ellen W. Freeman, PhD, principle investigator. Hormone assays conducted at the Clinical and Translational Research Center at the University of Pennsylvania were supported by the National Institute of Health #RR024132. Continuation of data collection in Year 18 was funded by the National Institute of Aging, RO1 AG048839, Neill Epperson, MD, principal investigator.

Author details
[1]Department of Obstetrics/Gynecology and Department of Psychiatry, 3701 Market Street, Suite 820 (Mudd Suite), Philadelphia, PA 19104, USA. [2]Center for Clinical Epidemiology and Biostatistics, Perelman School of Medicine, University of Pennsylvania, U.S, Philadelphia, USA.

References
1. ACOG. Practice Bulletin No. 141: management of menopausal symptoms. Obstet Gynecol. 2014;123:202–16.
2. Waksberg J. Sampling methods for random digit dialing. J Am Stat Assoc. 1978;73(361):40–6.
3. Faddy MJ, Gosden RG, Gougeon A, Richardson SJ, Nelson JF. Accelerated disappearance of ovarian follicles in mid-life: implications for forecasting menopause. Hum Reprod. 1992;7:1342–6.
4. Treloar AE. Menstrual cyclicity and the premenopause. Maturitas. 1981;3:249–64.
5. McKinlay SM, Brambilla DJ, Posner JG. The normal menopause transition. Maturitas. 1992;14:103–15.
6. Freeman EW, Sammel MD, Gracia CR, et al. Follicular phase hormone levels and menstrual bleeding status in the approach to menopause. Fertil Steril. 2005;83:383–92.
7. Freeman EW, Sammel MD, Liu L, Martin P. Psychometric properties of a menopausal symptom list. Menopause. 2003;10(3):258–65.
8. Ainsworth BE, Jacobs Jr DR, Leon AS, Montoye HJ, Sallis JF, Paffenbarger Jr RS. Compendium of physical activities. Med Sci Sports Exer. 1993;25:71–80.
9. Grisso JA, Main DM, Chiu GY, Snyder ED, Holmes JH. Effects of physical activity and life style factors on uterine contraction frequency. Amer J Perinatol. 1992;9:489–92.
10. Leigh TJ, Bird HA, Hindmarch I, Constable PDL, Wright V. Factor analysis of the St. Mary's Hospital sleep questionnaire. Sleep. 1988;11(5):448–53.
11. Ellis BW, Johns MW, Lancaster R, Raptopoulos P, Angelopoulos N, Priest. RG, et al. The St. Mary's Hospital sleep questionnaire; a study of reliability. Sleep. 1981;4(1):93–7.
12. Leon AC, Olfson M, Portera L, Farber L, Sheehan DV. Assessing psychiatric impairment in primary care with the Sheehan Disability Scale. Int J Psychiatry Med. 1997;27(2):93–105.
13. Freeman EW, Sammel MD, Lin H, et al. Symptoms associated with menopausal transition and reproductive hormones in midlife women. Obstet Gynecol. 2007;110(2):230–40.
14. Freeman EW, Sammel MD, Lin H, Gracia CR, Kapoor S. Symptoms in the menopausal transition. Obstet Gynecol. 2008;111(1):127–36.
15. Regier DA, Narrow WE, Rae DS, Manderscheid RW, Locke BZ, Goodwin FK. The de facto US mental and addictive disorders service system: epidemiologic catchment area prospective 1-year prevalence rates of disorders and services. Arch Gen Psychiatry. 1993;50(2):85–94.
16. Spitzer RL, Williams JBW, Gibbon M, First MB. Instruction Manual for the Structured Clinical Interview for DSM-III-R (SCID). New York: Biometrics Research; 1988.
17. Spitzer RL, Williams JBW, Kroenke K, et al. Utility of a new procedure for diagnosing mental disorders in primary care: the PRIME-MD 1000 study. JAMA. 1994;272(22):1749–56.
18. Spitzer RL, Williams JBW, Kroenke K, Hornyak R, McMurray J. Validity and utility of the PRIME-MD Patient Health Questionnaire in assessment of 3000 obstetric gynecologic patients: the PRIME-MD Patient Health Questionnaire Obstetrics Gynecology Study. Am J Obstet Gynecol. 2000;183(3):759–69.
19. Kroenke Kl, Spitzer RL, Williams JB. The PHQ-9: validity of a brief depression severity measure. J Gen Intern Med. 2001;16(9):606–13.
20. Radloff LS. The CES-D scale: a self-report depression scale for research in the general population. Appl Psychol Meas. 1977;1(3):385–401.
21. Harlow BL, Coen LS, Otto MW, Spiegelman D, Cramer DW. Prevalence and predictors of depressive symptoms in older premenopausal women: the Harvard Study of Moods and Cycles. Arch Gen Psychiatry. 1999;56(5):418–24.
22. Zung WWK. A rating instrument for anxiety disorders. Psychosomatics. 1971;12:371–9.
23. Cohen S, Kamarck T, Mermelstein R. A global measure of perceived stress. J Health Soc Behav. 1983;24:385–96.
24. Endicott J, Nee J, Harrison W, Blumenthal R. Quality-of-life enjoyment and satisfaction questionnaire - a new measure. Psychopharmacol Bull. 1993;29(2):321–6.
25. Utian WH, Janata JW, Kingsberg SA, Schluchter M, Hamilton JC. The Utian Quality of Life (UQOL) Scale: development and validation of an instrument to quantify quality of life through and beyond menopause. Menopause. 2002;9(6):402–10.
26. Ware JE, Kosinski M, Keller SD. A 12-item short-form health survey: construction of scales and preliminary tests of reliability and validity. Med Care. 1996;34(3):220–33.
27. Pien GW, Sammel MD, Freeman EW, Lin H, DeBlasis TL. Predictors of sleep quality in women in the menopausal transition. Sleep. 2008;31(7):991–9.
28. Freeman EW, Sammel MD, Gross SA, Pien GW. Poor sleep in relation to natural menopause: a population-based 14-year follow-up of mid-life women. Menopause. 2015;22(7):719–26.
29. Hollander LE, Freeman EW, Sammel MD, Berlin JA, Grisso JA, Battistini M. Sleep quality, estradiol levels and behavioral factors in late reproductive age women. Obstet Gynecol. 2001;98(3):391–7.
30. Levine DW, Bailey ME, Rockhill B, Tipping D, Naughton MJ, Shumaker SA. Validation of the Women's Health Initiative Insomnia Rating Scale in a multicenter controlled clinical trial. Psychosom Med. 2005;67(1):98–104.
31. Maislin G, Pack AI, Kribbs NB, et al. A survey screen for prediction of apnea. Sleep. 1995;18(3):158–66.
32. Rosen R, Brown C, Heiman J, et al. The female sexual function index (FSFI): a multidimensional self-report instrument for the assessment of female sexual function. J Sex Marital Ther. 2000;26:191–208.
33. Weissman MM, Bothwell S. Assessment of social adjustment by patient self-report. Arch Gen Psychiatry. 1976;33(9):1111–5.
34. Buschke H, Fuld PA. Evaluating storage, retention and retrieval in disordered memory and learning. Neurology. 1974;24:1019–25.
35. Wechsler D. Wechsler Adult Intelligence Scale - Revised. San Antonio, TX: Psychological Corp; 1991.
36. Salthouse TA. Influence of processing speed on adult age differences in working memory. Acta Psychol. 1992;79:155–70.
37. Rebbeck TR, Troxel AB, Wang Y, et al. Estrogen sulfation genes, hormone replacement therapy, and endometrial cancer risk. J Natl Cancer Inst. 2006;98:1311–20.
38. Shatalova EG, Walther S, Favorova OO, et al. Genetic polymorphisms in human SULT1A1 and UGT1A1 genes associated with breast tumor characteristics: a case-series study. Breast Cancer Res. 2005;7:R909–21.
39. Ainsworth BE, Sternfeld B, Richardson MT, Jackson K. Evaluation of the Kaiser Physical Activity Survey in women. Med Sci Sports Exerc. 2000;32(7):1327–38.
40. Jackson S, Donovan J, Brookes S, Eckford S, Swithinbank L, Abrams P. The Bristol Female Lower Urinary Tract Symptoms Questionnaire: development and psychometric testing. Br J Urol. 1996;77:805–12.
41. Willett WC, Sampson L, Stampfer MJ, et al. Reproducibility and validity of a semi-quantitative food frequency questionnaire. Am J Epidemiol. 1985;122(1):51–65.
42. Soules MR, Sherman S, Parrott E, et al. Executive summary: Stages of Reproductive Aging Workshop (STRAW). Fertil Steril. 2001;76:874–8.
43. Gracia CR, Sammel MD, Freeman EW, et al. Defining menopause status: creation of a new definition to identify the early changes of the menopause transition. Menopause. 2005;12(2):128–35.
44. Freeman EW, Sammel MD, Boorman DW, Zhang R. Longitudinal pattern of depressive symptoms around natural menopause. JAMA Psychiatry. 2014;71(1):36–43.
45. Freeman EW, Sammel MD, Lin H, Gracia CR. Obesity and reproductive hormone levels in the transition to menopause. Menopause. 2010;17(4):718–26.

46. Butts SF, Sammel MD, Greer C, Rebbeck TR, Boorman DW, Freeman EW. Cigarette, genetic background and menopausal timing: the presence of single nucleotide polymorphisms in cytochrome P450 genes is associated with increased risk of natural menopause in European-American smokers. Menopause. 2014;21(7):694–701.
47. Nelson DB, Sammel MD, Freeman EW, Liu L, Langan E, Gracia CR. Predicting participation in prospective studies of ovarian aging. Menopause. 2004;11(5):543–8.
48. Freeman EW, Sammel MD, Lin H, Liu Z, Gracia CR. Duration of menopausal hot flushes and asssociated risk factors. Obstet Gynecol. 2011;117(5):1095–104.
49. Freeman EW, Sammel MD, Sanders RJ. Risk of long-term hot flashes after natural menopause: evidence from the Penn Ovarian Aging Study cohort. Menopause. 2014;21(9):924–32.
50. Freeman EW, Sammel MD, Liu L, Gracia CR, Nelson DB, Hollander L. Hormones and menopausal status as predictors of depression in women in transition to menopause. Arch Gen Psychiatry. 2004;61(1):62–70.
51. Freeman EW, Sammel MD, Lin H, Nelson DB. Associations of hormones and menopausal status with depressed mood in women with no history of depression. Arch Gen Psychiatry. 2006;63(4):375–82.
52. Gracia CR, Freeman EW, Sammel MD, Lin H, Nelson DB. The relationship between obesity and race on inhibin B during the menopause transition. Menopause. 2005;12(5):559–66.
53. Butts SF, Freeman EW, Sammel MD, Queen K, Lin H, Rebbeck TR. Joint effects of smoking and gene variants involved in sex steroid metabolism on hot flashes in late reproductive-age women. J Clin Endocrin Metab. 2012;97(6):1032–42.
54. Gracia CR, Freeman EW, Sammel MD, Lin H, Mogul M. Hormones and sexuality during transition to menopause. Obstet Gynecol. 2007;109(4):831–40.
55. Gracia CR, Sammel MD, Freeman EW, Liu L, Hollander L, Nelson DB. Predictors of decreased libido in women during the late reproductive years. Menopause. 2004;11(2):144–50.
56. Epperson CN, Sammel MD, Freeman EW. Menopause effects on verbal memory: findings from a longitudinal community cohort. J Clin Endocrin Metab. 2013;58(9):3829–38.
57. Freeman EW, Sammel MD, Lin H, Gracia CR. Anti-mullerian hormone as a predictor of time to menopause in late reproductive age women. J Clin Endocrin Metab. 2012;97(5):1673–80.
58. Freeman EW, Sammel MD, Lin H, Boorman DW, Gracia CR. Contribution of the rate of change of antimullerian hormone in estimating time to menopause for late reproductive-age women. Fertil Steril. 2012;98(5):1254–9.

12

Stress and the menopausal transition in Campeche, Mexico

Lynnette Leidy Sievert[1]*[ID], Laura Huicochea-Gómez[2], Diana Cahuich-Campos[2], Dana-Lynn Ko'omoa-Lange[3] and Daniel E. Brown[4]

Abstract

Background: Stress has been implicated as a factor in the presence and severity of symptoms during the menopausal transition. Our primary aim was to test the hypothesis that stress-sensitive biological measures and self-reported stress would be positively associated with a greater likelihood and intensity of hot flashes. Our secondary aim was to examine measures of stress in relation to the most often reported symptoms in Campeche, Mexico. We also hypothesized ethnic differences (Maya versus non-Maya) in relation to measures of stress and symptom reports.

Methods: Participants aged 40–60 ($n = 305$) were drawn from multiple sites across the city of San Francisco de Campeche to achieve a generally representative sample. Measures included C-reactive protein (CRP), an indicator of inflammation; Epstein-Barr virus antibodies (EBV-Ab), an indicator of immune function; the Perceived Stress Scale (PSS); a symptom checklist; anthropometric measures; and a questionnaire that elicited symptoms, ethnicity (based on language, birthplace, and last names of the woman, her parents, and her grandparents) and ten dimensions of socioeconomic status (SES). The relationships between symptoms and stress-sensitive biological and self-reported measures were examined in bivariate analyses, and with logistic and linear regressions.

Results: The twelve most common symptoms reported, in descending order of frequency, were tiredness, muscle and joint pain, nervous tension, problems concentrating, feeling depressed, difficulty sleeping, headaches, feeling of ants crawling on the skin, loss of interest in sex, urinary stress incontinence, hot flashes, and night sweats. PSS scores were significantly associated with the likelihood of seven symptoms (yes/no), and with the intensity of ten symptoms after controlling for ethnicity, SES, education, cohabitation status, parity, smoking, body mass index, and menopausal status. The stress-sensitive biological measures of immune function (EBV-Ab and CRP) were not significantly associated with midlife symptoms. The PSS was associated with more symptoms among the Maya (e.g., feeling nervous/tense and having difficulty concentrating) than non-Maya.

Conclusion: PSS scores were associated with the intensity, but not the likelihood, of hot flashes. Other symptoms were also associated with self-reported stress but not with physiological measures. Maya/non-Maya differences may indicate that either symptoms or stress were experienced and/or reported in culture-specific ways.

Keywords: Menopause, Stress, Hot flashes, Night sweats, Fatigue, Sleep difficulties, Depression

* Correspondence: leidy@anthro.umass.edu
[1]Department of Anthropology, Machmer Hall, 240 Hicks Way, UMass Amherst, Amherst, MA 01003-9278, USA
Full list of author information is available at the end of the article

Background

The menopausal transition is often characterized by hot flashes and night sweats [1], fatigue and body aches [2], difficulty sleeping [3], and transient depression [4]. Some symptoms can be attributed to the changing hormone levels associated with the loss of ovarian follicles, including fluctuating estradiol and increases in follicle stimulating hormones [5, 6]. However, some symptoms may be better explained by combining physiological information with the social changes that coincide with this time of life. For example, a woman's children are likely to be adolescents with their own challenges, husbands may be undergoing transition in social status such as retirement or struggling with health issues, and parents may be in need of substantial levels of care [7, 8].

During the menopausal transition, stress may be a contributor to trouble sleeping, depression [9, 10], and/ or symptoms that may have a psychosomatic component [11]. For example, in cross-cultural work among women aged 45–55, Sievert et al. [12] found that *job* change was associated with an increased likelihood of nervous tension, difficulty concentrating, headaches, and fatigue in the U.S., but not in Spain. In Spain, but not the U.S., *household* change was associated with depressed mood and difficulty concentrating. These differences show that stress is variable and context dependent. It appears that job change may be experienced as more stressful in the U.S., whereas household change may be more stressful in Spain.

Specific to hot flashes, stress has been identified as a determinant in some [13–17], but not all [12, 18, 19] studies of factors associated with hot flashes. In a laboratory setting, where symptomatic women were exposed to a variety of stressors, there were 57% more self-reported hot flashes during stress periods compared to non-stress periods [20]. In the Study of Women's Health Across the Nation (SWAN), after adjusting for ethnicity, lifestyle, and other confounding variables, self-reported perceived stress was significantly associated with self-reported vasomotor symptoms (adjusted odds ratio 1.4, 95% confidence interval 1.2–1.6) [15], and significantly related to a longer persistence of self-reported hot flashes into the postmenopausal period [13]. In a 13-year longitudinal study in Philadelphia, women who reported moderate or severe hot flashes during the study period had a higher baseline Perceived Stress Scale (PSS) score (21.9) compared to women with mild hot flashes (19.5) or no hot flashes (18.2, $p < 0.01$). Stress was not significantly associated with the duration of self-reported hot flushes in a multivariable model [14].

Cortisol is a stress-sensitive biological measure [21] that has been examined in relation to hot flashes. Two early laboratory studies showed an increase in cortisol levels during and after monitored hot flashes [22, 23]. In the Seattle Women's Health Study, women with increased urinary cortisol had significantly greater self-reported hot flash and cold sweat symptom severity compared to women without increased cortisol [24]. In Modena, Italy, women with self-reported severe hot flashes had significantly higher levels of 24-h urinary cortisol compared to women with none to moderate vasomotor symptoms [25]. Hot flash report has also been associated with higher salivary cortisol levels in the early afternoon [26]. In a small study where women with hot flashes were measured by an ambulatory monitor, objectively measured hot flashes were associated with significantly higher salivary cortisol levels at 15, 30, and 45 min post-waking compared to women without biometrically measured hot flashes [27].

Not all studies have shown a consistently positive relationship between hot flashes and cortisol levels. For example, hot flash report has not been associated with the cortisol awakening response or diurnal variation in cortisol levels [26, 28, 29]. One study found greater self-reported hot flash severity associated with a flatter diurnal slope in salivary cortisol [30].

Self-reported hot flashes and other symptoms have been shown to vary across ethnicity within the same country [31–33]. Self-reported stress has also been shown to vary with ethnicity. For example, Brown [34, 35] compared levels of stress across two Filipino-American ethnic groups to show that individuals from Visayan backgrounds self-reported significantly higher levels of stress compared to individuals of Ilocano descent. At the same time, there was no difference in the 24-h excretion rates of norepinephrine and epinephrine between the two groups. Brown also found that Filipino American women (mostly Ilocanos) were significantly more likely to record being anxious in a diary compared to European American women, but European Americans had higher elevations in ambulatory blood pressure when they did report anxiety [36]. Ethnic differences were also found in response to doing household chores: Filipino American women were more likely to report being anxious during chores than European Americans, but the European American women had higher diastolic BP while doing chores than the Filipino Americans [36]. Ethnic differences in the report of stress may reflect psychosocial differences [37], or culturally-based reporting biases [38]. For these reasons, the study reported here examined self-reported stress and symptom frequencies between Maya and non-Maya women.

Previous studies of menopause among Maya women in the Yucatán Peninsula of Mexico found an early mean recalled age at natural menopause of 44 years, compared to 52.5 years in the U.S. [39–41]. An in-depth ethnographic study documented an absence of self-reported hot flashes among rural Maya women [42]. According to

Beyene, Maya women explained menopause as something that occurred when a woman used up her menstrual blood ([43], page 119). These women perceived menopause to be "a life stage free of taboos and restrictions, offering increased freedom of movement" (p.120). Other investigators recorded higher levels of hot flash frequencies among urban (49%) and rural (41%) Maya women in the Yucatán peninsula [44].

This study administered the PSS, as used in the SWAN and Philadelphia studies, to measure self-reported stress. To our knowledge, this will be the first study to examine hot flashes and other symptoms at midlife in relation to Epstein-Barr virus antibodies (EBV-Ab) [45, 46]. Both C-reactive protein (CRP) and EBV-Ab have been positively associated with high stress levels [47, 48]. CRP is an acute-phase protein that is commonly used as a measure of general inflammation. Because chronic stress is associated with elevated inflammation levels [49], this protein has been used as a marker of both acute and chronic stress [50, 51]. With regard to EBV-Ab, most people are chronically infected with EBV. When an individual is stressed, down-regulation of the immune system allows the virus to replicate, and antibodies to the virus increase in the blood stream. Accordingly, an elevated EBV-Ab level has been used as a biological marker of stress [47, 52].

The primary aim of this study was to test the hypothesis that two biological measures potentially sensitive to stress and a self-reported measure of stress would be associated with a higher likelihood and intensity of hot flashes after controlling for potential confounders. Our secondary aim was to examine the stress-sensitive measures and self-reported stress in relation to the most commonly reported symptoms in Campeche, Mexico. Based on the results of other cross-cultural studies [12, 36] detailed above, we paid particular attention to ethnic differences in nervous tension, difficulties concentrating, headaches, fatigue, and depressed mood, as well as hot flashes and trouble sleeping. We hypothesized that all stress measures would be associated with the frequency and intensity of each of the 12 most-reported symptoms in bivariate analyses, and after controlling for potential confounders. We also hypothesized ethnic differences (Maya vs. non-Maya) in relation to measures of stress and symptom reports [38]. Other variables that could affect both stress measures and symptoms were collected, including age, menopausal status, level of education, socioeconomic status (SES), body mass index (BMI), ethnicity, marital status and cohabitation with husband or partner, parity, and smoking habits.

Methods
Sample
The study took place in San Francisco de Campeche, a city of approximately 250,000 people [53] located on the western coast of the Yucatan peninsula. Nearly 12% of the city's population speaks Maya [53]. Women aged 40–60 years were drawn from businesses, schools, the city market, and by presentations given in homes. The use of several recruitment methods assured a diverse, although not random, sample of the city's population. These participants make up the urban component of a larger study of menopause in the state of Campeche [54]. In the city, a total of 305 women participated in interviews and anthropometric measures, with a subsample of 162 participants providing finger stick blood samples. Of those 162 women, 109 provided sufficient blood for the assay of both CRP and EBV-Ab levels.

The study was approved by the Institutional Review Board of the University of Massachusetts Amherst; the Human Subjects Committee of the University of Hawaii at Hilo; and the Committee for Ethics in Research of the Secretary of Health in the State of Campeche, Mexico. All participants signed a letter of consent after lengthy explanation in Spanish.

Measures
All participants answered questions related to their age, education, parity, and smoking status. An SES index was created from 10 dimensions related to housing construction, household composition, and infrastructure, such as, access to drinking water and type of cooking fuel. Within the city of Campeche, the range in SES index was from 22 to 39. With regard to marital status, 96% of married women ($n = 160$) and 73% of women with a partner ($n = 26$; *union libre*) lived with their partner and, therefore, the variable of interest used in the analyses here was whether or not a woman cohabited with a husband or partner.

Maya/non-Maya ethnicity was assessed on the basis of each woman's two last names, whether she could speak or understand Maya, and place of birth. The same information was collected with regard to her parents and grandparents. Women were categorized as Maya, not Maya, or not able to be clearly defined on the basis of this information from all three generations. There were 40 participants for whom an ethnic was unclear because of missing information (e.g., not everyone knew the language spoken by their grandparents).

Menopausal status was defined by STRAW+ 10 stages: (1) regular menstruation, (2) changes in the number of days or quantity of blood, (3) more or less frequent menstruation, (4) a change in periods of more than 6 days, (5) 2 months or more have passed without a period, and (6) more than 12 months have passed without a period [55]. Stages 1 and 2 were categorized as pre-menopausal, stages 3 to 5 as peri-menopausal, and stage 6 as postmenopausal.

Stature was measured with a Seca 213 stadiometer to the nearest 0.1 cm. Weight was measured to the nearest 0.1 kg with a digital scale. BMI was computed as kg/m^2.

All participants completed the PSS that has been previously used in Mexican populations [56]. The PSS is a well validated 10-item questionnaire that directly queries levels of stress experienced in the past month, and the degree to which one's life is unpredictable, uncontrollable, and overloaded [57, 58].

Participants were asked about the presence or absence of 19 symptoms during the past 2 weeks including hot flashes (*Ha tenido calores o bochornos?*) and night sweats (*En la noche ha tenido sudoraciones?*). This "everyday symptom list" has been used in many studies [59–61], including in Mexico [62]. Symptom intensities were reported as: 0 = *nada*; 1 = *un poco*; 2 = *mucho*; and 3 = *muchisimo*. Twelve symptoms had a frequency of 45% or higher in the city of Campeche. The cut off of 45% was selected in order to include hot flashes and night sweats in the analyses below. The 12 symptom reports were totaled to derive a total number of symptoms reported for each individual. Also, the intensity of the 12 symptoms were totaled to derive a total symptom intensity score for each participant.

Blood was collected by finger stick onto Whatman #903 Protein Saver filter paper sample cards [47], dried for 4 h, and immediately frozen in the Huicochea laboratory at ECOSUR, Campeche. The cards were carried to the United States by LLS, and mailed overnight to the University of Hawaii at Hilo with ice packs. The cards were then transferred to freezer storage at – 30 °C until analysis.

To determine the presence of EBV – Viral Capsid Antigen (VCA) in dried blood spot samples, an EBV-VCA enzyme-linked immunosorbent assay (Diamedix Corporation, Miami Lakes, FL), was modified for sampling dried blood spots. Briefly, a sample of each blood spot was taken by punching a single 6 mm disc using a standard hand held hole puncher. The blood spot samples were incubated in elution buffer overnight, on a platform shaker at low speed. 100 uL of the cut-off calibrator, controls and samples were transferred to the antigen wells. The samples and controls were allowed to incubate at room temperature for 30 min. The contents of the wells were discarded, and the wells were washed three times with wash solution. 100 uL of conjugate was pipetted into each well, and allowed to incubate at room temperature for 30 min. The contents were discarded, and the wells were washed three times in wash solution. Next, 100 uL of the substrate was pipetted into each well, and the wells were incubated at room temperature for 30 min. After incubation with substrate, 100 uL of stop solution was pipetted into each well. The absorbance was determined at 450 nm. All controls and samples were assayed in duplicate [45].

To determine the index value for each participant, the following formula was used:

$$\frac{\text{Absorbance of sample}}{\substack{\text{Mean absorbance of} \\ \text{cut-off calibrator}}} = \text{Index value}$$

Samples with an index value ≥1.10 were determined to be positive for VCA IgG antibody.

CRP enzyme-linked immunosorbent assay (Abcam, Cambridge, MA) was used to quantitatively measure human CRP in blood spots following the methods of McDade et al. [63]. CRP values in blood spots were converted into the equivalent values of CRP in plasma by the following: $(CRP_{bloodspot} * 1.15) - 0.13 = CRP_{Plasma}$ [63]. None of the participants had a CRP_{Plasma} value greater than 10.0 mg/L, an indicator of an active infection which would have led to exclusion from analyses involving CRP and EBV-Ab [64].

Analyses

PSS scores, EBV-Ab levels, and CRP_{Plasma} levels were appraised for normal distribution. PSS scores were normally distributed and examined in relation to ethnic categories (Maya, not Maya, difficult to categorize) by ANOVA and in relation to each symptom (yes/no) by t-tests. EBV-Ab and CRP_{Plasma} levels were not normally distributed, and therefore were examined in relation to ethnic categories and in relation to each symptom by two-tailed Mann Whitney tests. Spearman correlations were examined between EBV-Ab values, CRP_{Plasma} levels, and PSS scores.

Logistic regressions were performed with each of the 12 symptoms (none vs. any level of symptom experience) as a dependent variable in a separate regression model. Analyses were carried out separately for each of the three stress measures – PSS scores, EBV-Ab values, and CRP_{Plasma} levels; therefore, there were three analyses carried out for each of the 12 symptoms. BMI, SES, education, ethnicity, cohabiting with a husband or partner, parity, smoking, and menopausal status were covariates. Because of the correlation among the covariates SES and education ($r = .465$, $p < 0.001$), and in order to achieve the best set of variables associated with each symptom, backward stepwise regression was carried out with a probability for entry set at 0.05 and probability for removal set to 0.10. Because of the multiple testing, we applied an adjusted *p*-value of $p \leq 0.001$ to determine significance. Logistic regressions were repeated separately for women categorized as Maya and non-Maya.

Linear regressions with backwards elimination were carried out for all participants with intensity of symptom reports (*nada, un poco, mucho, muchisimo*) as dependent variables and PSS scores, EBV-Ab values, CRP_{Plasma} levels,

BMI, SES, education, ethnicity, cohabiting with a husband or partner, parity, smoking, and menopausal status as co-variates. As described above, analyses for each symptom were carried out separately for the three stress variables, and analyses were repeated separately for women categorized as Maya and non-Maya, respectively.

Results

Table 1 presents some characteristics of the sample by ethnicity. The Maya had a significantly lower SES index than non-Maya, but there were otherwise no significant ethnic differences in the listed characteristics. There were no significant differences in the PSS score between Maya and non-Maya women ($t = 1.3$, ns); Maya women had significantly higher EBV-Ab (two-tailed Mann Whitney test, $p < 0.05$), but there was no significant ethnic difference in CRP_{Plasma} levels. There were no significant ethnic differences in the frequency of symptoms, the total number of reported symptoms, or the total symptom intensity scores (two-tailed t-tests, ns). Figure 1 shows the frequency of reported symptoms for the entire sample.

For all women in the sample, there was a significant correlation between EBV-Ab values and CRP_{Plasma} levels (Spearman $\rho = 0.57$, $p < 0.001$), but PSS scores were not significantly correlated with either EBV-Ab values ($\rho = -0.08$, ns) or CRP_{Plasma} levels ($\rho = -0.02$, ns). Similar correlation results among stress measures were obtained when the ethnic groups were considered separately.

Table 2 presents results for bivariate analyses of the relation between stress measures and reported symptoms (none vs. any level of symptom experience) for all participants. The table gives means and standard deviations of the PSS scores, and medians of the CRP_{Plasma} and EBV-Ab levels. For nine of the 12 symptoms, women who reported the symptom had a significantly higher PSS score compared to women who did not report the symptom ($p \leq 0.001$). Women with hot flashes and headaches had higher PSS scores, with p-values of 0.004 and 0.006, respectively – slightly above the conservative Bonferroni correction of $p \leq 0.001$. EBV-Ab and CRP_{Plasma} values were not significantly higher among women reporting any symptom.

The total number of reported symptoms for each individual was significantly correlated with the PSS score

Table 1 Participant information. Means ± standard deviations, numbers of participants, or percentages shown

	Maya	Non-Maya	Could not classify	All
N	144	121	40	305
Age at interview Mean ± s.d.	47.9 ± 5.0	46.9 ± 5.0	47.5 ± 5.0	47.5 ± 5.0
BMI (kg/m²) Mean ± s.d.	31.3 ± 5.2	30.3 ± 5.8	29.1 ± 5.3	30.6 ± 5.5
SES Index[a] Range 22–39. Mean ± s.d.	32.8 ± 2.4	33.4 ± 2.3	33.4 ± 2.4	33.1 ± 2.4
Education (yrs) Mean ± s.d.	12.8 ± 4.4	13.8 ± 4.0	13.3 ± 4.4	13.2 ± 4.2
Menopause status (%)				
Pre-menopausal	40.3	47.9	42.5	43.6
Perimenopausal	20.8	24.0	22.5	22.3
Post – menopausal	38.9	28.1	35.0	34.1
% cohabiting with husband or partner	59.0	57.0	70.0	59.7
Parity Mean ± s.d.	2.0 ± 1.1	2.1 ± 1.2	2.0 ± 1.4	2.0 ± 1.2
Smoking (%)	10.4	14.9	12.5	12.5
PSS score Mean ± s.d. n = 305	1.55 ± 1.6	1.04 ± 0.6	1.58 ± 1.7	1.35 ± 1.3
EBV-Ab level* Mean ± s.d. n = 162	4.59 ± 1.4	4.06 ± 1.7	3.83 ± 1.6	4.30 ± 1.6
CRP_{plasma} level Mean ± s.d. n = 157	16.78 ± 5.2	17.65 ± 5.9	17.95 ± 4.5	17.28 ± 5.4
Total symptom score (range 0–12, based on 12 most common symptoms)	7.4 ± 3.0	7.4 ± 2.7	6.9 ± 3.1	7.3 ± 2.9
Total symptom intensity score (range 0–33, based on 12 most common symptoms)	10.9 ± 6.4	10.4 ± 6.0	9.3 ± 5.5	10.5 ± 6.0

[a]Ethnic difference, Maya versus non-Maya, $p < 0.05$

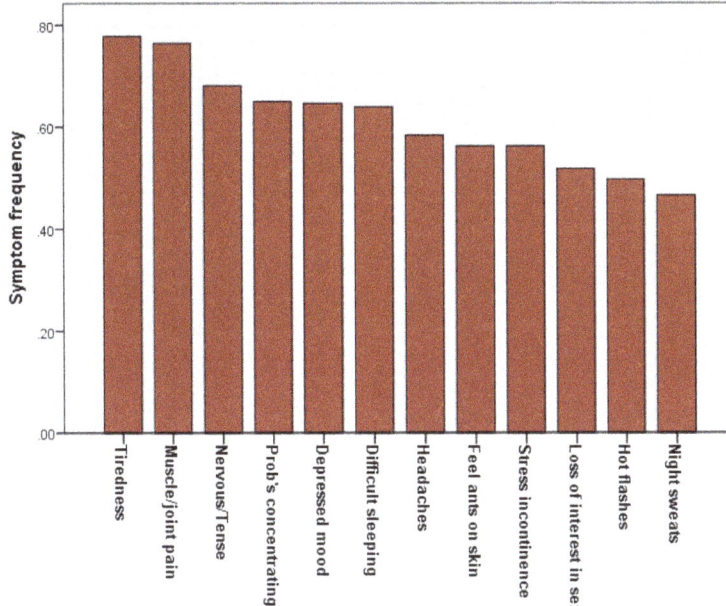

Fig. 1 Frequency of the 12 most often reported symptoms among Maya and non-Maya women living in the city of Campeche, Mexico (n = 305)

(two-tailed Spearman correlations, $\rho = 0.42$, $p < 0.001$), but not with CRP_{Plasma} ($\rho = -0.02$, ns) nor EBV-Ab ($\rho = -0.08$, ns) levels. The total symptom intensity score was significantly correlated with the PSS score ($\rho = 0.46$, $p < 0.001$) and EBV-Ab values ($\rho = 0.17$, $p < 0.05$).

Table 3 presents the covariates that remained in the models following backwards stepwise logistic regression for each symptom among all participants. PSS score was significantly, positively associated with the report of

tiredness, muscle/joint pain, feeling nervous/tense, problems concentrating, depressed mood, difficulty sleeping, and loss of interest in sex after controlling for BMI, SES, education, ethnicity, cohabiting with a husband or partner, parity, smoking, and menopausal status. Odds Ratios for PSS ranged from 1.10 (95% CI 1.04–1.15) for loss of interest in sex to 1.22 (95% CI 1.13–1.32) tiredness. Hot flashes, night sweats, and the feeling of ants crawling on the skin had p-values of 0.007, 0.004,

Table 2 Bivariate comparisons of stress levels by symptom complaints. Means ± standard deviations for PSS scores or medians for CRP_{Plasma} and EBV-Ab levels shown

Symptom	PSS score by symptom		EBV-Ab value by symptom		CRPPlasma level by symptom	
	No	Yes	No	Yes	No	Yes
Tiredness or lack of energy	13.9 ± 4.2	18.2 + 5.3***	0.81	1.00*	5.28	5.69
Muscle and joint pain	15.1 ± 4.6	17.9 ± 5.5***	1.00	0.96	5.61	5.64
Nervous or tense	15.3 ± 4.5	18.2 ± 5.5***	0.93	1.00	5.28	5.68
Problems concentrating	15.4 ± 4.5	18.3 ± 5.6***	0.94	0.99	5.57	5.65
Depressed mood or sadness	15.3 ± 4.3	10.4 ± 5.0***	0.93	1.00	4.86	5.72*
Difficulty sleeping	15.1 ± 5.0	18.6 ± 5.2***	0.86	1.01	5.34	5.68
Headaches	16.3 ± 4.7	18.0 ± 5.8**	0.94	1.00	5.48	5.69
Feeling of ants crawling on skin	16.0 ± 4.7	18.3 ± 5.7***	0.82	0.94*	5.33	5.48
Urinary stress incontinence with effort or laughter	16.4 ± 4.9	17.9 ± 5.7*	0.93	0.98	5.34	5.68
Loss of interest in sexual relations	16.3 ± 5.2	18.4 ± 5.4***	1.00	0.96	5.65	5.65
Hot flashes	16.4 ± 5.2	18.2 ± 5.4**	0.94	0.98	5.59	5.67
Night sweats	16.4 ± 5.0	18.5 ± 5.7***	0.84	1.02	5.34	5.68

Two tailed t-tests or Mann-Whitney tests, *$p <$ 0.05; **$p <$ 0.01; ***$p \leq$ 0.001

Table 3 Logistic regression analyses of symptom reports. 95% Confidence Intervals shown for Odds Ratios

With PSS scores			With CRP$_{Plasma}$			With EBV–Ab		
Variable	Odds Ratio (95% CI)	Signif.	Variable	Odds Ratio (95% CI)	Signif.	Variable	Odds Ratio (95% CI)	Signif.
Tiredness								
PSS Score	1.22 (1.13–1.32)	**<0.001**	[none remained in model]			Parity	1.41 0.94–2.10	<0.1
Parity	1.36 (1.02–1.83)	<0.05						
Muscle and Joint Pain								
PSS Score	1.11 (1.04–1.18)	**<0.001**	SES	0.80 0.64–1.01	<0.1	[none remained in model]		
Education	0.95 (0.80–0.95)	<0.01						
Nervous or Tense								
PSS Score	1.12 (1.06–1.18)	**<0.001**	Cohabiting (ref)			EBV-Ab	1.76 (1.00–3.12)	=0.05
Parity	1.36 (1.06–1.74)	<0.05	not cohabiting	0.41 (0.19–1.01)	<0.05	Cohabiting (ref)		
BMI	0.96 0.91–1.01	<0.1				not cohabiting	0.39 (0.18–0.85)	<0.05
Problems concentrating								
PSS Score	1.14 (1.08–1.21)	**<0.001**	Menopause Pre- (Ref)			Non-smoker (ref)		
			Peri-	3.99 (1.31–12.09)	<0.05	Smoker	3.50 (0.97–12.59)	<0.1
			Post-	1.57 (0.65–3.80)	ns			
			BMI	1.09 (1.00–1.19)	<0.05			
Depressed mood								
PSS Score	1.14 (1.07–1.20)	**<0.001**	BMI	1.10 (1.02–1.18)	<0.05	BMI	1.09 (1.01–1.18)	<0.05
BMI	1.07 (1.02–1.13)	=0.01				Education	0.92 (0.83–1.01)	<0.1
Difficulty sleeping								
PSS Score	1.18 (1.11–1.25)	**<0.001**	Education	0.85 (0.76–0.96)	=0.01	Education	0.91 (0.81–1.01)	<0.1
Cohabiting (ref)			Menopause Pre- (Ref)			BMI	0.94 (0.87–1.01)	<0.1
Not cohabiting	2.04 (1.12–3.70)	<0.05	Peri-	1.21 (0.49–2.98)	ns			
			Post-	3.56 (1.37–9.25)	<0.05			
Ethnicity						Ethnicity		
Maya (ref)						Maya (ref)		
Non-Maya	0.53 (0.30–0.92)	<0.05				Non-Maya	0.34 (0.16–0.74)	<0.01

Table 3 Logistic regression analyses of symptom reports. 95% Confidence Intervals shown for Odds Ratios *(Continued)*

With PSS scores			With CRP$_{Plasma}$			With EBV–Ab		
Variable	Odds Ratio (95% CI)	Signif.	Variable	Odds Ratio (95% CI)	Signif.	Variable	Odds Ratio (95% CI)	Signif.
Parity	1.25 (0.97–1.61)	< 0.1						
Headaches								
PSS Score	1.06 (1.01–1.11)	< 0.05	CRP$_{Plasma}$	1.19 (0.97–1.45)	p< 0.1	[none remained in model]		
Education	0.93 (0.87–0.99)	< 0.05	Ethnicity Maya (ref)					
			Non–Maya	2.24 (1.07–4.67)	< 0.05			
Cohabiting (ref)								
Not cohabiting	0.63 (0.38–1.05)	< 0.1						
Feeling of ants crawling on skin								
PSS Score	1.08 (1.03–1.13)	= 0.002	CRP$_{Plasma}$	1.22 1.00–1.49	< 0.1	Education	0.90 (0.81–1.00)	= 0.05
			Menopause Pre- (ref)					
			Peri-	2.89 (1.08–7.76)	< 0.05			
			Post-	1.58 (0.69–3.66)	ns			
Stress Incontinence								
PSS Score	1.05 (1.00–1.10)	< 0.05	[none remained in model]			[none remained in model]		
Menopause Pre- (ref)								
Peri-	0.72 (0.38–1.38)	ns						
Post-	0.54 (0.30–0.95)	< 0.05						
Loss of interest in sex								
PSS Score	1.10 (1.04–1.15)	**< 0.001**	Cohabiting (ref)			Cohabiting (ref)		
			not cohabiting	0.30 (0.14–0.64)	= 0.002	not cohabiting	0.48 (0.23–1.01)	= 0.05
Cohabiting (ref)						SES	0.83 (0.69–0.99)	< 0.05
Not cohabiting	0.26 (0.15–0.43)	**< 0.001**						
Ethnicity Maya (ref)								
Non-Maya	0.60 (0.36–1.02)	< 0.1						
Hot flashes								
PSS Score	1.07 (1.02–1.12)	= 0.007	[none remained in model]			Cohabiting (ref)		
						not cohabiting	0.54 (0.26–1.13)	= 0.1

Table 3 Logistic regression analyses of symptom reports. 95% Confidence Intervals shown for Odds Ratios (Continued)

With PSS scores			With CRP$_{Plasma}$			With EBV–Ab		
Variable	Odds Ratio (95% CI)	Signif.	Variable	Odds Ratio (95% CI)	Signif.	Variable	Odds Ratio (95% CI)	Signif.
Menopause Pre- (ref)						Menopause Pre- (ref)		
Peri-	1.90 (0.99–3.66)	< 0.1				Peri-	2.12 (0.94–4.77)	< 0.1
Post-	1.73 (0.97–3.08)	< 0.1				Post-	2.22 (0.91–5.43)	< 0.1
Parity	1.23 (0.99–1.53)	< 0.1						
Night sweats								
PSS Score	1.07 (1.02–1.13)	= 0.004	CRP$_{Plasma}$	1.26 (1.01–1.57)	< 0.05			
Cohabiting (ref)			Cohabiting (ref)			Cohabiting (ref)		
Not cohabiting	0.40 (0.23–0.69)	**= 0.001**	not cohabiting	0.28 (0.12–0.63)	= 0.002	not cohabiting	0.24 (0.11–0.53)	**< 0.001**
Menopause Pre- (ref)			Menopause Pre- (ref)			Menopause Pre- (ref)		
Peri-	2.06 (1.05–4.06)	< 0.05	Peri-	2.37 (0.92–6.10)	ns	Peri-	3.03 (1.27–7.21)	< 0.05
Post-	2.12 (1.16–3.88)	< 0.05	Post-	2.60 (1.05–6.42)	< 0.05	Post-	2.02 (0.78–5.22)	ns

Variables entered into the logistic models: ethnicity, SES, education, cohabitation status, parity, smoking, body mass index, and menopausal status. Significance set to $p < = 0.001$

and 0.002, respectively – slightly above the conservative Bonferroni correction of $p \leq 0.001$. EBV-Ab and CRP_{Plasma} levels were not significantly associated with any of the symptoms.

Along with the PSS score, not cohabiting with a husband or partner significantly decreased report of the loss of interest in sex and the likelihood of night sweats. Along with the PSS score, number of children was positively associated with the risk of tiredness and nervousness, although not at the level of $p \leq 0.001$. Overall, the PSS score was the variable most likely to be associated with symptom frequencies.

When the logistic regressions were carried out separately by ethnicity, for Maya, the PSS score was significantly associated with tiredness, feeling nervous/tense, difficulty concentrating, depressed mood, and night sweats ($p \leq 0.001$); for non-Maya, the PSS score was significantly associated with reported tiredness, depressed mood, and sleep difficulties (not shown). CRP_{Plasma} levels and EBV-Ab values were not significantly associated with any symptom reports for Maya or non-Maya when ethnic groups were examined separately.

As shown in Table 4, the PSS score was significantly associated with the intensity (*nada = 0 to muchisimo = 3*) of ten of the 12 reported symptoms, including hot flashes and night sweats ($p \leq 0.001$). CRP_{Plasma} levels and EBV-Ab values were not significantly associated with the intensity of any symptom reports. When regressions were carried out separately by ethnicity, among Maya participants, the PSS score was significantly associated with the intensity of feeling tired, muscle/joint pain, feeling nervous/tense, difficulty concentrating, depressed mood, difficulty sleeping, and night sweats ($p \leq 0.001$); for non-Maya, the PSS score was significantly associated with the intensity of the same symptoms except for night sweats. Among the Maya, the association between the PSS score and hot flashes approached significance ($p = 0.002$). CRP_{Plasma} levels were not associated with symptoms among the Maya or non-Maya. EBV-Ab values were not significantly associated with any reported symptom intensity among the Maya or non-Maya.

Along with the PSS score, level of education was negatively associated with the intensity of muscle and joint pain. Cohabiting with a husband or partner was positively associated with the intensity of the loss of interest in sex. Progression through menopause was associated with the increased intensity of night sweats.

Discussion

In this urban population of women aged 40 to 60 from Campeche, Mexico, hot flashes and night sweats were not the most commonly reported symptoms. This finding is consistent with other studies that have found aches and stiffness [32, 60, 65], lack of energy [59], and tiredness or fatigue [61, 66] to be more common than hot flashes.

Correlations between self-report measures and biological markers of stress tend to be small or moderate [38]. In the case of this Campeche sample, there were no significant relationships between self-reports of stress (PSS score) and the potentially stress-sensitive biological measures (EBV-Ab and CRP levels), although the two measures of immune function were positively and significantly correlated. None of the measures used in this study were solely measuring stress; there are many factors that can influence immune system activity, and the PSS measures perceptions of stress which can be quite variable in different individuals [38]. It may be that biological measures were elevated in relation to immunological stress, but that immunological activity did not correlate with the impact of stress on the participants within the context of their lives. It may be that these particular biomarkers were not sensitive enough, or that the biomarkers could not effectively measure stress as perceived by the person.

Self-reported PSS was found to be significantly associated with nine of the most common symptoms in bivariate analyses, and with seven symptoms after controlling for potential covariates, whereas neither CRP nor EBV-Ab were associated with symptoms. PSS scores were also associated with the intensity of ten reported symptoms, including hot flashes and night sweats. No other variable in the logistic or linear models was associated with so many midlife symptoms. Our findings are similar to the relationship reported by SWAN researchers who found that the PSS score was significantly associated with vasomotor symptoms [15].

When logistic regressions were carried out separately by ethnicity, the PSS score was significantly associated with five of the reported symptoms among Maya women, including night sweats ($n = 144$). However, among non-Maya women ($n = 121$) the PSS score was significantly associated with only three of the symptoms. These ethnic differences may reflect cultural differences in either the experience or reporting of vasomotor and other symptoms [38, 67]. For Maya women, symptoms may be a means of expressing feelings of stress [11], more so than for non-Maya women.

In results reported here, Maya and non-Maya women did not differ in mean PSS scores; however, Maya women with higher PSS scores were more likely to report a higher intensity of hot flashes ($p = 0.002$) and the presence of and a higher intensity of night sweats ($p \leq 0.001$). It is of interest to note that earlier literature found an absence of hot flash report among Maya women in the Yucatán peninsula [42, 43, 68]. In contrast, the study presented here did not find an ethnic

Table 4 Linear regression analyses of symptom reports

With PSS scores				With CRP$_{Plasma}$				With EBV-Ab			
Variable	Beta	t	Signif.	Variable	Beta	t	Signif.	Variable	Beta	t	Signif.
Tiredness											
PSS Score	0.39	6.8	**<0.001**	CRP$_{Plasma}$	0.19	2.3	<0.05	Education	−0.20	−2.3	<0.05
Education	−.11	2.0	<0.05								
Muscle and Joint Pain											
PSS Score	0.31	5.4	**<0.001**	Education	−0.27	−3.2	<0.01	Education	−0.26	−2.3	<0.01
Education	−0.22	−3.8	**<0.001**								
Nervous or Tense											
PSS Score	0.38	6.8	**<0.001**	CRP$_{Plasma}$	0.17	2.1	<0.05	EBV-Ab	0.18	2.1	<0.05
Cohabiting	0.10	1.7	<0.1	Cohabiting	0.15	1.8	<0.1	Smoker	0.19	2.3	<0.05
Smoker	0.16	2.9	<0.01	Smoker	0.20	2.4	<0.05				
Difficulty Concentrating											
PSS Score	0.33	5.6	**<0.001**	BMI	0.23	2.7	<0.01	[No variables left in model]			
Parity	0.12	2.1	<0.05	Parity	0.14	1.7	<0.1				
Depressed mood											
PSS Score	0.51	9.7	**<0.001**	CRP$_{Plasma}$	0.19	2.3	<0.05	Education	−0.18	−2.1	<0.05
Parity	0.13	2.5	<0.05	Education	−0.18	−2.2	<0.05				
				Parity	0.18	2.1	<0.05				
Difficulty sleeping											
PSS Score	0.39	6.9	**<0.001**	Menopause status	0.27	3.3	**<0.001**	Education	−0.22	−2.6	<0.05
Menopause status	0.13	2.2	<0.05	Education	−0.21	−2.6	<0.05				
Head aches											
PSS Score	0.26	4.5	**<0.001**	Ethnicity	−0.19	−2.2	<0.05	[No variables left in model]			
Cohabiting	0.12	2.0	<0.05	Smoker	−0.16	−1.8	<0.1				
Smoker	−0.12	−2.0	<0.1								
Feeling of Ants Crawling on the Skin											
PSS Score	0.24	3.9	**<0.001**	CRP$_{Plasma}$	0.21	2.4	<0.05	Education	−0.30	−3.7	**<0.001**
SES	−0.10	−1.7	<0.1	BMI	−0.18	−2.0	<0.05				
Menopause status	0.10	1.7	<0.1								

Table 4 Linear regression analyses of symptom reports (Continued)

	With PSS scores				With CRP$_{Plasma}$				With EBV-Ab			
	Variable	Beta	t	Signif.	Variable	Beta	t	Signif.	Variable	Beta	t	Signif.
Stress Incontinence												
	PSS Score	0.15	2.4	< 0.05	Cohabiting	0.16	1.9	< 0.1	BMI	0.24	2.9	< 0.01
	BMI	0.13	2.1	< 0.05					Cohabiting	0.18	2.1	< 0.05
	Cohabiting	0.11	1.8	< 0.1					Menopause status	−0.14	−1.7	< 0.1
Loss of interest in sex												
	PSS Score	0.18	2.9	< 0.01	Cohabiting	0.31	3.7	**< 0.001**	Cohabiting	0.22	2.6	< 0.05
	Education	−0.11	−1.8	< 0.1					SES	−0.18	−2.1	< 0.05
	Cohabiting	0.27	4.6	**< 0.001**								
	Menopause status	0.14	2.4	< 0.05								
	Ethnicity	0.10	1.7	< 0.1								
Hot flashes												
	PSS Score	0.23	3.8	**< 0.001**	[No variables left in model]				SES	−0.19	−2.3	< 0.05
	Menopause status	0.13	2.2	< 0.05					BMI	0.17	2.0	< 0.05
	BMI	0.15	2.6	< 0.01					Menopause status	0.15	1.8	< 0.1
Night sweats												
	PSS Score	0.24	4.2	**< 0.001**	CRP$_{Plasma}$	0.19	2.4	< 0.05	Menopause status	0.23	2.8	< 0.01
	Menopause status	0.22	3.7	**< 0.001**	Menopause status	0.30	3.7	**< 0.001**	Education	−0.21	−2.7	< 0.01
	Education	0.15	2.5	< 0.05	Education	−0.22	−2.7	< 0.01	Cohabiting	0.28	3.4	**< 0.001**
	Cohabiting	0.12	2.1	< 0.05	Cohabiting	0.22	2.7	< 0.01				

Variables entered into the linear models: ethnicity, SES, education, cohabitation status, parity, smoking, body mass index, and menopausal status. Significance set to $p <= 0.001$

difference in hot flash report, but instead found a greater likelihood of vasomotor symptoms among the Maya in relation to higher perceived levels of stress. This bears further investigation.

This study provides only modest support for the idea that immune biomarkers applied as stress-sensitive measures are associated with the frequency of symptoms at midlife. The relationship between CRP_{Plasma} levels and the occurrence of depressed mood did not reach significance, although there was a suggestion of a relationship in bivariate and linear regression analyses ($p < 0.05$). The association between CRP levels and depressed mood has been previously noted [69].

In agreement with our findings, one other previous study did not find a relationship between CRP and hot flashes [70]. In SWAN, women who had a higher frequency of hot flashes had significantly higher levels of CRP and other biological markers of inflammation, but there was no significant association between night sweat frequency and inflammatory markers [71].

EBV-Ab values were not significantly associated with hot flashes or night sweats in terms of yes/no frequency or intensity of report. To our knowledge, this is the first study to examine symptoms at midlife in relation to levels of EBV-Ab. Although CRP_{Plasma} and EBV-Ab have been used as stress-sensitive biological measures in the study of stress in the past [47, 50, 51], in this study neither CRP_{Plasma} nor EBV-Ab levels were associated with symptoms at midlife to the same extent as the self-reported stress measure, PSS.

Self-reports of stress have been associated with the frequency of hot flashes, both with short-term reports such as hassles scales [72] and reports of chronic stress [73]. However, there may well be differences in the association between stress and hot flashes depending upon the manner in which hot flashes are measured. For example, in a prospective study of mood and hot flashes, negative mood was associated with fewer objectively measured hot flashes but was associated with more frequent self-reported hot flashes [19]. In this study, PSS scores were significantly associated with the intensity of vasomotor symptoms when correction for multiple testing was applied, and PSS scores tended to be associated with the likelihood of vasomotor symptoms ($p = 0.007$ and $p = 0.004$ for hot flashes and night sweats), unlike the physiological measures of stress.

In general, women who reported high levels of perceived stress were also more likely to report a broad array of symptoms. Some of these symptoms are specific to menopause, such as night sweats, but many are more general concerns of men and women of a broad age range. These symptoms are associated with multiple factors. For example, not cohabiting with a husband or partner significantly decreased report of the loss of interest in sex.

Self-reported stress is clearly implicated as associated with symptoms, especially among the Maya in this sample. It is, however, unclear to what degree stress may be a causal factor in inducing these symptoms, or if instead the symptoms are a causal factor in the stress levels. There could be a reciprocal effect, with stress inducing symptoms that in turn lead to greater perceptions of stress. Few women reported either no symptoms (1.4%) or all 12 symptoms (5.4%), suggesting that there is not a simple relation between being under stress and having all symptoms; different women suffer from different symptoms, and these are likely to differ in the importance of stress levels for their occurrence. It is unclear why the stronger association between perceived stress and vasomotor symptoms is present among Maya but not non-Maya participants. The women may differ in beliefs about how stress should be reported, since ethnic differences in self-reports of stress are found in other populations [38].

This study has limitations. While the sample is likely to broadly represent the population of women at midlife in Campeche due to the multiple strategies used for contacting potential participants, it is not a random sample. The sample size is small, with 305 women providing PSS scores, and only 162 and 157 women with EBV-Ab and CRP measures, respectively. We did not find the expected relationship between the PSS and the two biomarkers. Also, this paper has relied upon self-reports of hot flashes and night sweats as well as other symptoms. As noted, a previous study has shown a difference in the relation between stress and either subjectively reported or objectively measured hot flashes [19]. Finally, this study is cross-sectional and, therefore, cannot derive causation from associations between the variables used in analyses.

Conclusions

In support of our primary hypothesis, perceived stress was associated with the intensity of hot flashes and night sweats. In logistic and linear regressions, perceived stress was the variable most consistently associated with each of the 12 symptoms studied. This was not true for the potentially stress-sensitive biological measures of EBV-Ab or CRP_{Plasma}. There were ethnic differences in the associations between measures of stress and symptom frequency and intensity. Maya women demonstrated a relationship between perceived stress and five symptoms, including night sweats, while the non-Maya demonstrated no association between between perceived stress and vasomotor symptoms, suggesting that either symptoms or stress were experienced and/or reported in culture-specific ways.

Acknowledgements
We are indebted to the women who participated and authorities of the city of Campeche. Special thanks to Drs. Alfonso Cobos Toledo, Secretario de Salud; Carlos Juárez López, Secretario Técnico del Comité de Ética en Investigación; and Liliana Montejo León, Directora Operativa del Comité de Ética de Investigación. For assistance with fieldwork, we thank Isai Delgado, Gía del Pino, Guadalupe Islas Monter, Lizbeth de las Mercedes Rodríguez, Giselle O'Connor, Elena Pasqual, and Alba Valdéz Tah. In addition, we thank Drs. Jorge Jiménez Madrigal, Diana Edith Arceo Sánchez, Miguel Briceño Dzib, Enrique Fernando Reyes Pascual; Lic. Francisco Góngora Ramírez, and especially Lic. Marlene Narváez Rosado. Authorities who facilitated the interviews by giving us the needed space include Dra. Landy del Socorro Ortíz Aldana, Ing. Jorge Marín Farías Maldonado, M. en C. Lirio Suárez Améndola, Antrop. Marco Carvajal, Dra. Lizbeth Rodríguez, Lic. Lidia Elena Berrón Osorio, Lic. Ana Verónica Lemus Castillo, Lic. José Dolores Uribe Castro, Ing. Leidy Elena Legorreta Barrancos, Ing. Rosario Suárez Améndola, Ing. José Luis Herrera Martínez, Lic. Cecilia Zúñiga Rosel, Lic. Lorenzo Alberto Can Sánchez, Lic. Yolanda Isabel Segovia Cuevas, Ing. José Raúl Ochoa Aguedo, Ing. Agustín Balvanera Aguilar, Lic. Román Acosta Estrella, Lic. Ricardo Ocampo Fernández, Lic. Margarita Alfaro Waring. Finally, we thank Prof. Martha del Carmen Preciat Castilla and Lic. Rosa Angélica Prevé Quintero for their enthusiastic support of this study.

Funding
Supported by NSF BCS-1156368.

Authors' contributions
LLS, LHG, and DB designed this study; data collection was carried out and supervised by LHG and DCC in collaboration with LLS and DB; DLK carried out laboratory assays; DB and LLS carried out all analyses; LLS and DB drafted the manuscript; all authors read and approved the final manuscript.

Competing interests
The authors declare that they have no competing interests.

Author details
[1]Department of Anthropology, Machmer Hall, 240 Hicks Way, UMass Amherst, Amherst, MA 01003-9278, USA. [2]Departamento de Sociedad y Cultura, El Colegio de la Frontera, ECOSUR, Campeche, Mexico. [3]Department of Pharmaceutical Science, University of Hawai'i at Hilo, Hilo, HI, USA. [4]Department of Anthropology, University of Hawai'i at Hilo, Hilo, HI, USA.

References
1. Freedman RR. Menopausal hot flashes: mechanisms, endocrinology, treatment. J Steroid Biochem Mol Biol. 2014;142:115–20.
2. World Health Organization. Research on the menopause in the 1990s, WHO technical report series, 866. Geneva: World Health Organization; 1996.
3. Kravitz HM, Ganz PA, Bromberger J, Powell LH, Sutton-Tyrrell K, Meyer PM. Sleep difficulty in women at midlife: a community survey of sleep and the menopausal transition. Menopause. 2003;10:19–28.
4. de Kruif M, Spijker AT, Molendijk ML. Depression during the perimenopause: a meta-analysis. J Affect Disord. 2016;206:174–80.
5. Ryan J, Burger H, Szoeke C, Lehert P, Ancelin M-L, Dennerstein L. A prospective study of the association between endogenous hormones and depressive symptoms in postmenopausal women. Menopause. 2009;16(3):509–17.
6. Ford K, Sowers M, Crutchfield M, Wilson A, Jannausch M. A longitudinal study of the predictors of prevalence and severity of symptoms commonly associated with menopause. Menopause. 2005;12(3):308–17.
7. Dennerstein L. Well-being, symptoms and the menopausal transition. Maturitas. 1996;23:147–57.
8. Darling CA, Coccia C, Senatore N. Women in midlife: stress, health and life satisfaction. Stress Health. 2012;28:31–40.
9. Staner L. Sleep and anxiety disorders. Dialogues Clin Neurosci. 2003;5(3):249–58.
10. Hammen C. Stress and depression. Annu Rev Clin Psychol. 2005;1:293–319.
11. Sievert LL, Obermeyer CM. Symptom clusters at midlife: a four-country comparison of checklist and qualitative responses. Menopause. 2012;19(2):133–44.
12. Sievert LL, Obermeyer CM, Saliba M. Symptom groupings at midlife: cross-cultural variation and association with job, home, and life change. Menopause. 2007;14(4):798–807.
13. Avis NE, Crawford SL, Greendale G, Bromberger JT, Everson-Rose SA, Gold EB, Hess R, Joffe H, Kravitz HM, Tepper PG, Thurston RC, Study of Women's Health Across the Nation. Duration of menopausal vasomotor symptoms over the menopause transition. JAMA Intern Med. 2015;175(4):531–9.
14. Freeman EW, Sammel MD, Lin H, Liu Z, Gracia CR. Duration of menopausal hot flushes and associated risk factors. Obstet Gynecol. 2011;117(5):1095–104.
15. Gold EB, Block G, Crawford S, Lachance L, FitzGerald G, Miracle H, Sherman S. Lifestyle and demographic factors in relation to vasomotor symptoms: baseline results from the study of Women's Health Across the Nation. Am J Epidemiol. 2004;159(12):1189–99.
16. Kuh DL, Wadsworth M, Hardy R. Women's health in midlife: the influence of the menopause, social factors and health in earlier life. Br J Obstet Gynaecol. 1997;104(8):923–33.
17. Thurston RC, Bromberger J, Chang Y, Goldbacher E, Brown C, Cyranowski JM, Matthews KA. Childhood abuse or neglect is associated with increased vasomotor symptom reporting among midlife women. Menopause. 2008;15:16–22.
18. Binfa L, Castelo-Branco C, Blümel JE, Cancelo MJ, Bonilla H, Muñoz I, Vergara V, Izaguirre H, Sarrá S, Ríos RV. Influence of psycho-social factors on climacteric symptoms. Maturitas. 2004;48(4):425–31.
19. Thurston RC, Blumenthal JA, Babyak MA, Sherwood A. Emotional antecedents of hot flashes during daily life. Psychosom Med. 2005;67(1):137–46.
20. Swartzman LC, Edelberg R, Kemmann E. Impact of stress on objectively recorded menopausal hot flushes and on flush report bias. Health Psychol. 1990;9:529–45.
21. Pollard TM, Ice GH. Measuring hormonal variation in the hypothalamic pituitary adrenal (HPA) axis: cortisol. In: Ice GH, James GD, editors. Measuring stress in humans: a practical guide for the field. Cambridge: Cambridge University Press; 2007. p. 122–57.
22. Cignarelli M, Cicinelli E, Corso M, et al. Biophysical and endocrinemetabolic changes during menopausal hot flashes: increase in plasma free fatty acid and norepinephrine levels. Gynecol Obstet Investig. 1989;27:34–7.
23. Meldrum DR, Defazio JD, Erlik Y, et al. Pituitary hormones during the menopausal hot flash. Obstet Gynecol. 1984;64:752–6.
24. Woods NF, Carr MC, Tao EY, Taylor HJ, Mitchell ES. Increased urinary cortisol levels during the menopausal transition. Menopause. 2006;13(2):212–21.
25. Cagnacci A, Cannoletta M, Caretto S, Zanin R, Xholli A, Volpe A. Increased cortisol level: a possible link between climacteric symptoms and cardiovascular risk factors. Menopause. 2011;18(3):273–8.
26. Reed SD, Newton KM, Larson JC, Booth-LaForce C, Woods NF, Landis CA, Tolentino E, Carpenter JS, Freeman EW, Joffe H, Anawalt BD, Guthrie KA. Daily salivary cortisol patterns in midlife women with hot flashes. Clin Endocrinol. 2016;84(5):672–9.
27. Rubin LH, Drogos LL, Kapella MC, Geller SE, Maki P. Cortisol awakening response differs for midlife women with objective vasomotor symptoms versus without vasomotor symptoms. Menopause. 2014;21(12):1362. [abstract]
28. Gerber LM, Sievert LL, Schwartz JE. Hot flashes and midlife symptoms in relation to levels of salivary cortisol. Maturitas. 2017;96:26–32.

29. Greenberg GP, Sievert LL. Is there a relationship between hot flashes, night sweats, and the cortisol awakening response? Am J Hum Biol. 2018;30(2): e23110. [abstract]

30. Gibson CJ, Thurston RC, Matthews KA. Cortisol dysregulation is associated with daily diary-reported hot flashes among midlife women. Clin Endocrinol. 2016;85(4):645–51.

31. Avis NE, Stellato R, Crawford S, et al. Is there a menopausal syndrome? Menopausal status and symptoms across racial/ethnic groups. Soc Sci Med. 2001;52:345–56.

32. Lerner-Geva L, Boyko V, Blumstein T, Benyamini Y. The impact of education, cultural background, and lifestyle on symptoms of the menopausal transition: the Women's Health at Midlife Study. J Women's Health (Larchmt). 2010;19:975–85.

33. Sievert LL, Morrison L, Brown DE, Reza AM. Vasomotor symptoms among Japanese-American and European-American women living in Hilo, Hawaii. Menopause. 2007;14:261–9.

34. Brown DE. Physiological stress and culture change in a group of Filipino-Americans: a preliminary investigation. Ann Hum Biol. 1982;9(6):553–63.

35. Brown DE, James GD, Nordloh L. Comparison of factors affecting daily variation of blood pressure in Filipino-American and Caucasian nurses in Hawaii. Am J Phys Anthropol. 1998;106(3):373–83.

36. Brown DE, Sievert LL, Morrison LA, Rahberg N, The RAM. Relation between hot flashes and ambulatory blood pressure: the Hilo Women's health study. Psychosom Med. 2011;73:166–72.

37. Dressler WW, Oths KS, Gravlee CC. Race and ethnicity in public health research: models to explain health disparities. Annu Rev Anthropol. 2005;34:231–52.

38. Brown DE. Stress biomarkers as an objective window on experience. In: Sievert LL, Brown DE, editors. Biological measures of human experience across the lifespan: making visible the invisible. New York: Springer; 2016. p. 117–41.

39. Beyene Y, Martin MC. Menopausal experiences and bone density of Mayan women in Yucatan, Mexico. Am J Hum Biol. 2001;13:505–11.

40. Canto-de-Cetina TE, Canto-Cetina P, Polanco-Reyes L. Encuesta de sintomas del climaterio en areas semirurales de Yucatan. Revista de Investigacion Clinica. 1998;50:133–5.

41. Gold EB, Crawford SL, Avis NE, Crandall CJ, Matthews KA, Waetjen LE, Lee JS, Thurston R, Vuga M, Harlow SD. Factors related to age at natural menopause: longitudinal analyses from SWAN. Am J Epidemiol. 2013;178:70–83.

42. Beyene Y. Cultural significance and physiological manifestations of menopause: a biocultural analysis. Cult Med Psych. 1986;10:47–71.

43. Beyene Y. From menarche to menopause: reproductive histories of peasant women in two cultures. Albany: State University of New York Press; 1989.

44. Malacara JM, Canto-de-Cetina T, Bassol S, Gonzalez N, Cacique L, Vera-Ramirez ML, Nava LE. Symptoms at pre- and postmenopause in rural and urban women from three states of Mexico. Maturitas. 2002;43:11–9.

45. Eick G, Urlacher SS, McDade TW, Kowal P, Snodgrass JJ. Validation of an optimized ELISA for quantitative assessment of Epstien-Barr virus antibodies from dried blood spots. Biodemography Soc Biol. 2016;62(2):222–33.

46. McDade TW, Stallings JF, Angold A, Costello EJ, Burleson M, Cacioppo JT, Glaser R, Worthman CM. Epstein-Barr virus antibodies in whole blood spots: a minimally invasive method for assessing an aspect of cell-mediated immunity. Psychosom Med. 2000;62(4):560–7.

47. McDade TW. Measuring immune function: markers of cell-mediated immunity an inflammation in dried blood spots. In: Ice GH, James GD, editors. Measuring stress in humans: a practical guide for the field. Cambridge: Cambridge University Press; 2007. p. 181–207.

48. Wium-Andersen MK, Orsted DD, Nielsen SF, Nordestgaard BG. Elevated C-reactive protein levels, psychological distress, and depression in 73,131 individuals. JAMA Psychiatry. 2013;70(2):176–84.

49. Black PH, Garbutt LD. Stress, inflammation and cardiovascular disease. J Psychosom Res. 2002;52:1–23.

50. Low CA, Matthews KA, Hall M. Elevated CRP in adolescents: roles of stress and coping. Psychosom Med. 2013;75(5):449–52.

51. Steptoe A, Hamer M, Chida Y. The effects of acute psychological stress on circulating inflammatory factors in humans: a review and meta-analysis. Brain Behav Immun. 2007;21:901–12.

52. McDade TW. Status incongruity in Samoan youth: a biocultural analysis of culture change, stress, and immune function. Med Anthropol Q. 2002;16(2):123–50.

53. INEGI. Anuario estadístico y geográfico de Campeche, 2014. Instituto Nacional de Estadística y Geografía. Aguascalientes: INEGI; 2014. www.inegi.org.mx

54. Huicochea Gómez L, Sievert LL, Cahuich Campos D, Brown DE. An investigation of life circumstances associated with the experience of hot flashes in Campeche, Mexico. Menopause. 2017;24(1):52–63.

55. Harlow SD, Gass M, Hall JE, Lobo R, Maki P, Rebar RW, Sherman S, Sluss PM, de Villiers TJ, STRAW+ 10 Collaborative Group. Executive summary of the Stages of Reproductive Aging Workshop+ 10: addressing the unfinished agenda of staging reproductive aging. Menopause. 2012;19(4):387–95.

56. González Ramírez MT, Landero Hernández R. Factor structure of the perceived stress scale (PSS) in a sample from Mexico. Spanish J Psychol. 2007;10:199–206.

57. Cohen S, Kamarck T, Mermelstein R. A global measure of perceived stress. J Health Soc Behav. 1983;24:386–96.

58. Cohen S, Williamson G. Perceived stress in a probability sample of the United States. In: Spacapan S, Oskamp S, editors. Social psychology of health. Newbury Park: Sage; 1988. p. 31–67.

59. Avis NE, Kaufert PA, Lock M, McKinlay SM, Vass K. The evolution of menopausal symptoms. Bailliere's Clin Endocrinol Metab. 1993;7:17–32.

60. Dennerstein L, Smith AMA, Morse C, Burger H, Green A, Hopper J, Ryan M. Menopausal symptoms in Australian women. Med J Aust. 1993;159:232–6.

61. Obermeyer CM, Reher D, Saliba M. Symptoms, menopause status, and country differences: a comparative analysis from DAMES. Menopause. 2007;14:788–97.

62. Sievert LL, Espinosa-Hernandez G. Attitudes toward menopause in relation to symptom experience in Puebla, Mexico. Women Health. 2003;38(2):93–106.

63. McDade TW, Burhop J, Dohnal J. High-sensitivity enzyme immunoassay for C-reactive protein in dried blood spots. Clin Chem. 2004;50(3):652–4.

64. Pearson TA, Mensah GA, Alexander RW, Anderson JL, Cannon RO 3rd, Criqui M, Fadl YY, Fortmann SP, Hong Y, Myers GL, Rifai N, Smith SC Jr, Taubert K, Tracy RP, Vinicor F. Markers of inflammation and cardiovascular disease: application to clinical and public health practice: a statement for healthcare professionals from the Centers for Disease Control and Prevention and the American Heart Association. Circulation. 2003;107(3):499–511.

65. Melby MK. Factor analysis of climacteric symptoms in Japan. Maturitas. 2005;52:205–22.

66. Hemminki E, Topo P, Kangas I. Experience and opinions of climacterium by Finnish women. Eur J Obstet Gynecol. 1995;62:81–7.

67. Brown DE. General stress in anthropological fieldwork. Am Anthropol. 1981;83(1):74–92.

68. Martin MC, Block JE, Sanchez SD, Arnaud CD, Beyene Y. Menopause without symptoms: the endocrinology of menopause among rural Mayan Indians. Am J Obstet Gynecol. 1993;168:1839–45.

69. Valkanova V, Ebmeier KP, Allan CL. CRP, IL-6 and depression: a systematic review and meta-analysis of longitudinal studies. J Affect Disord. 2013;150(3):736–44.

70. Bechlioulis A, Naka KK, Kalantaridou SN, Kaponis A, Papanikolaou O, Vezyraki P, Kolettis TM, Vlahos AP, Gartzonika K, Mavridis A, Michalis LK. Increased vascular inflammation in early menopausal women is associated with hot flush severity. J Clin Endocrinol Metab. 2012;97(5):E760–4.

71. Thurston RC, El Khoudary SR, Sutton-Tyrrell K, Crandall CJ, Gold E, Sternfeld B, Selzer F, Matthews KA. Are vasomotor symptoms associated with alterations in hemostatic and inflammatory markers? Findings from the study of Women's Health Across the Nation. Menopause. 2011;18(10):1044–51.

72. Gannon L, Hansel S, Goodwin J. Correlates of menopausal hot flashes. J Behav Med. 1987;10(3):277–85.

73. Gannon L, Luchetta T, Pardie L. Perimenstrual symptoms: relationships with chronic stress and selected lifestyle variables. J Behav Med. 1989;15(4):149–59.

Changes in androstenedione, dehydroepiandrosterone, testosterone, estradiol, and estrone over the menopausal transition

Catherine Kim[1]* [iD], Siobàn D. Harlow[2], Huiyong Zheng[2], Daniel S. McConnell[2] and John F. Randolph Jr.[3]

Abstract

Background: Previous reports have noted that dehydroepiandrosterone-sulfate (DHEAS) increases prior to the final menstrual period (FMP) and remains stable beyond the FMP. How DHEAS concentrations correspond with other sex hormones across the menopausal transition (MT) including androstenedione (A4), testosterone (T), estrone (E1), and estradiol (E2) is not known. Our objective was to examine how DHEAS, A4, T, E1, and E2 changed across the MT by White vs. African-American (AA) race/ethnicity.

Methods: We conducted a longitudinal observational analysis of a subgroup of women from the Study of Women's Health Across the Nation observed over 4 visits prior to and 4 visits after the FMP ($n = 110$ women over 9 years for 990 observations). The main outcome measures were DHEAS, A4, T, E1, and E2.

Results: Compared to the decline in E2 concentrations, androgen concentrations declined minimally over the MT. T (β 9.180, $p < 0.0001$) and E1 (β 11.365, $p < 0.0001$) were higher in Whites than in AAs, while elevations in DHEAS (β 28.80, $p = 0.061$) and A4 (β 0.2556, $p = 0.052$) were borderline. Log-transformed E2 was similar between Whites and AAs (β 0.0764, $p = 0.272$). Body mass index (BMI) was not significantly associated with concentrations of androgens or E1 over time.

Conclusion: This report suggests that the declines in E2 during the 4 years before and after the FMP are accompanied by minimal changes in DHEAS, A4, T, and E1. There are modest differences between Whites and AAs and minimal differences by BMI.

Keywords: Dehydroepiandrosterone-sulfate, Androstenedione, Testosterone, Estrone, Menopause

Background

The menopausal transition (MT) represents a marked shift in women's sex steroid profile, of which changes in estradiol (E2) are the best studied [1]. On average, women's E2 concentrations begin to change more rapidly about 2 years prior to the final menstrual period (FMP) and stabilize several years after the FMP [2]. The rapidity of decline and average E2 levels may be predicted by race/ethnicity and body mass index (BMI) at the beginning of the transition [3, 4]. The most pronounced differences occur between African-American (AA) and White women, the former group having more gradual changes than the latter group [4]. Presumably in part due to adipose tissue production of E2, women with higher BMI have more gradual changes than women with lower BMI [3, 4].

The adrenal gland is the primary source of dehydroepiandrosterone-sulfate (DHEAS) and androstenedione (A4) and also contributes to circulating testosterone (T) [5]. Aromatase catalyzes A4 and T into estrogens, i.e. A4 into estrone (E1) and T into estradiol (E2). Previous reports have suggested that, prior to the FMP, adrenal DHEAS production increases even as

* Correspondence: cathkim@umich.edu
[1]Departments of Medicine and Obstetrics & Gynecology, University of Michigan, 2800 Plymouth Road, Building 16, Room 430W, Ann Arbor, MI 48109, USA
Full list of author information is available at the end of the article

peripheral E2 decreases [6–10]. As adrenal sex hormones exist in equilibrium with ovarian sex hormones in the peripheral circulation, it is plausible that adrenal hormone metabolism also changes over the MT [11]. This is consistent with the hypothesis that increasing adrenal sex hormone production and aromatization may be concurrent with decreasing ovarian estrogen production [12]. It is also possible that DHEAS production may also eventually decline over time resulting lower peripheral A4 and E1 concentrations.

Few longitudinal studies examine changes in a comprehensive array of adrenal sex hormones across the MT. Since concentrations of circulating DHEAS increase in the 5th decade of life [6–10] and concentrations among women in their 8th decade of life are low [13], DHEAS must decline in the postmenopause. However, it is uncertain when in the postmenopause this might occur. In addition, few reports examine concentrations of A4 or E1 during the MT and whether ratios of A4:E1 change over the MT, consistent with changes in aromatase activity or consistent with increased A4 production and concomitant increases in aromatization. No reports examine whether E1 concentrations change across the MT. In addition, studies have not examined whether these patterns differ by BMI, as has been reported for E2, or between Whites and AAs.

Therefore, using data from the Study of Women's Health Across the Nation (SWAN), we characterized serum adrenal and ovarian sex steroid changes over the MT. We assessed concentrations of DHEAS, A4, T, E2, and E1 annually in the 4 years before and the 4 years after the FMP. We assessed whether concentrations changed in relation to the FMP during this time period and whether patterns differed between White and AA race/ethnicity, and BMI. We hypothesized that concentrations of DHEAS and A4 would increase slightly over the 4 years prior to and after the FMP, consistent with augmented adrenal androgen production. We hypothesized that AA women would be less likely to have adrenal sex hormone changes over the MT, as previous reports have suggested that AA women have less fluctuation in DHEAS concentrations than White women [4]. We also hypothesized that women with higher BMI would be more likely to have more gradual increases in DHEAS and A4 over the MT, since previous SWAN reports have suggested that women with higher BMI have more gradual declines in E2 than women with lower BMI [3].

Methods

The study protocol of SWAN has been described previously: briefly, eligibility criteria for the SWAN cohort study enrollment included the following: age 42–52 years,

no surgical removal of uterus and/or both ovaries; not currently using exogenous hormone medications that were known to affect ovarian function; at least one menstrual period as well as one of the following five other racial/ethnic groups. These groups included women who were White, AA, Chinese and Japanese, and Hispanic. A total of 3302 women were recruited. Institutional review boards approved the study protocol at each site; signed, written informed consent was obtained from all participants. The current study included a subsample of White and AA women who met inclusion criteria. We focused upon these 2 racial/ethnic groups as they had sufficient numbers of subjects with a documented final menstrual period (FMP) and complete hormone data for 4 years before and after the FMP, they were the largest number of participants in SWAN, the largest racial/ethnic differences in sex steroids have previously been observed between these 2 populations, and funds restricted examination of other racial/ethnic groups [3].

Other inclusion criteria included having a BMI of 22–30 kg/m^2, a natural FMP i.e. no history of hysterectomy or oophorectomy, no exogenous hormone therapy use, and at least 9 sequential annual samples spanning 4 years before and 4 years after the FMP, for a total of 110 women with 990 observations. Compared to White participants in SWAN generally, White women in the current report were similarly aged at baseline, were more likely to report excellent or very good self-reported health, and had similar smoking status. Compared to AA participants who did not meet inclusion criteria, AA women in the current report had similar age, self-rated health, and smoking status. Due to the inclusion criteria designed to limit outliers of BMI, both White and AA women in the current report had lower BMI than women who did not meet inclusion criteria.

Annual fasting blood samples were collected. Two attempts were made to collect a follicular phase sample. When follicular phase samples were not available or when a woman stopped menstruating, a random fasting sample was collected within 90 days of the baseline recruitment date. All serum hormones were measured at the CLASS/RSP Central Laboratory at the University of Michigan (Ann Arbor, MI). A4 was measured using a commercially available enzyme-linked immunosorbent assay (ELISA) from Diagnostic Systems Laboratories (DSL). The assay measures analyte concentrations from 0.1 to 10 ng/mL with a minimum detectable concentration of 0.1 ng/mL, and a sensitivity of 0.03 ng/mL. The inter-assay coefficient of variation (CV) is 3.9% at 0.98 ng/mL and 3.0% at 6.1 ng/mL. The intra-assay CV is 2.1% at 0.98 ng/mL, 1.3% at 6.1 ng/mL. DHEAS was measured using an automated, ACS:180-based chemiluminescent assay developed in the CLASS laboratory and based upon the Bayer Diagnostics ACS:180. The detection level of this assay is approximately 1.9 μg/dL. The intra-assay CV is 8.02% (n = 261) and inter-assay CV is 11.34% (53.32 μg/dL, n = 37) and 9.74% (250.21 μg/dL, n = 37). The CLASS laboratory modified the ACS:180 total testosterone chemiluminescent assay to measure with greater precision samples in the low ranges found in women in the peri- and postmenopause. To accomplish this, sample volume was increased while evaluating the consequences of this change on volumes of subsequent reagents. The limit of detection of this assay is <5.15 ng/dL. The limit of quantification (lowest reported value) is set at the lowest standard, 5.15 ng/dL. The intra-assay CV is 11.78% (24.4 ng/dL, n = 30), 4.6% (191.2 ng/dL, n = 30) and 9.1% (414.2 ng/dL, n = 30). The inter-assay CVs are 11.34% (53.3 ng/dL, n = 37) and 9.7% (250.2 ng/dL, n = 37). E1 was measured using a commercially available ELISA from DSL. This method features a wide dynamic standard range of 0.05 to 90 ng/mL, and a minimum detectable concentration of 0.01 ng/mL. Inter-assay CVs were 12.7% at 1.2 ng/mL and 10.8% at 9.2 ng/mL, and intra-assay CVs were 6.7% at 1.2 ng/mL and 2.9% at 9.2 ng/mL. E2 concentrations were measured using the Estradiol-6 III immunoassay performed on the ADVIA Centaur instrument (Siemens HealthCare Diagnostics). Inter-assay CVs are 11.0% (102.9 pg/mL) and 7.0% (225.9 pg/mL) and 3.8% (615.9 pg/mL). Intra-assay CVs are 3.9% (102.9 pg/mL), 5.0% (225.9 pg/mL) and 1.4% (615.9 pg/mL). Follicle stimulating hormone (FSH) was measured with a two-site chemiluminescence (sandwich) immunoassay with a minimum detectable concentration of 0.3 mIU/mL. Inter- and intra-assay CVs are 8.1% and 3.5%, respectively.

Statistical analyses

For the purposes of this analysis, BMI was analyzed in tertiles (< 25 kg/m², 25–26.9 kg/m², >27 kg/m²) and by White vs. AA race/ethnicity. Distributions of DHEAS, A4, T, E2, and E1 were examined at each year in relation to time before and after the FMP. Population hormone trajectories in relation to FMP and covariates were analyzed using linear mixed models. Piecewise linear mixed models were applied to test the rate of changes at each stage, i.e., pre-menopause (2 years before FMP), transition stage (+/- 2 years around FMP), and post-menopause (2 years after FMP). [2, 14, 15] For presentation in Figs. 1 and 2, data were stratified by race/ethnicity and BMI (normal vs. overweight and by tertile of BMI). In order to determine whether race/ethnicity or BMI was associated with serum hormone concentrations, we created semiparametric stochastic mixed models that accounted for the multiple repeated measures in women and adjusted for the time from the FMP. [16] Hormone distributions were also examined after log-transformation; log transformation did not alter the pattern of the results with the exception of E2, so non-transformed values are presented for other sex

hormones. Racial/ethnic differences in SHBG were also examined, but differences were minimal (results not shown). All analyses were performed with SAS Windows 9.2 (SAS Institute, Cary NC).

Results

Thirty-four AA and 76 White women were included. Participant characteristics are shown in Table 1. Forty-seven (42%) of women had BMIs of 22–24.9 kg/m² vs. 30 (27%) of women who had BMIs 25.0–26.9 kg/m² vs. 33 (30%) who had BMIs 27.0–30.0 kg/m². Women had lower median FSH concentrations at 4 years prior to their FMP (21.4 IU/L) compared to 4 years after their FMP (125.7 IU/L), consistent with the transition from premenopause to postmenopause.

Figure 1 displays the average concentrations of sex hormones across the FMP for White and AA women for each year of the MT. Declines in log E2 concentrations were the most marked out of all of the sex hormone changes in both Whites and AAs, but E2 declines were not accompanied by increases in E1 concentrations. The ratio of E1:A4 remained fairly constant across the MT. Table 2 shows median values for sex hormones at 4 years prior the FMP, the year of the FMP, and 4 years after the FMP for Whites and AAs, and Table 3 shows the association between race/ethnicity and hormone concentration after adjustment for FMP and repeated measures within women. Hormone concentrations were generally higher in Whites than AAs, although only T and E1 met criteria for significance and log E2 concentrations were similar between Whites and AAs.

Figure 2 shows the average concentration trajectories of sex hormones across the MT for women by BMI tertile. Table 2 shows median values for sex hormones at 4 years prior the FMP, the year of the FMP, and 4 years after the FMP by BMI tertile. BMI tertile was not associated with differences in DHEAS, A4, or E1 at different times in relation to the FMP. Table 4 shows the association between BMI as a continuous variable and hormone concentration after adjustment for FMP and repeated measures within women. Although BMI as a continuous variable was associated with slightly higher T concentrations, this association was of borderline statistical significance (p = 0.051). Otherwise, higher BMI was not associated with higher hormone concentrations.

Discussion

In a longitudinal analysis spanning 8 years across the MT, DHEAS concentrations were stable across the MT [6, 7]. We also note that A4, T, and E1 concentrations remain relatively stable as long as 4 years after the FMP. Moreover, the ratios of E1 and A4 remained fairly constant across the MT. Although A4 and E1 declined slightly, these changes did not mirror the dramatic declines in E2

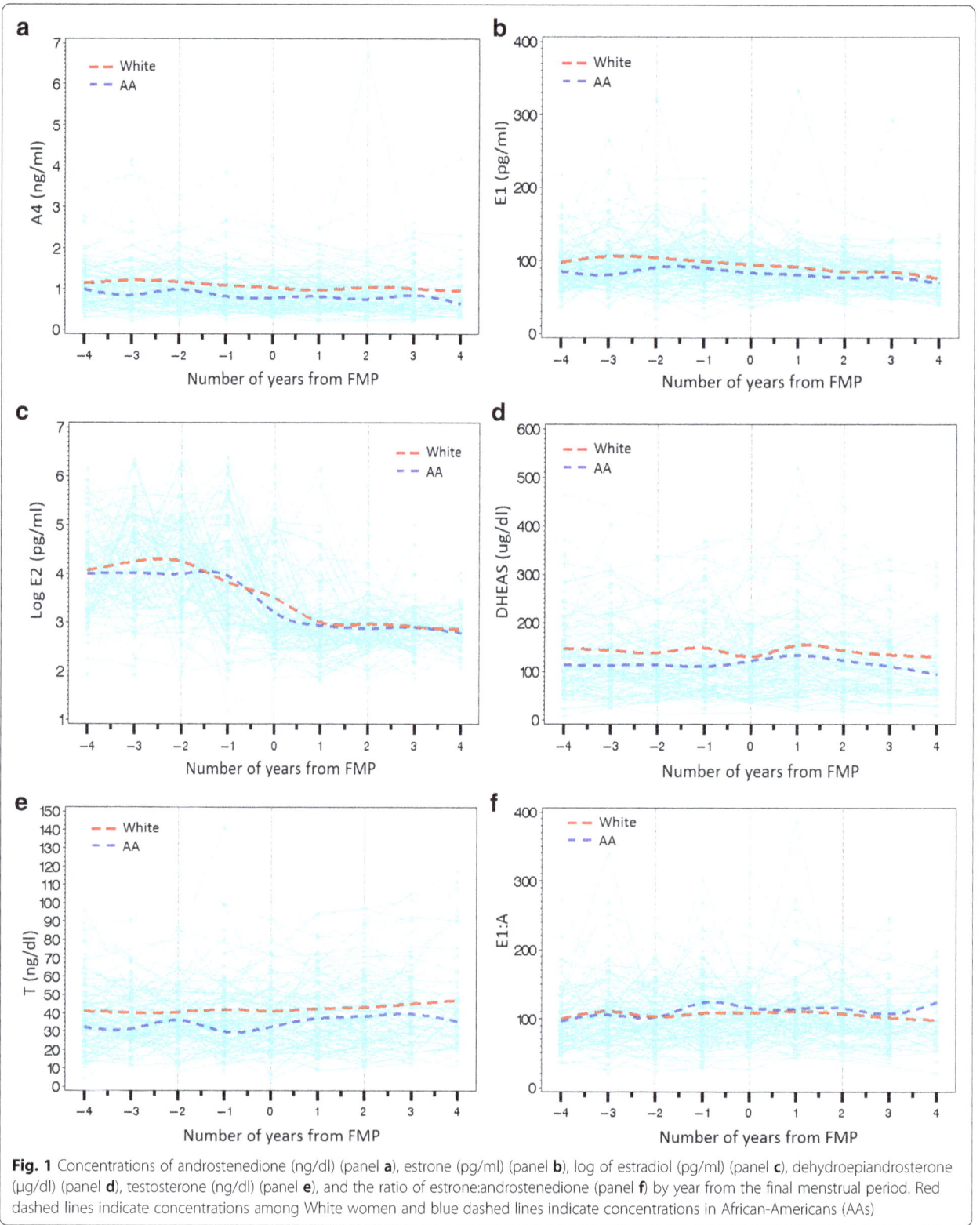

Fig. 1 Concentrations of androstenedione (ng/dl) (panel **a**), estrone (pg/ml) (panel **b**), log of estradiol (pg/ml) (panel **c**), dehydroepiandrosterone (μg/dl) (panel **d**), testosterone (ng/dl) (panel **e**), and the ratio of estrone:androstenedione (panel **f**) by year from the final menstrual period. Red dashed lines indicate concentrations among White women and blue dashed lines indicate concentrations in African-Americans (AAs)

production. We also found that AAs had slightly lower sex hormone concentrations than Whites. The racial/ethnic differences were likely not due to BMI, as the nature and rate of decline in DHEAS, A4, and E1 were similar by BMI.

Our results are consistent with previous reports that suggest that a rise in DHEAS concentrations prior to menopause is concurrent with the declines in peripheral levels of other sex steroids, as well as reports that note declines in

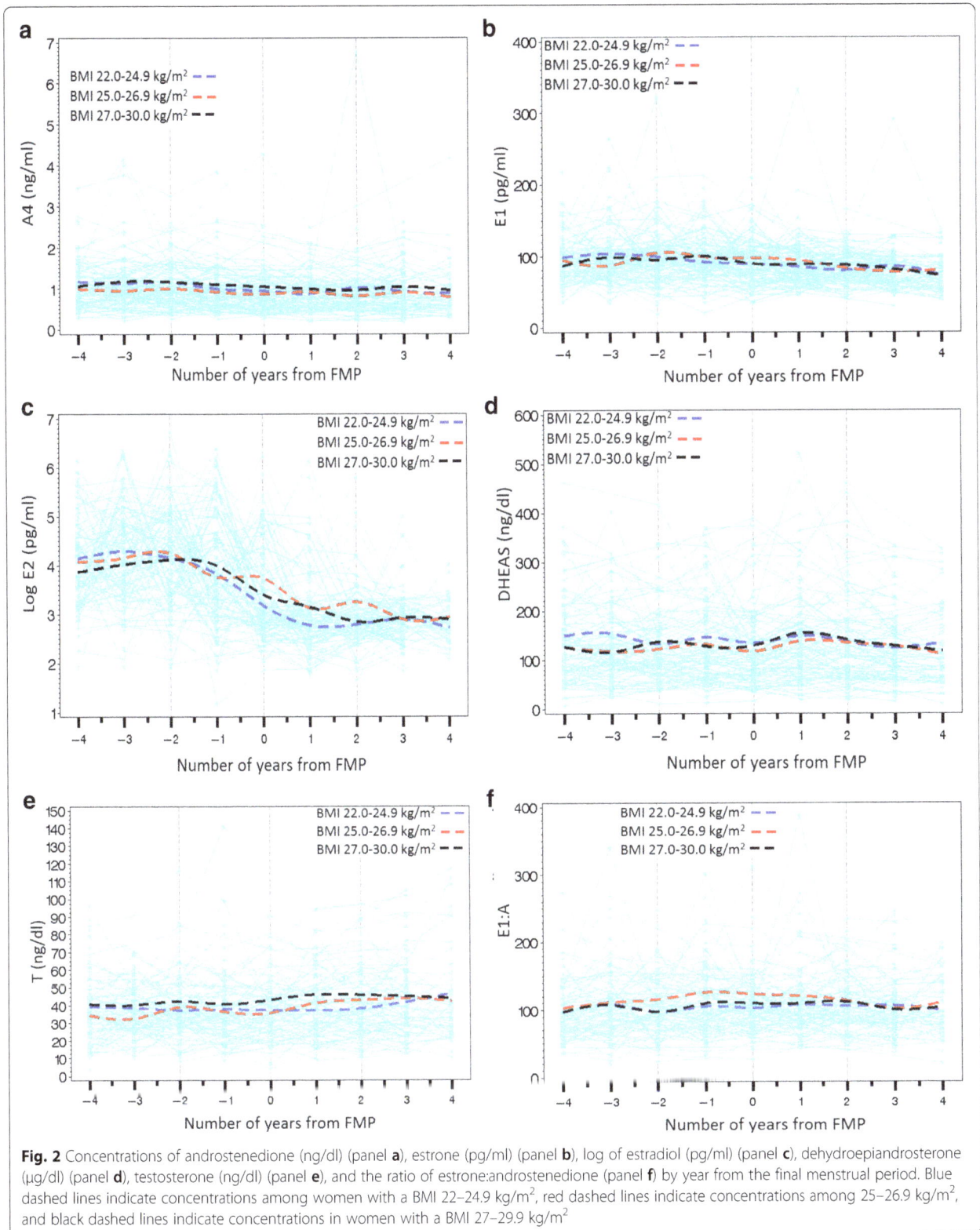

Fig. 2 Concentrations of androstenedione (ng/dl) (panel **a**), estrone (pg/ml) (panel **b**), log of estradiol (pg/ml) (panel **c**), dehydroepiandrosterone (µg/dl) (panel **d**), testosterone (ng/dl) (panel **e**), and the ratio of estrone:androstenedione (panel **f**) by year from the final menstrual period. Blue dashed lines indicate concentrations among women with a BMI 22–24.9 kg/m², red dashed lines indicate concentrations among 25–26.9 kg/m², and black dashed lines indicate concentrations in women with a BMI 27–29.9 kg/m²

DHEAS after the FMP [6–10]. Our report is novel in its inclusion of AAs, the breadth of sex hormones examined, the longitudinal analysis of androgens timed to the FMP, and the length of time spanning the MT.

With the marked decline in ovarian estrogen production in the postmenopause, the adrenal gland becomes a particularly important source of sex steroids, chiefly androgens. DHEA produced by the ovary and the adrenal gland

Table 1 Characteristics of the study population by race/ethnicity

	White women (n = 76)	African-American women (n = 34)
Age at baseline (years)	46.36 (2.47)	45.96 (2.05)
Age at final menstrual period (years)	52.03 (2.52)	51.96 (1.97)
Self-reported health (n, %)		
Excellent	29 (38.67%)	4 (12.50%)
Very good	36 (48.00%)	9 (28.13%)
Good	8 (10.67%)	15 (46.88%)
Fair/Poor	2 (2.67%)	4 (12.50%)
Body mass index (kg/m²)	25.61 (2.18)	25.71 (2.01)
Baseline smoking status (n,%)		
Never	40 (52.63%)	20 (60.61%)
Past	26 (34.21%)	7 (21.21%)
Current	10 (13.16%)	7 (21.21%)

is aromatized peripherally via A4 to bioactive estrogens such as E1. The adrenal gland is also an important source of T which is aromatized to E2. Adrenal-ovarian sex hormone production, conversion to other hormones, and clearance have been postulated to exist in equilibrium [6]. However, longitudinal studies testing this hypothesis are few. Previous reports in SWAN have noted that the majority of women had slight increases in DHEAS prior the FMP followed by declines after the FMP [6, 7], raising the possibility that increased production of DHEAS and/or conversion to other androgens could be a contributor to women's increased androgenicity postmenopause.

Our report extends this prior work: we confirm a modest perimenopausal increase in DHEAS levels, stable T concentrations, and minimal declines in A4 up to 4 years after the FMP. Additionally, since DHEAS and A4 changes do not mirror each other over the transition, it is unlikely that the fluctuations in DHEAS are due to increased peripheral conversion into A4. Similarly, as E1:A4 ratios were stable over time, it is also unlikely that aromatization of A4 to E1 changes significantly over the MT, assuming that A4 production remains the same, although it is possible that both A4 production and aromatization increased concomitantly. Other reports have not reported changes in DHEAS, A4, and T across the menopause. In a cohort of 59 Norwegian women, Overlie and colleagues noted that A4 levels corresponded with both E1 and E2 levels, consistent with the shift from ovarian to adrenal sex hormone production in the postmenopause. However, A4 levels declined in the premenopause, and no significant changes were observed in DHEAS [17]. In a cohort of Swedish women, Rannevik and colleagues also observed that A4 correlated with postmenopausal E1 and E2 concentrations, but concentrations of DHEAS and A4 declined minimally [18].

Our report and previous SWAN studies may have found modest perimenopausal elevations in DHEAS due to larger sample size and our ability to follow women over a longer period of time prior to and after the FMP. Thus, changes in the estrogen/androgen ratio are driven by declines in circulating estrogens, and this relative increase in androgenicity may drive some of the phenotypic changes characteristic of later menopause, such as increased hirsutism [19]. Although speculative, it is possible that such effects are exerted at the tissue level, due to the differential binding of A4 and E2 [20]. Changes in the estrogen/androgen ratio may also be driven by the adrenal response to changing LH concentrations: studies in humans have noted the presence of luteinizing hormone (LH) receptors in the adrenal cortex [21], and mouse models note increases in LH receptors in response to increasing LH levels [22], thus explaining how the adrenal gland might increase sex hormone production even as ovarian response to LH declines.

Previous publications have also reported racial/ethnic differences in androgens, although the direction of reported associations is inconsistent. In a cross-sectional study, Spencer and colleagues noted that even after adjustment for age, BMI, and insulin resistance, AA women had lower DHEAS, A4, and T concentrations than White women [23]. In contrast, Kim and colleagues noted minimal differences in a glucose-intolerant population [24]. Thus, the source of racial/ethnic differences in DHEAS, A4, E1, and T remain speculative. Previous analyses using SWAN data have noted that AAs had the lowest overall DHEAS levels and lowest rates of decline with chronologic age [6, 7]. In those reports, concentrations of A4 were not examined, and thus it was unclear whether racial/ethnic differences in DHEAS concentrations were due to increased adrenal androgen production vs. decreased metabolism of DHEAS into A4. Our report suggests that racial/ethnic differences in A4 metabolism are unlikely to contribute to racial/ethnic differences in DHEAS concentrations.

Previous reports have also suggested that weight may be a significant modifier of adrenal sex hormone production, possibly by affecting E2 concentrations, which in turn might lead to compensatory increases in E1. However, we did not find significant effect modification by tertile of BMI for the sex hormones examined in this report. Our report agrees with that of population-based studies examining cross-sectional associations between DHEAS, A4, and BMI in postmenopausal women [25, 26]. Although E2 and T correlate with waist circumference and BMI in women, the association between BMI and other sex hormones has been relatively weak. One explanation for our conflicting results is that we examined non-obese women within a narrow range of BMI. It is also possible that BMI and waist circumference do not reflect adipose tissue

Table 2 Median (interquartile range) serum hormone levels of women 4 years prior to their final menstrual period (FMP), at the time of their FMP, and 4 years after their FMP ($n = 110$)

	4 years prior to FMP	Year of the FMP	4 years after the FMP
DHEAS (μg/dl)	127.5 (100.4)	108.2 (89.1)	98.6 (105.9)
African-American	103.2 (82.4)	104.8 (113.5)	98.2 (66.7)
White	130.2 (109.7)	109.6 (79.2)	102.1 (123.3)
p-value	0.116	0.583	0.156
BMI 22.0–24.9 kg/m^2	133.0 (118.2)	108.2 (92.8)	125.1 (128.8)
BMI 25.0–26.9 kg/m^2	110.0 (63.1)	110.3 (58.2)	98.2 (70.6)
BMI 27.0–30.0 kg/m^2	107.2 (69.3)	84.4 (110.8)	95.6 (56.8)
p-value	0.316	0.730	0.772
A4 (ng/ml)	1.03 (0.67)	0.84 (0.58)	0.70 (0.59)
African-American	1.03 (0.72)	0.75 (0.33)	0.61 (0.38)
White	1.01 (0.71)	0.91 (0.65)	0.78 (0.62)
p-value	0.338	0.066	0.075
BMI 22.0–24.9 kg/m^2	1.10 (0.70)	0.86 (0.57)	0.77 (0.59)
BMI 25.0–26.9 kg/m^2	0.99 (0.59)	0.83 (0.52)	0.70 (0.61)
BMI 27.0–30.0 kg/m^2	0.94 (0.53)	0.81 (0.64)	0.68 (0.58)
p-value	0.348	0.800	0.883
T (ng/dl)	35.9 (24.8)	36.3 (21.0)	38.3 (24.4)
African-American	34.6 (18.7)	30.9 (20.0)	33.6 (26.2)
White	36.7 (30.2)	38.7 (20.2)	38.8 (29.6)
p-value	0.095	0.020	0.111
BMI 22.0–24.9 kg/m^2	37.8 (32.8)	36.3 (22.1)	38.8 (24.8)
BMI 25.0–26.9 kg/m^2	31.2 (18.2)	36.2 (20.5)	40.1 (29.9)
BMI 27.0–30.0 kg/m^2	36.4 (19.7)	37.2 (28.3)	37.7 (24.2)
p-value	0.418	0.566	0.831
E2 (pg/ml)	53.0 (74.8)	21.6 (39.8)	16.6 (8.0)
African-American	53.5 (65.5)	18.7 (10.3)	16.6 (14.9)
White	51.6 (79.8)	24.4 (54.8)	16.6 (7.9)
p-value	0.741	0.155	0.692
BMI 22.0–24.9 kg/m^2	59.5 (99.0)	18.8 (27.4)	14.4 (5.3)
BMI 25.0–26.9 kg/m^2	41.7 (123.8)	21.0 (127.6)	18.1 (7.0)
BMI 27.0–30.0 kg/m^2	51.6 (46.6)	24.3 (32.9)	17.5 (9.2)
p-value	0.533	0.166	0.090
E1 (pg/ml)	89.4 (39.4)	87.0 (38.6)	69.9 (31.0)
African-American	77.8 (44.5)	85.4 (34.5)	64.8 (30.6)
White	99.4 (38.4)	88.4 (40.4)	72.7 (29.9)
p-value	0.069	0.232	0.369
BMI 22.0–24.9 kg/m^2	97.0 (42.3)	86.9 (45.9)	67.9 (23.9)
BMI 25.0–26.9 kg/m^2	94.4 (41.8)	100.0 (42.0)	82.8 (42.9)
BMI 27.0–30.0 kg/m^2	80.5 (26.7)	80.3 (34.2)	65.5 (34.5)
p-value	0.111	0.317	0.633

Table 3 Associations between race/ethnicity and hormone levels from semiparametric stochastic mixed models, beta-coefficient (standard error) and p-value

	Beta-coefficient (standard error)	p-value
DHEAS (μg/dl)	28.80 (15.34)	0.061
A4 (ng/ml)	0.2556 (0.1315)	0.052
T (ng/dl)	9.180 (1.652)	<0.00001
ln E2	0.0764 (0.0695)	0.272
E1 (pg/ml)	11.365 (0.7306)	<0.00001
E1:A4	−6.527 (7.040)	0.354

Reference group is African-American women; a beta-coefficient greater than 0 indicates higher sex hormone levels in white women

deposition, as examination of associations between visceral adiposity and sex steroids using radiographic imaging has found stronger associations [27].

Strengths of the current report include the longitudinal design, inclusion of AAs, examination of a comprehensive list of adrenal sex hormones, high assay sensitivity for low androgen concentrations, and observation for 9 years during the MT for 990 observations. Limitations include a limited sample size, and thus small fluctuations in hormone concentrations may not have been detected. Our ability to adjust for confounders, particularly racial-ethnic differences in adipose tissue deposition, was also limited. It is possible that self-rated health and smoking status contributed to racial/ethnic differences along with unmeausured confounders, but we had limited power to adjust for these possibilities. We did not use LC/MS for measurement of E2 concentrations, which are low after the FMP; however, our objective was to show relative change over the MT, rather than to establish a definitive absolute value for E2. Finally, we did not conduct adrenal and ovarian vein sampling, and thus cannot definitively distinguish between ovarian and adrenal production of androgens and estrogens.

Conclusions

Our report supports the importance of adrenal androgens as the primary source of estrogens in the postmenopause

Table 4 Associations between body mass index (BMI) and hormone levels from semiparametric stochastic mixed models, beta-coefficient (standard error) is the unit hormone increase per kg/m²

	Beta-coefficient (standard error)	p-value
DHEAS (μg/dl)	0.0000 (0.0000)	1.00
A4 (ng/ml)	−0.0026 (0.0289)	0.929
T (ng/dl)	0.7359 (0.3758)	0.051
ln E2	0.0230 (0.0151)	0.128
E1 (pg/ml)	−0.3466 (0.912)	0.704
E1:A4	0.0274 (1.5409)	0.354

and the increased androgenicity of the postmenopausal hormonal milieu. It is also possible that ovarian production of E1 remains even as E2 declines. Modest increases in DHEAS concentrations are not accompanied by measurably increased levels of A4, T, or E1. Concentrations of these hormones appear to be lower in AAs than White women in the perimenopause, and these racial/ethnic differences are unlikely due to BMI. Examination of the mechanisms for lower DHEAS, A4, and T concentrations in AA women is needed, particularly prior the FMP when declines in other sex hormones occur. Examination of whether these differences contribute to vasomotor symptoms or altered risk of chronic disease risk by race/ethnicity, particularly in other groups besides Whites and AAs, is needed.

Abbreviations
A4: Androstenedione; AAs: African-Americans; BMI: Body mass index; DHEAS: Dehydroepiandrosterone sulfate; E1: Estrone; E2: Estradiol; FMP: Follicle stimulating hormone; FSH: Follicle stimulating hormone; LC/MS: Liquid chromatography mass spectrometry; LH: Luteinizing hormone; MT: Menopausal transition; T: Testosterone

Acknowledgments
We thank the study staff at each site and all the women who participated in the Study of Women's Health Across the Nation (SWAN). This publication was supported in part by the National Center for Research Resources and the National Center for Advancing Translational Sciences, National Institutes of Health through UCSF-CTSI Grant UL1 RR024131.

Authors' contributions
CK interpreted the data regarding hormone distributions and wrote the manuscript. HZ performed the analysis, interpreted the data, and revised the manuscript. DM performed the assays and revised the manuscript. SH collected the data, guided the analyses, and revised the manuscript. JR guided the analyses and revised the manuscript. All authors read and approved the final manuscript.

Funding
The Study of Women's Health Across the Nation (SWAN) has grant support from the National Institutes of Health (NIH), Department of Health and Human Services, through the National Institute on Aging (NIA), the National Institute of Nursing Research (NINR) and the NIH Office of Research on Women's Health (ORWH) (Grants U01NR004061, U01AG012505, U01AG012535, U01AG012531, U01AG012539, U01AG012546, U01AG012553, U01AG012554, and U01AG012495). The content of this manuscript is solely the responsibility of the authors and does not necessarily represent the official views of the NIA, NINR, ORWH, or the NIH.

Competing interests
The authors declare that they have no competing interests.

Author details

[1]Departments of Medicine and Obstetrics & Gynecology, University of Michigan, 2800 Plymouth Road, Building 16, Room 430W, Ann Arbor, MI 48109, USA. [2]Department of Epidemiology, University of Michigan, Ann Arbor, MI, USA. [3]Department of Obstetrics & Gynecology, University of Michigan, Ann Arbor, MI, USA.

References

1. Santoro N, Randolph J Jr. Reproductive hormones and the menopause transition. Obstet Gynecol Clin N Am. 2011;38:455–66.
2. Sowers M, Zheng H, McConnell D, Nan B, Harlow S, Randolph J Jr. Estradiol rates of change in relation to the final menstrual period in a population-based cohort of women. J Clin Endocrinol Metab. 2008;93(10):3847–52.
3. Randolph J Jr, Zheng H, Sowers M, Crandall C, Crawford S, Gold E, et al. Change in follicle-stimulating hormone and estradiol across the menopausal transition: effect of age at the final menstrual period. J Clin Endocrinol Metab. 2011;96(3):746–54.
4. Tepper P, Randolph J, McConnell D, Crawford S, El Khoudary S, Joffe H, et al. Trajectory clustering of estradiol and follicle-stimulating hormone during the menopausal transition among women in the study of Women's health across the nation. J Clin Endocrinol Metab. 2012;97(8):2872–80.
5. Davison S, Bell R, Donath S, Montalto J, Davis S. Androgen levels in adult females: changes with age, menopause, and oophorectomy. J Clin Endocrinol Metab. 2005;90(7):3847.
6. Lasley B, Santoro N, Randolph J Jr, Gold E, Crawford S, Weiss G, et al. The relationship of circulating dehydroepiandrosterone, testosterone, and estradiol to stages of the menopausal transition and ethnicity. J Clin Endocrinol Metab. 2002;87(8):3760–7.
7. Crawford S, Santoro N, Laughlin G, Sowers J, McConnell D, Sutton-Tyrrell K, et al. Circulating dehydroepiandrosterone sulfate concentrations during the menopausal transition. J Clin Endocrinol Metab. 2009;94(8):2945–51.
8. Lasley B, Chen J, Stanczyk F, El Khoudary S, Gee N, Crawford S, et al. Androstenediol complements estrogenic bioactivity during the menopausal transition. Menopause. 2012;19(6):650–7.
9. McConnell D, Stanczyk F, Sowers M, Randolph J Jr, Lasley B. Menopausal transition stage-specific changes in circulating adrenal androgens. Menopause. 2012;19(6):658–63.
10. Lasley B, Crawford S, Laughlin G, Santoro N, McConnell D, Crandall C, et al. Circulating dehydroepiandrosterone sulfate levels in women with bilateral salpingo-oophorectomy during the menopausal transition. Menopause. 2011;18(5):494–8.
11. Lasley B, Crawford S, McConnell D. Adrenal androgens and the menopausal transition. Obstet Gynecol Clin N Am. 2011;38(3):467–75.
12. Lobo R, Pickar J, Stevenson J, Mack W, Hodis H. Back to the future: hormone replacement therapy as part of a prevention strategy for women at the onset of menopause. Atherosclerosis. 2016;254:282–90.
13. Cappola A, O'Meara E, Guo W, Bartz T, Fried L, Newman A. Trajectories of dehydroepiandrosterone sulfate predict mortality in older adults: the cardiovascular health study. J Gerontol A Biol Sci Med Sci. 2009;64(12):1268–74.
14. Randolph J Jr, Sowers M, Bondarenko I, Harlow S, Luborsky J, Little R. Change in estradiol and FSH across the early menopausal transition: effects of ethnicity and age. J Clin Endocrinol Metab. 2004;89(4):1555–61.
15. Sowers M, Zheng H, McConnell D, Nan B, Harlow S, Randolph J Jr. Follicle stimulating hormone and its rate of change in defining menopause transition stages. J Clin Endocrinol Metab. 2008;93(10):3958–64.
16. Zhang D, Lin X, Raz J, Sowers M. Semiparametric stochastic mixed models for longitudinal data. J Am Stat Assoc. 1998;93(442):710–9.
17. Overlie I, Moen M, Morkrid L, Skjaeraasen J, Holte A. The endocrine transition around menopause–a five year prospective study with profiles of gonadotropins, estrogens, androgens, and SHBG among healthy women. Acta Obstet Gynecol Scand. 1999;78(7):642–7.
18. Rannevik G, Jeppsson S, Johnell O, Bjerre B, Laurell-Borulf Y, Svanberg L. A longitudinal study of the perimenopausal transition: altered profiles of steroid and pituitary hormones, SHBG and bone mineral density. Maturitas. 2008;61(102):67–77.
19. Shifren J, Gass M. North American Menopause Society recommendations for clinical Care of Midlife Women Working Group. The North American Menopause Society recommendations for clinical care of midlife women. Menopause. 2014;21(10):1038–62.
20. Miller K, Al-Rayyan N, Ivanova M, Mattingly K, Ripp S, Klinge C, et al. DHEA metabolites activate estrogen receptors alpha and beta. Steroids. 2013;78(1):15–25.
21. Pabon J, Li X, Lei Z, Sanfilippo J, Yussman M, Rao C. Novel presence of luteinizing hormone/chorionic gonadotropin receptrs in human adrenal glands. J Clin Endocrinol Metab. 1996;81:2397–400.
22. Lasley B, Crawford S, McConnell D. Ovarian adrenal interactions during the menopausal transition. Minerva Ginecol. 2013;65(6):641–51.
23. Spencer J, Klein M, Kumar A, Azziz R. The age-associated decline of androgens in reproductive age and menopausal black and white women. J Clin Endocrinol Metab. 2007. epub ahead of print.
24. Kim C, Golden S, Mather K, Laughlin G, Kong S, Nan B, et al. Racial/ethnic differences in sex hormone levels among postmenopausal women in the diabetes prevention program. J Clin Endocrinol Metab. 2012;97(11):4051–60.
25. Kische H, Gross S, Wallaschofski H, Volzke H, Dorr M, Nauck M, et al. Clinical correlates of sex hormones in women: the study of health in Pomerania. Metabolism. 2016;65(9):1286–96.
26. Daan N, Jaspers L, Koster M, Broekmans F, de Rijke Y, Franco O, et al. Androgen levels in women with various forms of ovarian dysfunction: associations with cardiometabolic features. Hum Reprod. 2015;30(10):2376–86.
27. Mongraw-Chaffin M, Anderson C, Allison M, Ouyang P, Szklo M, Vaidya D, et al. Association between sex hormones and adiposity; qualitative differences in women and men in the multi-ethnic study of atherosclerosis. J Clin Endocrinol Metab. 2015;100:E596–600.

14

The Seattle Midlife Women's Health Study: a longitudinal prospective study of women during the menopausal transition and early postmenopause

Nancy Fugate Woods[1][*] and Ellen Sullivan Mitchell[2]

Abstract

Background: The need for longitudinal, population-based studies to illuminate women's experiences of symptoms during the menopausal transition motivated the development of the Seattle Midlife Women's Health Study.

Methods: Longitudinal, population-based study of symptoms women experienced between the Late Reproductive stage of reproductive aging and the early postmenopause. Data collection began in 1990 with 508 women ages 35–55 and continued to 2013. Entry criteria included age, at least one period in past 12 months, uterus intact and at least 1 ovary. Women were studied up to 5 years postmenopause. Data collection included yearly health questionnaires, health diaries, urinary hormonal assays, menstrual calendars and buccal cell smears.

Results: Contributions of the study included development of a method for staging the menopausal transition; development of bleeding criteria to differentiate bleeding episodes from intermenstrual bleeding from menstrual calendars; identification of hormonal changes associated with menopausal transition stages; assessment of the effects of menopausal transition factors, aging, stress-related factors, health factors, social factors on symptoms, particularly hot flashes, depressed mood, pain, cognitive, sexual desire, and sleep disruption symptoms, and urinary incontinence symptoms; identification of naturally occurring clusters of symptoms women experienced during the menopausal transition and early postmenopause; and assessment of gene polymorphisms associated with events such as onset of the early and late menopausal transition stages and symptoms.

Conclusions: Over the course of the longitudinal Seattle Midlife Women's Health Study, investigators contributed to understanding of symptoms women experience during the menopausal transition and early postmenopause as well as methods of staging reproductive aging.

Keywords: Menopausal transition, Staging reproductive aging, Menopause, Midlife cohort, Symptoms, Endocrine changes

Background

During the 1970s and 1980s attention to women's health research increased in the US, culminating in several important milestones, among them establishment of the Office of Women's Health Research in the National Institutes of Health in 1991 and development of the first US Women's Health Research Agenda [1]. In 1993 the National Institutes of Health/National Institute on Aging, National Institute of Child Health and Development, and collaborating organizations convened a workshop on Menopause to provide focus for future research about midlife women and menopause. This work was preceded by the landmark longitudinal study of the menopausal transition (MT): the Massachusetts Women's Health Study begun in 1982 [2], a longitudinal study developed to expand knowledge about the experiences of a community-based population of women as they traversed the MT. This focus on a community-based population was in

* Correspondence: nfwoods@uw.edu
[1]Department of Biobehavioral Nursing, University of Washington, Seattle, WA 98195, USA
Full list of author information is available at the end of the article

contrast to earlier studies of clinical populations. Another early effort by Matthews and colleagues recruited women from the state of Pennsylvania (The Healthy Women Study) to determine the natural history of the MT, and behavioral and biological changes that occurred during the MT and postmenopause (PM) and their effects on cardiovascular disease risk [3].

The Seattle Midlife Women's Health Study (SMWHS) was built on the foundational studies of the 1980s, including our longitudinal studies of perimenstrual symptoms that focused on women after they had reached age 40 years [4–6]. The SMWHS originated as one component of a Center for Women's Health Research (CWHR) at the University of Washington School of Nursing in 1989. Funded by the National Institute of Nursing Research, the CWHR was created by an interdisciplinary cadre of investigators to support research development in women's health [7].

Overview of the SMWHS
The initial phase of SMWHS from September 1989 to July 1996, as part of the CWHR, was designed to test a model relating MT status, stress exposure, socialization for midlife, personal and social factors modulating midlife experiences, reproductive health history, and health behaviors to health status and health-seeking behavior in midlife women between the ages of 35 and 55. A model including menopausal changes, socialization for midlife, health status, stressful life context, and vasomotor symptoms guided analysis of depressed mood symptoms, an outcome of interest [8]. The model was generalized to other symptoms, for example, by testing outcomes including hot flashes, sleep, cognitive, mood, and pain symptoms, to name a few. (The Aims for Phase 1 are included in Table 1)

Based on results of the initial study, additional funding was obtained for the SMWHS from July 1996 to February 2001. This second funding phase focused on the MT and its relationship to symptoms, altered ovarian function, perceived stress and stress arousal, as well as symptom management. A major addition to the measures for this study included hormonal assays (urinary estrone, FSH, testosterone, cortisol and catecholamines). (Aims for Phase 2 are included in Table 1).

A third funding phase spanned 2002 through 2006. Phase 3 of SMWHS continued to focus on symptoms as the primary endpoints. In addition to linking the symptoms to endocrine patterns, the effect of gene polymorphisms in estrogen synthesis, metabolism and receptor genes was added to the aims. (Detailed aims for Phase 3 are given in Table 1).

A fourth and final phase of data collection, after the end of major funding, continued from 2007 to 2013. The focus of this phase was to complete the data collection for the study. Women who had not yet reached 5 years PM, were not taking any estrogen and had an intact uterus were entered into this final phase. Aims for this phase were a combination of the aims for the three prior phases of funding. The model guiding the longitudinal analysis of symptom data across all 4 phases is depicted in Fig. 1.

Two small grants supported the fourth phase of the study. The first was "Menopausal Transition Symptom Clusters: Genetic, Endocrine, and Social Correlates" that focused on the secondary analyses of symptom data, particularly on multiple co-occurring symptoms called symptom clusters that women experienced during the MT and early PM. Symptom data were analyzed to identify clusters of symptoms women experienced and to relate them to stress, health behaviors, health status, endocrine patterns, and gene polymorphisms. (Aims for this study are in Table 1). A second small grant during the fourth phase of the study, Urinary Incontinence during the Menopausal Transition and Early Postmenopause, was awarded by Pfizer, Inc, Medical Division, that supported the secondary analysis of urinary incontinence data over time. (Aims for this study are in Table 1).

In addition, research support was provided by intramural funds to develop a scannable health diary form, for a pilot study of gene polymorphisms related to symptoms, and to complete collection of data from women as they experienced the early PM (Research Intramural Funding Program, University of Washington School of Nursing).

Methods
Design
A prospective, repeated measures design was used to study a population-based sample of women who were about to begin or had begun the transition to menopause at the time of entry into the study. Data were collected throughout the study at intervals described below for a total of 23 years. The study was divided into 4 phases based on the aims associated with each funding period. Each phase expanded the aims of the previous phase.

Sample
From early 1990 to early 1992, 508 women were enrolled. This original population-based sample from the Seattle area was obtained by telephone screening of all households in over 20 census tracts selected for mixed ethnicity and mixed income. There were 13,120 households enumerated. Of the 11,222 households able to be contacted (85.5 % of those enumerated), 1,428 women between the ages of 35 and 55 were screened (12.7 % of those contacted) and 820 were eligible (57.4 % of those screened). In addition to age, a woman was eligible if

Table 1 Aims for the Seattle Midlife Women's Health Study by Phase

Phase 1: 1990–1996

The aim of Phase I was to test a model relating menopausal status, stress exposure, socialization for midlife, personal and social factors modulating midlife experiences, reproductive health history, and health behaviors to health status and health-seeking behavior in midlife women between the ages of 35 and 55.

Phase 2: 1996–2001

Aim 1. Describe the **progression through stages of the perimenopause** (pre transition, early transition, middle transition, late transition, and postmenopause as determined from annual health updates and daily menstrual calendars) for women over a nine year period with respect to:
a) **Symptoms**, including vasomotor, dysphoric mood, insomnia, somatic, and discomfort symptoms, recorded in a daily health diary for three days monthly (coinciding with hormone assays);
b) **Altered ovarian function** (estrone, testosterone (T), and FSH), measured in first morning urine samples at monthly intervals;
c) **perceived stress** (stressful life events, income inadequacy) measured annually and perceived stress measured 3 days each month in the health diary;
d) **stress arousal** (urinary levels of cortisol and catecholamines) measured in the first morning urine samples at monthly intervals; and
e) **symptom management**, including use of health services and hormone replacement therapy assessed annually in a health update questionnaire and interview.
Aim 2. Test the following **hypotheses regarding symptoms** during the three stages of the transition to menopause (early to middle to late):
a) women who experience more severe **vasomotor symptoms** during the transition to menopause will have: higher levels of perceived stress, lower levels of estrone, and higher levels of catecholamines and cortisol;
b) women who experience more severe **dysphoric mood symptoms** during the transition to menopause will have: higher levels of perceived stress, higher levels of cortisol, and norepinepherine, and a lower estrogen:androgen ratio;
c) women who experience more sever **insomnia symptoms** during the transition to menopause will have: higher levels of perceived stress, lower levels of estrone, and higher levels of catecholamines.
Aim 3. Test the relationship within individual women among HPO axis hormones (estrone, FSH, testosterone), indicators of physiologic stress arousal (cortisol and catecholamines), daily stress ratings, and symptoms (especially vasomotor, dysphoric mood, and insomnia), measured monthly over a nine year period, using auto-correlation and cross-correlation techniques.
Aim 4. To estimate the stability of symptom patterns women have recorded in daily health diaries each year with symptom patterns women experience during the menopausal transition (over the period of 1991 to 1995, 1996–2000 and 2001–2005).

Phase 3: 2002–2006

Aim 1. Describe and compare women in the menopausal transition (early, middle and late transition), in the early postmenopause, and those who use HRT, on indicators of pituitary-ovarian hormone changes, perceived stress, physiologic stress arousal, vasomotor, dysphoric mood, somatic, discomfort and insomnia symptoms.
Aim 1 Hypotheses:
Hypothesis 1: Women in late transition will have higher levels of urinary FSH, cortisol and norepinepherine, higher perceived stress and higher vasomotor symptom severity than women in early or middle transition.
Hypothesis 2: Women in the postmenopause will have lower levels of urinary estrone and testosterone, lower perceived stress and higher levels of FSH and vasomotor symptoms than women in the three menopausal transition stages.
Hypothesis 3: There will be no group differences among women in the three menopausal transition stages for urinary estrone,

Table 1 Aims for the Seattle Midlife Women's Health Study by Phase *(Continued)*

testosterone and epinephrine, depressed mood or the 5 symptom clusters except for vasomotor symptoms.
Hypothesis 4: Women on HRT will have higher estrone levels and lower perceived stress, urinary cortisol, and vasomotor symptoms than women who are not on HRT, those in the menopausal transition or those who are postmenopausal.
Aim 2. Compare women in the menopausal transition and early postmenopause with different *estrogen metabolism and catabolism gene polymorphisms* with respect to estradiol and estrone levels, age of onset of middle and late menopausal transition stage and menopause, and heaviness of menstrual blood flow.
Aim 3. Compare women in the menopausal transition and early postmenopause with different *estrogen receptor gene polymorphisms* with respect to estradiol and estrone levels, age of onset of middle and late menopausal transition stage and menopause, and heaviness of menstrual blood flow.

Phase 4: 2007–2013

Continuation of aims from Phases 1 –3.
Additional aims for the Symptom Cluster Study that was part of Phase 4.
1. Identify symptom clusters (SC) SMWHS participants experienced during the late reproductive, early menopausal transition stages and early postmenopause using latent class analysis to complement the preliminary analyses of the late stage SCs;
2. Determine the consistency of SCs with the clusters identified for the late menopausal transition stage across the late reproductive stage, early menopausal transition stage and early postmenopause;
3. Test models hypothesizing the relationship between SC groups and profiles of:
a) gene polymorphisms in the estrogen synthesis pathways (CYP 19 and 17 HSD) and genes polymorphisms in neuroendocrine pathways modulated by estrogen (5HTTLPR, NPY, BDNF);
b) hypothalamic-pituitary-ovarian (HPO) biomarkers (E, T, FSH), and hypothalamic-pituitary-adrenal (HPA – cortisol) and autonomic nervous system (ANS- epinephrine, norepinephrine) biomarkers;
c) reproductive aging stages (late reproductive, early and late menopausal transition, and early postmenopause);
d) socio-behavioral risk factors (e.g. high stress, role burden, low income adequacy, employment, education, social support);
e) symptom vulnerability factors (e.g. history of sexual abuse, low mastery, self-consciousness, low self esteem); and outcomes of well-being and interference with work and relationships;
4. Based on a systematic review of controlled clinical trials for managing hot flashes, identify treatment effects on co-occuring symptoms and reported adverse treatment effects, including sleep disturbances, mood, pain and cognitive symptoms;
5. Synthesize results of the empirical analyses (aims 1–3) and systematic review (aim 4) to develop novel symptom cluster management protocols to be tested in a future feasibility study.
Additional aims for Urinary Incontinence Study that was part of Phase 4.
1. Determine the influence of age and menopausal transition factors on the experience of urinary incontinence (stress, urge and any incontinence) among midlife women;
2. Assess the influence of lifespan health factors and life context (personal and social resources and stress) on urinary incontinence; and
3. Determine the relationship between urinary incontinence and well-being, symptoms (fatigue, disrupted sleep, anxiety and depressed mood) and interference with daily living (work and relationships).

she had an intact uterus and at least one ovary, had at least one menstrual period within the past 12 months, was not pregnant or lactating, and could read and understand English. Of the 820 women eligible, 620 agreed to participate (75.6 % of those eligible) and 508 actually began the study and provided initial cross–

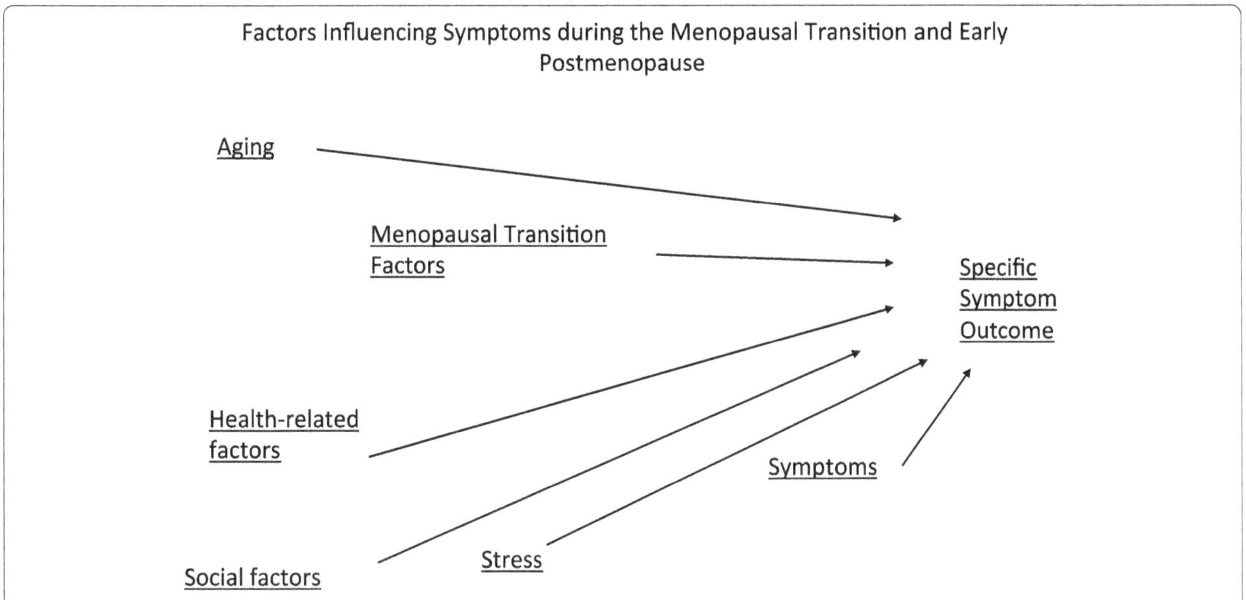

Fig. 1 General Model Guiding SMWHS Symptom Analyses Across Time

sectional data (81.9 % of those who initially agreed to participate) (See Table 2). 390 of the 508 women entered the longitudinal component of the study (76.8 % of the cross-sectional sample) by agreeing to provide data over time. A description of the characteristics of the women who agreed to participate in the longitudinal component ($N = 390$) and those who only completed the initial cross sectional component ($N = 118$) is shown in Table 3. Those who entered the longitudinal component compared to those who did not enter were more likely to be partnered, not a parent and not Black. There were no significant differences for education, employment, age, BMI, income and stress level.

For entry into the second major funding phase of the study (mid-1996), women still enrolled at the end of the previous phase of this longitudinal project, plus those who had dropped out of phase 1 but had contributed at least two years of data, were contacted by phone about participating in this second phase. A total of 300 women were contacted in mid-1996 and screened for continuing eligibility (5 years or less PM or, if taking hormones, age less than 60 years old, uterus intact and at least one ovary intact). Of

Table 2 Smwhs sample identification and screening

Sampling Identification	N and (% of total enumerated)
Households enumerated	13,120 (100 %)
Households contacted by phone	11,222 (86 %)
Women in households 35–55 years of age screened	1,428 (11 %)
Women eligible after screening	820 (6 %)
Women who agreed to participate	620 (5 %)
Women who actually began study	508 (4 %)

those 300 women screened, 243 were eligible and agreed to enroll in phase 2 (62 % of the 390 who began the longitudinal component). In addition, between 2000 and 2002, 174 women provided a buccal cell smear for genotyping. See Fig. 2 for retention across the entire project.

For entry into the third major funding phase of the study (2001–2006) all eligible women (5 years or less PM or, if taking hormones, age less than 60, uterus intact and at least one ovary) who were still participating ($N = 160$) were contacted and screened (66 % of those who entered phase 2). Of these 160 women, 144 (90 %) agreed to continue for a third phase. At the end of phase three 67 women were still eligible and participating.

Research funds from the UW School of Nursing Research Intramural Funding Program were obtained in 2007 to continue data collection from those still eligible for the study. Of these 67 women, 64 were eligible and agreed to continue participation in the fourth and final phase until no longer eligible. This part of the study continued until February 2013 when all data collection was completed. Of the original 508 women who entered the study, by the end of the study in 2013, 173 had dropped due to personal reasons (34 %), 162 were lost to contact (32 %) and 173 became ineligible sometime during the study (34 %).

Retention efforts

Numerous efforts were taken to retain the eligible sample throughout the study. These include the following:

- yearly birthday card with a personal note
- yearly thank you checks through the first two funding periods

Table 3 Baseline Sample Characteristics for women who participated in the Longitudinal Component Compared with women who participated only in the Cross Sectional Component (1990–1991)

Characteristic	Women in Longitudinal Component (n = 390) Mean (SD)	Women in Cross Sectional Component (n = 118) Mean (SD)	p value*
Age (years)	41.5 (4.3)	41.4 (4.4)	0.43
Years of education	15.7 (2.8)	15.3 (3.2)	0.15
Family gross income ($)	37360 (15,800)	35,500 (17,460)	0.27
Number live births	1.97 (1.4)	1.57 (1.4)	.006
Perceived stress	2.2 (0.55)	2.3 (0.55)	0.31
Characteristic	N (Percent)	N (Percent)	p value**
Currently employed			
Yes	336 (86.1)	102 (86.4)	0.94
No	54 (13.8)	16 (13.6)	
Race/ethnicity			
African American	32 (8.2)	26 (22.0)	.001
Asian /Pacific Islander	34 (8.7)	9 (7.6)	
Caucasian	311 (79.7)	80 (67.8)	
Other (Hispanic, Mixed)	13 (3.3)	3 (2.5)	
Marital Status			
Married/partnered	277 (71.0)	71 (60.2)	0.03
Never partnered/ divorced/widowed	113 (29.0)	47 (39.8)	
Never married/partnered	21 (7.2)	14 (6.5)	

*Independent t-test
**Chi-square test

- personal and consistent contact by the research staff
  - reminder postcards about data collection
  - in-person pick-up of urine and diaries at a community site or at home
  - reminder phone calls about pick-up of data
- flexibility regarding schedules; negotiating alternatives
- periodic sharing of findings with women
- yearly newsletter, The Midlife Times
- two Health Fairs at community sites
- a web site
- a certification of appreciation after 10 years of participation
- easy access to research staff via phone and email

Data collection

In the first phase of the study all measures were pencil and paper measures. This included measures of symptom severity, stress, personal and social resources, socialization for midlife and aging, reproductive health experiences including menstrual cycle changes, social environmental demands, and personal health practices. These measures were obtained in an annual daily health diary across two to three menstrual cycles, an annual health questionnaire and a menstrual calendar.

In the second phase of the study measures of pituitary-ovarian and pituitary-adrenal function were added. These additional measures were obtained by collecting monthly first AM urine specimens on day 6 of the menstrual cycle, if the woman was still cycling. Women were instructed not to eat, drink, smoke, take medications or exercise before each urine collection. The health diary was collected on 3 consecutive days (days 5, 6 and 7) to coordinate with the time of the urine collection (day 6). For those with very erratic bleeding and those no longer having periods a consistent 3 days of the month was used for data collection. This procedure was used from late 1996 through 2000.

The data collection time for the diary and urine specimens was modified from 2001 through 2005. The timing was changed from monthly to quarterly for both the diary and urine collections. During all phases of the study the yearly health questionnaire and menstrual calendars were continued (See Table 4 for sample size for each measure by year).

In addition, buccal cell smears were obtained from 174 of these women between 2000 and 2002. Urine collections stopped at the end of 2005. From 2006 to the end of the study quarterly health diaries, yearly health questionnaires and menstrual calendars, if still bleeding, were obtained.

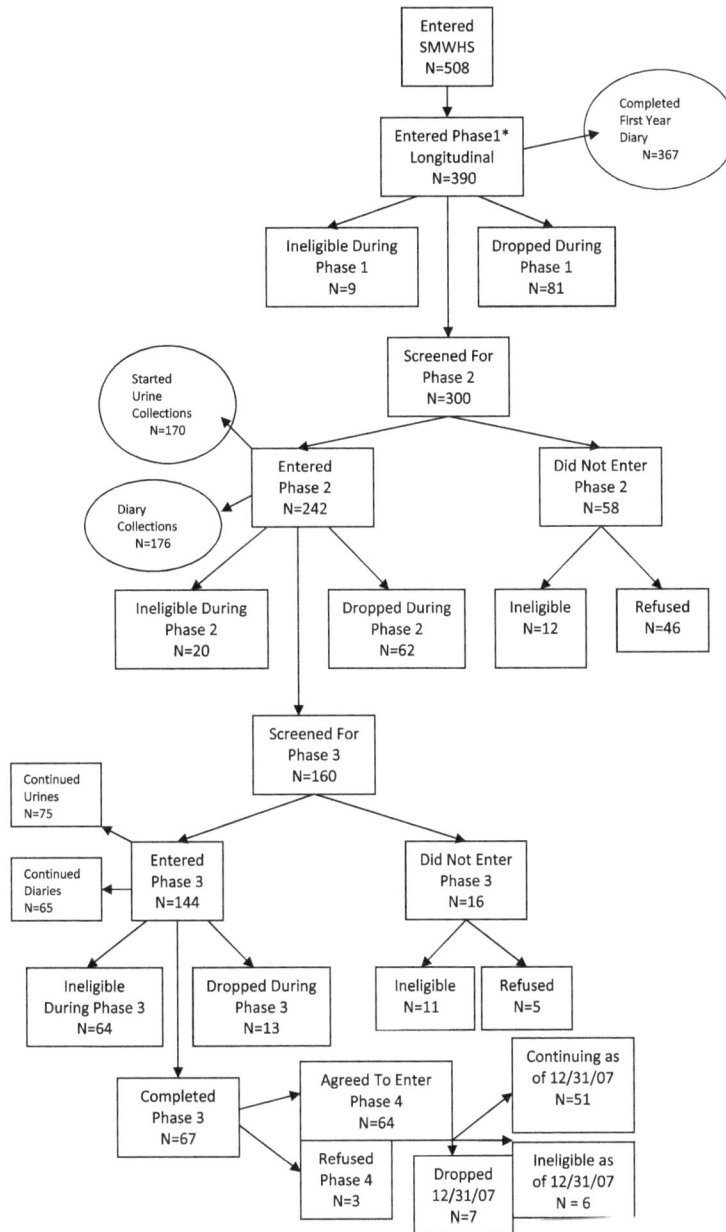

Fig. 2 Retention Flow Chart. *Funding phases

Data handling

Except for the interview at the start of the study, all data in phase 1 and phase 4 were collected by mail (yearly questionnaire, diaries, menstrual calendars). In phases 2 and 3 the diaries and urine samples were collected in person while the annual questionnaire and menstrual calendar were collected by mail. For the urine samples, after the first morning urine was collected by the participant it was immediately frozen in a home freezer at 0°. These specimens were either brought frozen to a community site by the participant at a prearranged time or were picked up by a research associate within 56 days

(8 weeks) of collection. Each specimen was kept frozen during transport and then taken to the University of Washington School of Nursing Biobehavioral Lab and placed in a –70° centigrade freezer. The specimens were then assayed by the laboratory staff. (See Additional file 1: Assay Descriptions and Laboratory Assay Procedure). A maximum of 56 days for home freezing was determined by the laboratory staff using various intervals and testing for sample degradation. The diaries were picked up in a similar manner as the urine during phases 2 and 3. If urine was not collected, the diaries were mailed to the study personnel.

Table 4 Frequencies for data sources (1990–2013)

	Questionnaire N	Diary N	Assay N (# specimens)
1990–1992	508	367	NA
1993	347	259	NA
1994	309	261	NA
1995	250	141	NA
1996	192	146	NA
1997	233	176	170 (1783)
1998	205	162	167 (1820)
1999	212	149	157 (1478)
2000	190	103	106 (1036)
2001	175	79	85 (340)
2002	157	65	74 (279)
2003	140	59	59 (236)
2004	110	46	54 (208)
2005	95	44	49 (179)
2006	84	30	NA
2007	57	20	NA
2008	47	18	NA
2009	37	15	NA
2010	31	10	NA
2011	20	10	NA
2012	17	5	NA
2013	12	5	NA

Measures

A blank **menstrual calendar** was mailed at the end of each calendar year for completion during the following year. Any occurrence of bleeding (B) or spotting (S) was recorded. Beginning in 1996, the amount of B on a scale of 1 (light flow) to 4 (very heavy/flooding) was recorded with each occurrence. Spotting was any bloody vaginal discharge that did not require any protection [9]. (See Additional file 1 for sample calendar). The menstrual calendars were returned at the start of the following year and reviewed for completeness.

Definitions of bleeding events used for the study, called standard bleeding events, were modifications of those recommended by WHO [9] [Gray, RH. WHO Meeting on the Analysis of Bleeding Patterns, Feb 28, 1978, unpublished]. A standard bleeding episode was defined as ≥2 days of B or a mix of ≥2 B and S days but not all S days with ≤2 bleed free days. A standard bleeding interval was any series of ≥4 consecutive bleed-free days bounded by bleeding episodes. A bleeding segment was a bleeding episode and the subsequent bleeding interval.

The WHO standard definitions did not differentiate bleeding episodes from intermenstrual bleeding (IMB)

or non-menses bleeding such as S or B days between consecutive bleeding episodes and within a bleeding interval. A limitation of the WHO standard definition of a bleeding episode (≥1 days B or S) was the creation of many very short bleeding segments. Short bleeding segments can overstate the incidence of irregularity, bias downward the age of onset of each MT stage and bias upward the duration of MT stages. To address this problem of short bleeding segments additional criteria were developed by the study staff and Sybil Crawford, PhD, to determine if a bleeding event with 1 B day or 1 or more S days only was an episode or IMB and whether 3 bleed free days between B or S days represented a bleeding interval or was part of the episode. The criteria were applied using the woman as the unit of analysis as recommended by Treloar [10] (See Additional file 1 for Nonstandard Bleeding Criteria). The basic premise behind these additional criteria was that the typical bleeding pattern of some women can reflect a slight variation from the standard definitions and that IMB or non-menses bleeding is a phenomenon that needs to be accounted for as part of a woman's bleeding pattern.

A reduction in the number of short bleeding segments was the result of this procedure. In the SMWHS sample. The majority of instances of 1 S day or ≥2 S days together occurred between episodes, in the bleeding interval (unpublished data).

After all the bleeding criteria were applied to the calendar data each calendar was assigned a subgroup for staging using staging criteria developed by the study personnel [11] and modified based on the findings of the ReSTAGE Collaboration [12] (See Additional file 1 for Staging Criteria).

A **health questionnaire** was mailed at the end of each year. This questionnaire obtained data about changes in health, the menstrual cycle, current health practices, medication use, stress, social support, mental health, symptoms and well-being. (See Additional file 1 for a summary of measures included in the annual health questionnaires).

A **health diary** was kept by a subset of the original 508 women. Initially this diary was kept daily for two to three menstrual cycles. It was completed once a year for three years (at the start of the study, 12 months later, and 24 months from the start). The data from this early diary was hand entered into the computer. In 1994 the diary was converted to a scannable format and for 1995 and 1996 was kept daily for two weeks once a year (around the time of the yearly health questionnaire). Beginning in late 1996 to the end of 2000 this scannable diary was kept for 3 days every menstrual cycle on days 5, 6, and 7, if there were identifiable menstrual periods, to correspond with the urine collection on day 6. Otherwise it was kept monthly on the same 3 days every month. Starting in 2001 the diary was completed once a quarter for the same 3 consecutive days instead of monthly. The diary included items such as symptoms commonly experienced by midlife women, medication use, stress levels and health practices (smoking, drinking alcohol, caffeine use, exercise, sleep). (See Additional file 1 for sample pages of the diary).

Urine specimens were obtained from a subset of women one time per menstrual cycle on day 6 or once a month if there were no identifiable periods. These urine collections began in late 1996 and continued until the end of 2005. This was a first morning specimen and was assayed for estrone glucuronide, FSH, total testosterone, cortisol, epinephrine and norepinephrine. (See Additional file 1 for assay descriptions).

A **buccal cell smear** was obtained for genetic analysis from 174 women sometime between 2000 and 2002. (See Additional file 1 for buccal cell smear collection procedure and Additional file 1 for genotyping sequencing).

Analytic strategies

A variety of analytic strategies was used over the course of the study. Examples include discriminant function analysis [9], confirmatory factor analysis and LISREL [8–14], content analysis with cross tabulations [15–17], ANOVA and regression analysis [18], cluster analysis [19], t-tests [20], time series analysis [21], general estimating equation [22] and numerous papers since 2006 using multilevel modeling (MLM) [23–35]. The analytic method called multi-level modeling (MLM) was used for most of the longitudinal analyses once most of the data were collected and processed (from 2006 on). For all MLM analyses age was used as the measure of time. This method was specifically adapted for the SMWHS data by a statistician (Don Percival, PhD) and was developed using an R program to account for specific characteristics of the data such as an unbalanced design, serial correlation, and missing data [30]. (See Additional file 1 for a detailed description of the MLM procedure).

Results

Selected results are presented to illustrate the contributions of each phase of the SMWHS. A complete list of publications from the Seattle Midlife Women's Health Study is appended to the References section.

Phase 1

Data collected during phase I of the study were used to amplify our understanding of women's views of midlife and menopause, as well as to evaluate models of women's health and health-seeking behavior during midlife. In response to open-ended questions, women described midlife as a time of many transitions: getting older and changing bodies, outlooks and relationships.

Personal achievements and employment were central to the lives of midlife women in this study [16]. Women viewed menopause as a period of transition. When women were asked about their anticipation of menopause they indicated it was a time of uncertainty that elicited mixed feelings [17]. Women also revealed their meanings of menopause as the cessation of periods, experiencing the end of fertility and reproductive capacity, hormonal changes, new or different life stage, changing emotions, changing bodies, symptoms, and part of the aging process. Few referred to menopause as a time of risk for disease or of need for health care.

A model of depressed mood symptoms was developed, evaluating 3 pathways to depressed mood, comparing the influence of the MT, stressful life context, and health status pathways in a multiethnic sample ($N = 337$). The stressful life context pathway was most influential in accounting for depressed mood. Health status had a direct effect on depressed mood and an indirect effect through perceived stress. The menopausal changes pathway had little explanatory power. At the time this model was tested, the majority of participants were in the Late Reproductive stage or the Early MT stage. Nonetheless, these results suggested the need for clinicians to look beyond menopausal status to the broader context of midlife women's lives [8].

The primary endpoint throughout the study was type and severity of symptoms women experienced and reported during the MT and early PM. When the symptoms women experienced during midlife were first examined, measured during the premenses week, several groups were identified, including: dysphoric mood, vasomotor, somatic, neuromuscular,and insomnia symptoms. Notably the stability of vasomotor and somatic symptoms was lowest over the three year period studied, but dysphoric mood, neuromuscular, and insomnia symptoms were relatively stable, suggesting their chronic experience in this cohort [13]. The variability of the vasomotor and somatic symptoms over the three year period led to a focus on the role of the MT and related hormonal changes during subsequent phases of the study.

During phase 1 women's health-seeking behavior was also investigated and was then tracked during subsequent phases. After publication of Women's Health Initiative findings in 2002 linking hormone therapy (HT) with increased risk of breast cancer, stroke, heart attacks and other health problems, the percent of women taking hormones during the MT decreased from 49 % in 1999 to 35 % in 2003 [23].

Phases 2, 3, and 4

Development of a staging system

Phase 2 of the study focused on the development of a staging system for the MT that eventually informed and was integrated with the Staging Reproductive Aging Workshop (STRAW) efforts [36], and later validated by the multi-country work of the Re-STAGE Collaboration [11, 37–39]. Mitchell led development of the MT staging system from detailed observation and analysis of menstrual calendar data over a seven year period (1990–1997) [11]. Development of the staging system for the MT provided a useful framework to organize subsequent analyses and demonstrate the influence of the MT stages on endocrine patterns, symptoms, and other aspects of the MT.

An important measurement issue related to staging reproductive aging was whether retrospective and prospective reporting of menstrual irregularity by women would influence staging efforts. Agreement between women's reporting on a menstrual calendar and questionnaires with retrospective reports was weak, thus we incorporated only prospective reporting on menstrual calendars in the SMWHS staging approach [40].

The original and modified stages and criteria for staging used by SMWHS were as follows:

Pretransition stage when cycles were regular with no change in length of periods, amount of flow or cycle length from the previous year. This stage was later called Late Reproductive stage to correspond to STRAW recommendations.

Early stage when cycles were still regular but there was a change in length of periods, amount of flow or cycle length from the previous year. This stage was later called Late Reproductive stage to correspond to STRAW recommendations.

Middle stage when cycles became irregular, i.e., start of consecutive cycles were 7 or more days apart. This stage was later called Early stage to correspond to STRAW recommendations.

Late stage when periods were skipped, i.e., twice the modal cycle length between consecutive cycles. The criteria for this stage were later changed to 60 or more days of amenorrhea between the start of consecutive periods to correspond to the findings from the ReSTAGE Collaboration [39].

The original focus of staging in the SMWHS was on the menopausal transition. When the Staging Reproductive Aging Workshop (STRAW) investigators proposed use of stages of reproductive aging across the lifespan, we adopted the STRAW staging approach derived from consensus of investigators who participated in the STRAW workship in 2001. Our initial staging system had included an early, middle, and late stage of the menopausal transition. Because the STRAW investigators believed that the menopausal

transition did not begin until cycle intervals became irregular, we adapted our staging to fit their recommendations. We no longer used our old definition of early menopausal transition, which included regular cycles with more subtle changes in the length of the period and cycle length, and instead adopted the STRAW definition of early stage. We also changed our pretransition stage to use the nomenclature of STRAW: late reproductive stage.

Age of onset of MT stages and the final menstrual period (FMP), and **duration** of the Early and Late MT stages were identified. On average, women ($N = 121$) entered Early stage at age 46.4 (SD = 3.4) and stayed in the stage ($N = 82$) for an average of 2.8 years (SD = 1.5). On average, women ($N = 130$) entered Late stage at age 49.4 (SD = 2.7) and stayed in this stage ($N = 84$) for an average of 2.5 years (SD = 1.3). The average age ($N = 114$) for the FMP (start of PM) for this cohort was 52.1 (SD = 2.9) years [37].

To identify an onset of each MT stage it was necessary to have bleeding data about the prior stage for the previous 12 months so the time of change could be identified. For example, using the staging criteria, if a woman was in Early stage for one year and the next year met the criteria for Late stage, the onset of Late stage could be identified. However, if she was in Late stage for one year but the prior 12 months of calendar data were not available, her onset of Late stage would be unknown. This same situation also would apply to onset of Early stage. Content analysis of women's descriptions of irregularity and skipping of periods revealed that using simple questions about these was not adequate to apply the staging criteria. Instead, it was important to use the menstrual calendars to collect actual bleeding data [40].

Hormonal changes across the menopausal transition

An inspection of changes in urinary **FSH** (follicle-stimulating hormone) levels across the MT showed a rise as women progressed from Early MT to Late MT stage and to early PM and urinary **estrone** levels rose slightly from the Early to the Late MT stage and then dropped substantially the final year before and the first year after the FMP. **Urinary testosterone** levels remained flat across all MT stages and early PM. When these 3 hormones were analyzed for an association with MT stage across time, early PM had a significant negative effect on estrone and both Late MT stage and early PM had a significant positive effect on FSH. Testosterone was not affected by stage (unpublished data). (See Figs. 3 a,b,c)

When these same hormone levels were graphed based on number of **years before and after FMP** (from 8 years before to 5 years after FMP) FSH began to rise at 3 years before FMP and steadily increased to 3 years after FMP

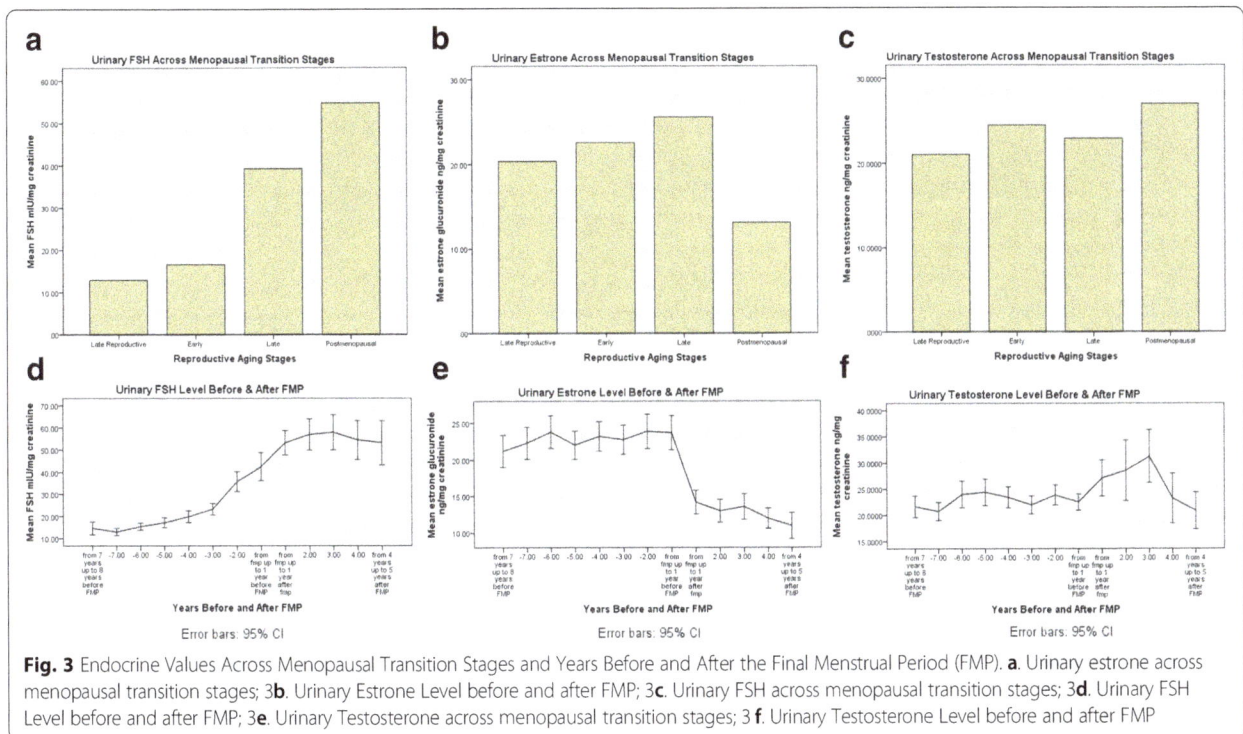

Fig. 3 Endocrine Values Across Menopausal Transition Stages and Years Before and After the Final Menstrual Period (FMP). **a**. Urinary estrone across menopausal transition stages; 3**b**. Urinary Estrone Level before and after FMP; 3**c**. Urinary FSH across menopausal transition stages; 3**d**. Urinary FSH Level before and after FMP; 3**e**. Urinary Testosterone across menopausal transition stages; 3 **f**. Urinary Testosterone Level before and after FMP

when it leveled off to at least 5 years FMP. Estrone showed a drop in level within 1 year before FMP and then slowly continued to decline to at least 5 years after FMP. Testosterone began to rise within 1 year before FMP, peaked at 3 year after FMP and declined steadily to at least 5 years after FMP (See Figs. 3 d,e,f).

Because of the important relationship of stress during midlife to symptoms, urinary **cortisol** was studied. The findings showed an increase in cortisol in the 7 to 12 months after onset of Late stage compared to the 7 to 12 months before onset of Late stage [20]. Also, women with increased cortisol levels during the Late stage had more severe hot flashes than those without a cortisol increase during the same stage [20]. In another study of cortisol using multilevel modeling there was a significant positive relationship between urinary epinephrine, norepinephrine, estrone, FSH, testosterone and hot flashes with cortisol levels in a univariate model. Health-related and social factors and symptoms other than hot flashes did not show a significant effect on cortisol levels. When the significant variables were combined in a multivariate model only estrone and FSH had a significant effect on cortisol [25].

An inspection of changes in urinary cortisol revealed a rise in the late MT stage, as seen in earlier analyses (See Fig. 4a) [15] and inspection revealed a gradual increase from 7 years before to 5 years after FMP (Fig. 4b). An inspection of urinary epinephrine and norepinephrine levels across MT stages showed a minimal change in epinephrine across stages and a slight rise in norepinephrine from

Early MT stage to early PM (Fig. 4 c and d). When a multilevel analysis of these catecholamines across MT stage was done no significant effect of stage was found on epinephrine or on norepinephrine (unpublished data). In contrast, when number of years before and after FMP were examined, epinephrine showed no definitive pattern while norepinephrine slowly rose from 8 years before FMP to 5 years after FMP (Fig. 4 e and f).

Well-being and the menopausal transition
General well-being as measured by the 4 item subscale of the General Well-Being Scale [41] was positively associated with satisfaction with social support and a sense of mastery [27]. A decrease in well-being was associated with negative life events. Being in Late Stage of MT was associated with a decrease in well-being only in the univariate analysis.

Symptom patterns across the menopausal transition
Because the primary end points throughout the SMWHS were symptoms, of interest was identifying effects of MT stages on various types of symptoms. In addition, we used a general model (See Fig. 1) to guide analyses of women's symptom experiences over time that included the following concepts and examples of indicators for each: menopausal transition factors, aging, health-related factors, stress-related factors, and other co-occurring symptoms. In the following paragraphs, findings related to each of the symptom groups studied are summarized.

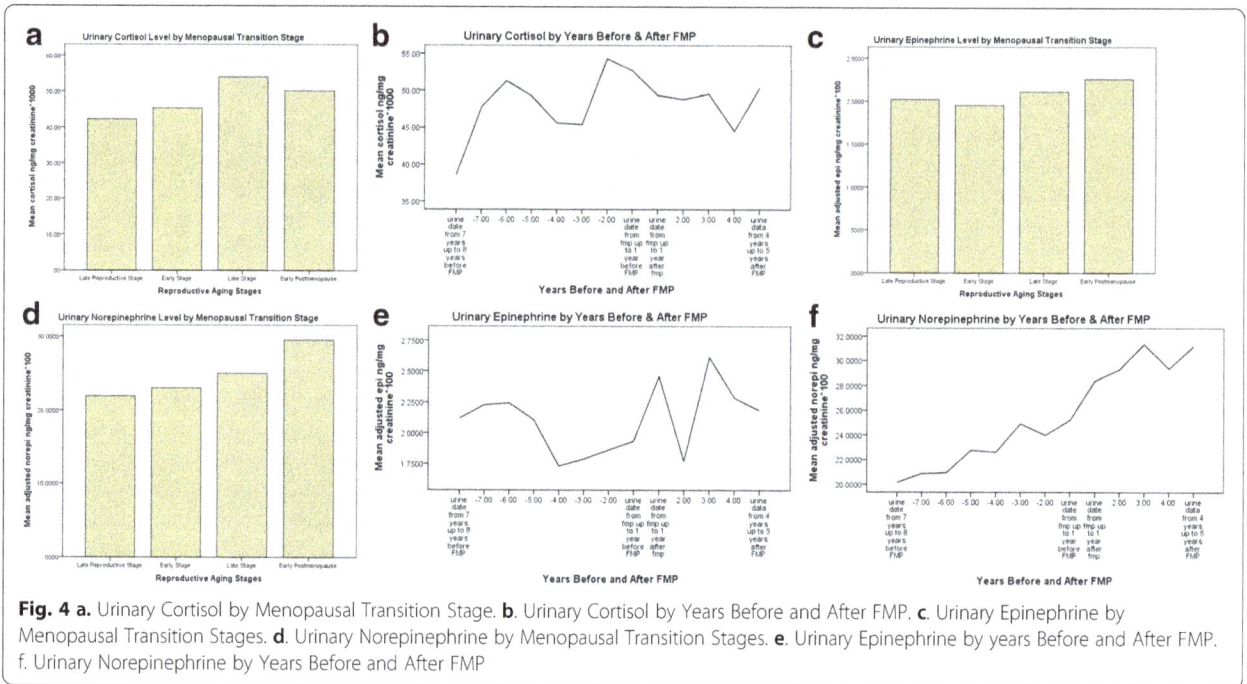

Fig. 4 a. Urinary Cortisol by Menopausal Transition Stage. **b**. Urinary Cortisol by Years Before and After FMP. **c**. Urinary Epinephrine by Menopausal Transition Stages. **d**. Urinary Norepinephrine by Menopausal Transition Stages. **e**. Urinary Epinephrine by years Before and After FMP. f. Urinary Norepinephrine by Years Before and After FMP

Hot flashes

An analysis of women using and not using hormone therapy (HT) revealed that increases in hot flash severity were associated with late transition stage, early postmenopause, use of HT, duration of early transition stage, age of entry into early PM and level of FSH. Age of entry into early transition and estrone levels were associated with decreased hot flash severity. Not associated with hot flash severity were being in early transition stage, age of entry into or duration of late transition stage and all of the psychosocial (anxiety, stress, depressed mood) and lifestyle variables (BMI, activity level, sleep, alcohol use). Use of HT ameliorated but did not eliminate severe hot flashes [23].

Hot flash severity persisted through the MT stages, peaking in the Late MT stage and diminishing only after the second year PM. Hot flash severity was associated with being older, being in the Late MT stage or early PM, beginning the Late MT stage at a younger age and reporting greater anxiety. In a model including only endocrine factors, hot flash severity was significantly associated with higher FSH and lower estrone levels [34].

Sleep symptoms

Severity of **nighttime awakening** was significantly associated with age, Late MT stage and early PM, higher FSH, lower E1G, more severe hot flashes, depressed mood, anxiety, joint pain, backache, and perceived stress, history of sexual abuse, poorer perceived health, and less alcohol use [30]. Severity of **problems going to sleep** was associated with hot flashes, depressed mood,

anxiety, joint pain, backache, perceived stress, history of sexual abuse, poorer perceived health, less alcohol use, and lower cortisol, but not with MT stages or hormone levels. Severity of **early morning awakening** was significantly associated with age, hot flashes, depressed mood anxiety, joint pain, backache, perceived stress, history of sexual abuse, poorer perceived health, but not MT stages, estrone, or FSH.

Depressed mood

Most women experienced the MT without a high level of depressed mood. A small group of women experienced worsening of their mood. Another small group experienced improvement in their mood [19]. Women with consistently depressed mood were more likely to have hot flashes, stress, history of premenstrual syndrome and postpartum blues than women with occasional depressed mood or those without depressed mood [19, 42].

Depressed mood symptoms (measured by CES-D scores) were associated with being in the Late MT stage, severity of hot flashes, life stress, family history of depression, history of postpartum blues, sexual abuse history, body mass index, and use of antidepressants. Hormonal levels and age of entry into and duration of Late MT stage were unrelated [24]. In another multivariate analysis, when covariates were examined individually, a decrease in depressed mood as a single symptom was associated with early PM, higher estrone, more exercise and being partnered. An increase in depressed mood was associated with perceived stress, a history of sexual abuse and more severe sleep disruption symptoms (problem getting to sleep, awakening at night, early morning awakening). FSH level, BMI, alcohol use, number of live births and hot flash severity were not associated with depressed mood. In a model with multiple covariates that individually had a significant effect, awakening at night no longer significantly increased depressed mood. Also, estrone level and early PM were no longer associated with a decrease in depressed mood [Mitchell, ES and Woods, NF Depressed Mood during the Menopausal Transition, Reproductive Aging and Life: Observations from the Seattle Midlife Women's Health Study. Unpublished].

Cognitive symptoms

Women in the Late Reproductive and Early MT stages and those who used hormones reported more problems with memory measured by the Memory Functioning Questionnaire than women in Late stage [18]. About 72 % of women reported problems remembering names at least some of the time. About 50 % had a problem remembering where they put things, recent phone numbers, things others told them (or they told others), keeping up correspondence and forgetting what they were doing. However, none of these events was considered a serious problem [18]. Many types of problems with memory were related to lower ratings of health and depressed mood. Problems with current memory and remembering past events were associated with higher levels of reported stress, which women attributed to the burden of meeting multiple role demands [18].

Memory changes most noted by women (mean age 47 years) who responded to open-ended questions about their memory were difficulty remembering words or numbers, i.e., verbal memory. These changes were attributed to increased role burden and stress, getting older, physical health, menstrual cycle changes/hormones, inadequate concentration, and emotional factors [15].

As individual covariates and in a multivariate model, age, anxiety, depressed mood, night-time awakening, perceived stress, perceived health, and employment were each significantly related to **difficulty concentrating**. Hot flashes, amount of exercise and history of sexual abuse had a significant effect as individual covariates but not in the final multivariate model. The best predictors of forgetfulness when analyzed as individual covariates and in the multivariate model were age, hot flashes, anxiety, depressed mood, perceived stress, perceived health and history of sexual abuse [32].

Pain symptoms

Pain symptoms rose slightly with age. A significant increase in **back pain** was reported during the Early and Late MT stages and early PM, but urinary E1G, FSH and testosterone levels were unrelated. Of the stress-related factors, perceived stress and lower overnight urinary cortisol levels were associated with more severe back pain; history of sexual abuse and catecholamines did not have a significant effect. Women most troubled by symptoms of hot flashes, depressed mood, anxiety, night-time awakening, and difficulty concentrating reported significantly greater back pain. Of the health-related factors, having worse perceived health, exercising more, using analgesics, and having a higher body mass index were associated with more back pain, but alcohol use and smoking did not have significant effects. Of the social factors, only having more years of formal education was associated with less back pain; parenting, having a partner, and employment did not have significant. Factors associated with joint pain included age but not menopausal transition-related factors. Symptoms of hot flashes, night-time awakening, depressed mood, and difficulty concentrating were each significantly associated with **joint pain**. Poorer perceived health, more exercise, higher body mass index, and greater analgesic use were all associated positively with joint pain. History of sexual abuse was the only stress-related factor significantly related to joint pain severity [29].

Sexual desire symptoms

Women's concerns about decreasing sexual desire during midlife prompted analysis of factors influencing sexual desire as recorded in the symptom diaries. Women reported a significant reduction in sexual desire during the Late MT stage and early PM. Those with higher urinary E1G and T reported significantly higher levels of sexual desire whereas those with higher FSH levels reported significantly lower sexual desire. Women using hormone therapy also reported higher sexual desire. Those reporting higher perceived stress reported lower sexual desire, but having a history of sexual abuse did not have a significant effect. Those most troubled by symptoms of hot flashes, fatigue, depressed mood, anxiety, difficulty getting to sleep, early morning awakening, and awakening during the night also reported significantly lower sexual desire, but there was no effect of vaginal dryness. Women with better perceived health and those reporting more exercise and more alcohol intake also reported greater sexual desire. Having a partner was associated with lower sexual desire [26].

Urinary incontinence symptoms

Stress urinary incontinence (SUI) was associated significantly with individual predictors of worse perceived health, history of ≥3 live births, being in the Early MT stage, having less formal education and being white. **Urge incontinence** (UUI) was associated significantly with individual predictors of increasing age, worse perceived health, BMI ≥30, history of ≥3 live births, and lower FSH levels. Both SUI and UUI were significantly associated with lower self-esteem and with age included in the models as a measure of time. UI effects on mood symptoms, attitudes toward aging and menopause, perceived health and consequences for daily life were not significant [22, 33].

Interference of symptoms with work and relationships
Women reported the effects of their symptoms on work and relationships in the symptom diary. Analyses of the extent to which symptoms interfered with daily living revealed that **interference with work** was significantly associated with perceived health, stress, hot flashes, depressed mood, anxiety, difficulty getting to sleep, awakening during the night, early morning awakening, backache, joint pain, forgetfulness and difficulty concentrating. **Interference with relationships** was significantly associated with age and individual covariates perceived health, estrone, perceived stress, depressed mood, anxiety, sleep symptoms, backache, joint pain, forgetfulness and difficulty concentrating [31].

Genetic influences and the menopausal transition
Polymorphisms in the estrogen synthesizing, metabolizing, and receptor genes were genotyped and associated with both symptoms and the timing of the events of the MT. Women with the CYP19 11r polymorphism reported more severe and frequent hot flashes during the Early and Late MT stages and early PM and higher E1G levels during Early and Late stages. [43]. In addition, polymorphisms in the 17 beta HSD gene (rs 5942 and rs 2389) were related to a symptom cluster incuding high severity hot flashes and moderate levels of 5 other symptom groups (sleep, mood, cognitive, pain symptoms). Moreover the rs2389 heterozygous allele had a significant positive effect on estrone and rs2830 homozygous mutant allele had a significant negative effect on FSH. The rs5942 17 HSD had no effect on either estrone or FSH (unpublished data).

Women with two CYP19 7r alleles had menarche earlier (11.5 y) than those with one CYP19 7r allele (13.1 y). Women with two CYP19 11r alleles were 2 years older at onset of Late stage than those with one CYP19 11r allele (50.7 y vs 48.6 y). Those with two CYP19 7r(−3) alleles were 2 years older at FMP than those without this allele (53.9 y vs 51.3 y). Women with the homozygous wild-type allele for HSDB1 (rs2830) were younger at FMP by 2 years than those with the heterozygous allele (50.8 y vs 52.9 y). Women with the heterozygous allele for CYP1B1*2 had a later age at menarche compared with women with the homozygous wild type (13 y vs 12.5 y). [44].

Stress and symptoms during the menopausal transition
Although some would contend that the MT is inherently stressful, factors that influenced the level of perceived stress among SMWHS participants were inadequate income to meet needs, lower levels of perceived health

status, role burden and current employment [28]. Of interest was that perceived stress was related to each of the symptoms studied: hot flashes, depressed mood, lower sexual desire, difficulty getting to sleep, night-time awakening, early morning awakening, forgetfulness, difficulty concentrating, but not urinary incontinence symptoms. Perceived stress was not related to MT stage nor to the endocrine assays measured, including E1G, FSH, cortisol, and the catecholamines.

Symptom clusters associated with the menopausal transition
Analyses of each of the symptoms studied indicated they were commonly associated with other symptoms, e.g. hot flashes with sleep problems, depressed mood, pain and cognitive symptoms. The realization that women experienced multiple, co-occurring symptoms (defined as symptom clusters) during the MT and early PM led to further study [45]. Three symptom clusters composed of hot flashes and five groups of symptoms that had been identified in prior factor analysis (depressed mood symptoms, sleep disruption symptoms, tension symptoms, cognitive symptoms, and pain symptoms) among this community-based cohort [46]. Cluster I was composed of low severity hot flashes with low severity sleep disruption symptoms, depressed mood symptoms, tension symptoms, cognitive symptoms and pain symptoms (75 %); Cluster II was high severity hot flashes with a moderate level of the 5 symptom clusters (12 %); and Cluster III was low severity hot flashes with moderate severity levels of the 5 symptom clusters (13 %). When each of the 3 clusters were compared with each other for estrone, FSH, testosterone, epinephrine and norepinephrine significant group differences were between Cluster I (low hot flash/low symptom clusters) and Cluster III (high hot flash/moderate symptom clusters), and between Cluster I and Cluster II (low hot flash/moderate symptom clusters). Cluster III had lower estrone, higher FSH, lower epinephrine and higher norepinephrine than Cluster I and Cluster II had lower epinephrine levels than Cluster I. Cortisol and testosterone had no significant group differences among the 3 clusters [47].

When perceived stress levels were compared among the 3 clusters, Clusters II and III had significantly higher levels than Cluster I (unpublished data). Finally, polymorphisms in estrogen synthesis, metabolism, and receptor genes were tested. Only the 17HSD polymorphisms (rs 5942 and rs 2389) significantly differentiated Cluster III from Cluster I. None of the polymorphisms differentiated Cluster II from I or Cluster II from III.

Conclusions and Discussion
Contributions of the SMWHS included:

- Development of a system for staging reproductive aging with emphasis on the period from the Late

Reproductive stage through the early PM and establishment of the validity of the staging system with the ReSTAGE Collaboration and contributions to the Staging Reproductive Aging Workshop and STRAW + 10 [48];

- Incorporation of the staging system into the study of endocrine changes during the MT stages and early PM, including demonstration of changes in estrone, FSH, testosterone, cortisol, epinephrine and norepinephrine by MT stages and PM;
- Integration of the staging system into models of symptoms including hot flashes, sleep disturbances, depressed mood, pain, cognitive symptoms, incontinence, and sexual desire;
- Confirmation of effects of the MT stages and early PM on the following symptoms: hot flashes, awakening during the night, back pain, and sexual desire, but not on depressed mood, cognitive symptoms, incontinence, or joint pain;
- Identification of functional effects of symptoms on interference with work and relationships, in particular, effects of depressed mood and difficulty concentrating on work and depressed mood, anxiety, difficulty concentrating, and awakening during the night on relationships;
- Demonstration of effects of gene polymorphisms CYP 19 11r, 17 beta HSD (rs 2389 and 5942) in estrogen synthesizing genes on hot flashes as well as CYP 19 7r, CYP 19 7r(−3), 17 beta HSD (rs 2830) and estrogen metabolizing gene CYP 1B1*2 on events related to menarche and the MT; and
- Identification of naturally occurring symptom clusters and their relationship to endocrine levels (estrone, FSH), perceived stress, epinephrine, norepinephrine levels, and 17 beta HSD genotypes.

Results of this study can be generalized to women experiencing the natural menopausal transition and early postmenopause and who were not using hormone therapy. Limitations of the SMWHS included a predominantly White and well-educated sample, despite efforts to include Asian American and African American women. Another limitation was the smaller sample size relative to larger studies, such as the Study of Women and Health Across the Nation (SWAN) The limitation of sample size was compensated in part by the more frequent occasions of measurement, with some measures obtained several times per year. In addition, SMWHS was a longitudinal population-based study that enabled analysis of patterns observed in symptoms over time, up to 23 years for some participants. Efforts to recruit and retain a multi-ethnic sample were effective initially, but with waning retention during the latter years of the study. In addition, the development and application of

specific criteria for staging the MT and analyzing data to examine effects of MT stages supported our ability to distinguish between endocrine factors, stress, and symptoms that were influenced by MT stages versus those who were not [44].

Issues for further study suggested by SMWHS included the importance of studying clusters of symptoms vs single symptoms and the need for interventions targeting multiple symptoms. We have begun examination of non-pharmacologic therapies that may be effective for clusters of symptoms vs individual symptoms [49–52]. In the interim, this research is being incorporated in the clinical education of women's health care providers [53].

Abbreviations
BMI: Body mass index; CYP: Cytochrome P450; E1G: Estrone; FMP: Final menstrual period; FSH: Follicle-stimulating hormone; HSD: Hydroxy steroid dehydrogenase; HT: Hormone therapy; MLM: Multi-level modeling; MT: Menopausal transition; PM: Postmenopause; SMWHS: Seattle Midlife Women's Health Study; STRAW: Staging Reproductive Aging Workshop; SUI: Stress urinary incontinence

Acknowledgements
We acknowledge the contribution of the participants who provided data for the Seattle Midlife Women's Health Study, some for over 20 years. Only the authors of this paper contributed to this manuscript.

Funding
- National Institute for Nursing Research, NIH, R01- NR 04141 need title
- National Institute for Nursing Research, NIH, P50-NR-02323, P30-NR04001 Center for Women's Health Research.
- National Institute of Environmental Health Sciences P30-07033 Center for Ecogenetics and Environmental Health.
- National Institute for Nursing Research R21-NR012218 Symptom Clusters during the Menopausal Transition and Early Postmenopause.
- Pfizer, Inc., Medical Division Research Grant (Pfizer, Inc, Medical Division. #WS1752232. Urinary Incontinence during the Menopausal Transition and Early Postmenopause.
- Research Intramural Funding Program, University of Washington School of Nursing.

Authors' contributions
Nancy Fugate Woods and Ellen Sullivan Mitchell both contributed to writing the manuscript. Both authors read and approved the final manuscript.

Authors' information
NFW and ESM: Study Design and Principal Investigator of the Seattle Midlife Women's Health Study. Over the course of the entire study NFW and ESM rotated roles as principal investigator.

Competing interests
The authors declare they have no competing interests.

Author details
[1]Department of Biobehavioral Nursing, University of Washington, Seattle, WA 98195, USA. [2]Department of Family and Child Nursing, University of Washington, Seattle, WA98195USA.

References
1. U. S. Public Health Services. Opportunities for Research on Women's Health. Bethesda: National Institutes of Health; 1992.
2. McKinlay S, Brambilla D, Posner J. The normal menopause transition. Maturitas. 1992;14(2):103–15.
3. Matthews K, Wing R, Kuller L, et al. Influences of natural menopause on psychological characteristics and symptoms of middle-aged healthy women. J Consult Clin Psychol. 1990;58:345–51.
4. Woods N, Lentz M, Mitchell ES, Heitkemper M, Shaver J. PMS after 40: Persistence of a stress-related symptom pattern. Res Nurs Health. 1997;20:329–40.
5. Woods NF, Lentz MJ, Mitchell ES, Shaver J, Heitkemper M. Luteal phase ovarian steroids, stress arousal, premenses perceived stress and premenstrual symptoms. Res Nurs Health. 1998;21:129–42.
6. Woods N, Lentz M, Mitchell E, Heitkemper M, Shaver J, Henker R. Perceived stress, physiologic stress arousal, and premenstrual symptoms: Group differences and intra-individual patterns. Res Nurs Health. 1998;21:511–23.
7. Woods NF, Shaver JF. The evolutionary spiral of a specialized center for women's health research. Image. 1992;24:229–34.
8. Woods NF, Mitchell ES. Patterns of depressed mood in midlife women: Observations from the Seattle Midlife Women's Health Study. Res Nurs Health. 1996;19:111–23.
9. Belsey EM, Farley TMM. The analysis of menstrual bleeding patterns: A review. Applied Stochastic Models Data Analysis. 1987;3:125–50.
10. Treloar AE. Variation of the human menstrual cycle through reproductive life. Int J Fertil. 1967;12:77–126.
11. Mitchell ES, Woods NF, Mariella A. Three stages of the menopausal transition: Toward a more precise definition. Menopause. 2000;7:334–49.
12. Harlow SD, Crawford S, Dennerstein L, Burger HG, Mitchell ES, Sowers MF for the ReSTAGE Collaboration. Recommendations from a multi-study evaluation of proposed criteria for Staging Reproductive Aging. Climacteric. 2007;10:112–9.
13. Mitchell ES, Woods NF. Symptom experiences of midlife women: Observations from the Seattle Midlife Women's Health Study. Maturitas. 1996;25:1–10.
14. Woods NF, Mitchell ES. Pathways to depressed mood for midlife women: Observations from the Seattle Midlife Women's Health Study. Res Nurs Health. 1997;20:119–29.
15. Mitchell ES, Woods NF. Midlife women's attributions about perceived memory changes: Observations from the Seattle Midlife Women's Health Study. J Womens Health Gend Based Med. 2001;10:351–62.
16. Woods NF, Mitchell ES. Women's images of midlife: Observations from the Seattle Midlife Women's Health Study". Health Care Women Int. 1997;18:439–53.
17. Woods NF, Mitchell ES. Anticipating menopause: Observations from the Seattle Midlife Women's Health Study. Menopause. 1999;6:167–73.
18. Woods NF, Mitchell ES, Adams C. Memory functioning among midlife women: Observations from the Seattle Midlife Women's Health Study. Menopause. 2000;7:257–65.
19. Woods NF, Mariella AM, Mitchell ES. Patterns of depressed mood across the menopausal transition: Approaches to studying patterns in longitudinal data. Acta Obstet Gynecol Scand. 2002;81:623–32.
20. Woods NF, Carr MC, Tao EY, Taylor HJ, Mitchell ES. Increased urinary cortisol levels during the menopausal transition. Menopause. 2006;13(2):212–21.
21. Woods NF, Smith-DiJulio K, Percival DB, Tao EY, Taylor HJ, Mitchell ES. Symptoms during the menopausal transition and early postmenopause and their relation to endocrine levels over time: Observations from the Seattle Midlife Women's Health Study. J Women's Health. 2007;16:667–77.
22. Mitchell ES, Woods NF. Correlates of Urinary Incontinence during the Menopausal Transition and Early Postmenopause: Observations from the Seattle Midlife Women's Health Study. Climacteric. 2013;16:653–62.
23. Smith-diJulio K, Percival DB, Woods NF, Tao EY, Mitchell ES. Hot flash severity in hormone therapy users/nonusers across the menopausal transition. Maturitas. 2007;58:191–200.
24. Woods NF, Smith-diJulio K, Percival DB, Tao EY, Mariella A, Mitchell ES. Depressed mood during the menopausal transition and early postmenopause: Observations from the Seattle Midlife Women's Health Study. Menopause. 2008;15:223–32.
25. Woods NF, Smith-DiJulio K, Percival DB, Mitchell ES. Cortisol Levels during the Menopausal Transition and Early Postmenopause: Observations from the Seattle Midlife Women's Health Study. Menopause. 2009;16:708–18.
26. Woods NF, Mitchell ES, Smith-DiJulio K. Sexual desire during the menopausal transition and early postmenopause Observations from the Seattle Midlife Women's Health Study. J Women's Health. 2010;19:2098–217.
27. Smith-DiJulio K, Woods NF, Mitchell ES. Well-being during the menopausal transition and early postmenopause: A longitudinal analysis. Menopause. 2008;15:1095–102.
28. Woods NF, Mitchell ES, Percival DB, Smith-DiJulio K. Is the menopausal transition stressful? Observations of perceived stress from the Seattle Midlife Women's Health Study. Menopause. 2009;16:90–7.
29. Mitchell ES, Woods NF. Pain symptoms during the menopausal and early postmenopause: Observations from the Seattle Midlife Women's Health Study. Climacteric. 2010;13:467–78.
30. Woods NF, Mitchell ES, Smith-DiJulio K. Sleep symptoms during the menopausal transition and early postmenopause Observations from the Seattle Midlife Women's Health Study. Sleep. 2010;33:539–49.
31. Woods NF, Mitchell ES. Symptom interference with work and relationships during the menopausal transition and early postmenopause: Observations from the Seattle Midlife Women's Health Study. Menopause. 2011;18:654–61.
32. Mitchell ES, Woods NF. Cognitive symptoms during the menopausal transition and early postmenopause: Observations from the Seattle Midlife Women's Health Study. Climacteric. 2011;14:252–61.
33. Woods NF, Mitchell ES. Consequences of incontinence for women during the menopausal transition and early postmenopause: Observations from the Seattle Midlife Women's Health Study. Menopause. 2013;20:915–21.
34. Mitchell ES, Woods NF. Hot flush severity during the menopausal transition and early postmenopause: beyond hormones. Climacteric. 2015;18:536–44.
35. Development Core Team. R: A Language and Environment for Statistical Computing. Vienna, Austria: R Foundation for Statistical Computing, 2005. Available at: http://www.R-project.org. Accessed 13 June 2007.
36. Soules MR, Sherman S, Parrott E, Rebar R, Santoro N, Utian W, Woods NF. Executive summary: Stages of Reproductive Aging Workshop (STRAW). Fertil Steril. 2001;76:874–78.
37. Harlow SD for the ReSTAGE Collaboration (in alphabetical order), Cain K, Crawford S, Dennerstein L, Little R, Mitchell ES, Nan B, Randolph J, Taffe J, Yosef M. Evaluation of four proposed bleeding criteria for the onset of late menopausal transition. J Clin Endocrinol Metab. 2006;91:3432–8. [PMID: 16772350] PMCID:PMC1950694.
38. Harlow SD, Mitchell ES, Crawford S, Nan B, Little R, Taffe J, ReSTAGE Collaboration. The ReSTAGE Collaboration: Defining Optimal Bleeding Criteria for the Onset of Early Menopausal Transition. Fertility Sterility. 2008;89:129–40.
39. Harlow S, Cain K, Crawford S, Dennerstein L, Little R, Mitchell E, Nan B, Randolph J, Taffe J, Yosef M. Evaluation of four proposed bleeding criteria for the onset of late menopausal transition. J Clin Endocrinol Metabol. 2006;91(9):3432–8.
40. Smith-DiJulio K, Mitchell ES, Woods NF. Concordance of retrospective and prospective reporting of menstrual irregularity by women in the menopausal transition. Climacteric. 2005;8:390–7.
41. Brook RH, Ware Jr JE, Davies-Avery A, Stewart AL, Donald CA, Rogers WH, et al. Overview of adult health measures fielded in Rand's health insurance study, ch 6. Findings Conclusions Medical Care. 1979;17:16–55.
42. Woods NF, Mariella A, Mitchell ES. Depressed mood symptoms during the menopausal transition: Observations from the Seattle Midlife Women's Health Study. Climacteric. 2006;9:195–203.
43. Woods NF, Mitchell ES, Tao Y, Viernes HM, Stapleton PL, Farin FM. Polymorphisms in the Estrogen Synthesis and Metabolism Pathways and Symptoms during the Menopausal Transition: Observations from the Seattle Midlife Women's Health Study. Menopause. 2006;13:902–10.
44. Mitchell ES, Farin FM, Stapleton PL, Tsai JM, Tao EY, Smith-DiJulio K, Woods NF. Association of estrogen-related polymorphisms with age at menarche,

age at final menstrual period and stages of the menopausal transition. Menopause. 2008;15:105–11.

45.   Cray LA, Woods NF, Herting JR, Mitchell ES. Symptom clusters during the late reproductive stage through the early postmenopause: Observations from the Seattle Midlife Women's Health Study. Menopause. 2012;2012(19):864–9.

46.   Cray LA, Woods NF, Mitchell ES. Identifying symptom clusters during the menopausal transition: Observations from the Seattle Midlife Women's Health Study. Climacteric. 2013;16:539–49.

47.   Woods NF, Cray L, Mitchell ES, Herting JR. Endocrine biomarkers and symptom clusters during the menopausal transition and early postmenopause: observations from the Seattle Midlife Women's Health Study. Menopause. 2014;21:646–52.

48.   Woods NF, Mitchell ES. Staging reproductive aging: contemporary research applications of Staging Reproductive Aging Workshop and Staging Reproductive Aging Workshop + 10. Menopause. 2013;20:717–8.

49.   Taylor-Swanson L, Thomas A, Ismail R, Schnall JG, Cray L, Mitchell ES, Woods NF. Effects of traditional Chinese medicine on symptom clusters during the menopausal transition. Climacteric. 2015;18:142–56.

50.   Ismail R, Taylor-Swanson L, Thomas A, Schnall JG, Cray L, Mitchell ES, Woods NF. Effects of herbal preparations on symptom clusters during the menopausal transition. Climacteric. 2015;18:11–28.

51.   Thomas AJ, Ismail R, Taylor-Swanson L, Cray L, Schnall JG, Mitchell ES, Woods NF. Effects of isoflavones and amino acid therapies for hot flashes and co-occurring symptoms during the menopausal transition and early postmenopause: a systematic review. Maturitas. 2015;78:263–76.

52.   Woods NF, Mitchell ES, Schnall JG, Cray L, Ismail R, Taylor-Swanson L, Thomas A. Effects of mind-body therapies on symptom clusters during the menopausal transition. Climacteric. 2014;17:10–22.

53.   Woods NF, Berg J, Mitchell ES. Midlife Women's Health. In: Alexander I, Kostos-Polsten E, Mallard VJ, Fogel C, Woods NF, editors. Women's Health Care in Advanced Practice Nursing. New York: Springer Publishing; 2017. pp. 155-190.

15

Is in utero exposure to maternal socioeconomic disadvantage related to offspring ovarian reserve in adulthood?

Maria E. Bleil[1*], Paul English[2], Jhaqueline Valle[2], Nancy F. Woods[3], Kyle D. Crowder[4], Steven E. Gregorich[5] and Marcelle I. Cedars[6]

Abstract

Background: Because the ovarian follicle pool is established in utero, adverse exposures during this period may be especially impactful on the size and health of the initial follicle endowment, potentially shaping trajectories of ovarian follicle loss and the eventual onset of menopause. Building on a robust literature linking socioeconomic status (SES) and menopausal timing, the current study examined adverse prenatal exposures related to maternal SES, hypothesizing that greater maternal socioeconomic disadvantage would be associated with lower ovarian reserve in the adult offspring.

Methods: In a healthy, community-based sub-sample ($n = 350$) of reproductive age participants in the OVA Study (2006–2011), prenatal maternal SES was examined in relation to two biomarkers of ovarian reserve, antimullerian hormone (AMH) and antral follicle count (AFC). Prenatal maternal SES was assessed indirectly using maternal addresses abstracted from participant birth certificates, geocoded, and linked to US Census-derived variables, including neighborhood-level characteristics: education (% of individuals with a HS diploma); poverty (% of families below the poverty line); unemployment (% of individuals > 16 years who are unemployed); and income (median family income).

Results: In separate covariate-adjusted linear regression models (following the backward elimination of main effects with $P > .10$), greater maternal neighborhood education was related to higher ovarian reserve as marked by higher levels of offspring AMH (beta = .142, $P < .001$) and AFC (beta = .092, $P < .10$) with models accounting for 19.6% and 21.5% of the variance in AMH and AFC, respectively. In addition, greater maternal neighborhood poverty was related to lower ovarian reserve as marked by lower offspring AMH (beta = −.144, $P < .01$), with the model accounting for 19.5% of the variance in AMH.

Conclusions: Maternal socioeconomic disadvantage measured indirectly at the neighborhood level was associated with lower ovarian reserve among the adult offspring, independently of offspring SES and other potential confounding factors. This suggests SES-related adversity exposures may have a detrimental impact on the size or health of the initial follicle endowment, leading to accelerated follicle loss over time.

Keywords: Ovarian reserve, Ovarian aging, Menopause, Antral follicle count (AFC), Antimullerian hormone (AMH), Socioeconomic status (SES), Poverty, Neighborhood

* Correspondence: mbleil@uw.edu
[1]Department of Family and Child Nursing, University of Washington, Box 357262, Seattle, WA 98195, USA
Full list of author information is available at the end of the article

Background

Younger age at menopause has been associated with an increase in cardiovascular risk for outcomes including ischemic heart disease, stroke, atherosclerosis, and cardiac-specific mortality which together account for a significant proportion of morbidity and mortality among women in the postmenopausal period [1–12]. The study of menopausal timing is limited, however, as menopause by definition is determined retrospectively after which time intervention is not possible [13]. Alternatively, recent methodological advances are enabling the examination of the real-time loss of ovarian follicles underlying variability in the timing of menopause, termed "ovarian aging" [14–16]. Using such methods by which the number of ovarian follicles remaining in the primordial pool (or ovarian reserve) is estimated, it is possible—for the first time—to characterize trajectories of ovarian aging over the life course. Recent work suggests, in parallel to findings in the menopausal timing literature, that even among younger, pre-menopausal women, more accelerated ovarian aging may be similarly associated with an increase in cardiovascular risk [17–21]. In this context, elucidating factors that explain variability in ovarian aging is of critical importance as it raises the possibility that such factors may be modified through intervention efforts specifically targeting the slowing of ovarian aging and/or the amelioration of its sequelae in at-risk women.

Socioeconomic status (SES) is one factor that has emerged has a reliable predictor of menopausal timing (see Gold [22]). Review of this literature shows almost one dozen studies reporting a prospective and independent effect of greater socioeconomic disadvantage on earlier menopause [23–33]. In summary, study findings suggest 1) indicators of lower SES predict earlier onset peri-menopause and menopause; 2) SES effects on earlier onset menopause are largely independent of confounding factors (e.g., smoking); and 3) the timing of lower SES exposures over time may be important. Regarding timing, studies show low SES across periods of childhood *and* adulthood conferred greatest risk, with women experiencing peri-menopause and menopause 1.2 and 1.7 years earlier, respectively, than their high SES counterparts [26, 33]. It remains unclear, however, whether it is the longer period of exposure that is important or whether there are sensitive developmental periods when exposures may be more impactful [34–39]. Notably, because the ovarian follicle pool is established in utero, exposures during this time may be especially relevant. In fact, a range of prenatal exposures (e.g., famine exposure, maternal pre-pregnancy diabetes, maternal smoking during pregnancy, multiple birth status, and both low and high birthweight) has been shown to predict earlier menopause in adult offspring [40–45] and, in the only study to examine a biomarker of ovarian aging (anti-mullerian hormone [AMH]), prenatal paternal smoking and

maternal gestational weight gain were related to lower AMH (indexing lower ovarian reserve) while pre-pregnancy maternal history of menstrual cycle irregularity was related to higher AMH (indexing higher ovarian reserve) in adolescent offspring [46]. To date, however, no studies have examined prenatal SES-related exposures in particular.

The biological underpinnings of ovarian aging and the eventual onset of menopause reflect a complex set of processes related to 1) the initial endowment of primordial follicles occurring in utero and 2) the continuous growth of follicles beginning at the time of the initial endowment and continuing until menopause (see McGee & Hsueh [47]). Follicle growth termed "folliculogenesis" describes the progression whereby dormant primordial follicles enter the pool of growing follicles, maturing through several stages of development with the majority of follicles ultimately lost through atresia (via apoptosis) [47]. Only at puberty are a subset of these follicles rescued (via high levels of circulating follicle stimulating hormone [FSH]) with one follicle becoming dominant in preparation for the release and potential fertilization of a mature oocyte [47]. Estimates indicate that approximately 5 million follicles are present at mid-gestation, decreasing to approximately 1 million follicles at birth, 400,000 at menarche, and 10,000 at the beginning of the menopausal transition [48–50]. To date, the methodological challenges of studying ovarian follicle formation and loss have been a barrier to understanding how particular exposures may influence the size and health of the initial follicle endowment as well as the rate of ovarian follicle loss over time. As evidenced by the literatures described above, the majority of studies of prenatal exposures have been limited to the examination of ovarian aging as indexed by markers of menopausal timing [40–45], with only one study examining prenatal exposures in relation to AMH, a biochemical marker of ovarian reserve [46].

Building on the literatures described above, the current study focused on the sensitive period of follicle formation in utero by examining adverse prenatal exposures related to maternal SES. We predicted greater maternal socioeconomic disadvantage would be associated with lower ovarian reserve in the adult offspring. This hypothesis was tested by leveraging a healthy, community-based sample of reproductive age participants in the Ovarian Aging (OVA) Study (2006–2011), an investigation in which ovarian aging was assessed using well established biomarkers of total ovarian reserve, including both a biochemical marker (AMH) and an ultrasound-derived marker (antral follicle count [AFC]). Prenatal maternal SES was assessed indirectly using maternal addresses abstracted from participant birth certificates, geocoded, and linked to US Census-derived variables, including neighborhood-level education, poverty, unemployment, and income. Effects of maternal neighborhood-level SES on ovarian reserve were estimated in multivariate models adjusted for current offspring SES (educational attainment) as well as other potential confounding factors, including maternal age and offspring characteristics (age, race/ethnicity, cigarette smoking, body mass index [BMI], menarcheal age, history of hormonal contraceptive use, and parity). The current study is unique insofar as two biomarkers of ovarian reserve (AFC, AMH) were examined and that the sample itself was healthy and regularly-cycling, eliminating confounding factors that were present in prior studies.

Methods
Participants
Women in the current sample were participants in the Ovarian Aging (OVA) Study, a community-based investigation of reproductive aging and its correlates [18, 51–53]. Women were recruited from Kaiser Permanente of Northern California, a large, integrated healthcare delivery system that provides medical care to approximately one third of the population of Northern California. The Kaiser Permanente membership compared to the population of Northern California is generally representative in its sociodemographic and health-related characteristics, especially when the comparison is limited to those with health insurance [54]. Selection criteria for the OVA Study were age 25–45 years; regular menses; having a uterus and both ovaries intact; self-identification as white, African American, Latina, Chinese, or Filipina; and ability to speak/read English, Spanish, or Cantonese. Exclusions were major medical illnesses (i.e., cardiovascular diseases, chronic kidney or liver disease, diabetes, invasive cancer, chemotherapy or radiation therapy, epilepsy, systemic lupus erythematosus, or HIV-positive status), use of medications affecting the menstrual cycle in the 3 months prior to study participation, and current pregnancy/breastfeeding.

The OVA Study protocol included an in-person medical history interview, transvaginal ultrasound, anthropometric assessment, blood draw, and self-report questionnaires. In addition, birth certificates were obtained for a subset of women born in the state of California. Maternal addresses were abstracted from the birth certificates, geocoded, and linked to tract-level neighborhood SES variables. Of 1019 total participants, 433 women were born in California. Of these 433 women, birth certificates for 417 women were located and addresses were abstracted for 409 women. Finally, of these 409 women, geocoding to the 2010 Census tract level was successful for 350 women, leaving a final sample of 350 women available for inclusion in the current analyses. Addresses that could not be geocoded to the tract level were the result of poor quality of the address data. Institutional review board approval was obtained from Kaiser Permanente, the University of California San Francisco, and the University of Washington.

Measures
Maternal neighborhood socioeconomic status (SES)
For a subset of participants in the OVA Study who were born in California, birth certificates were obtained from the California Department of Public Health Vital Records. Information on the birth certificates was abstracted, including maternal address and maternal age at the time of the participant's birth. Maternal addresses were then geocoded to 2010 Census tracts and crosswalks were used to map 2010 Census tracts to the appropriate earlier Census—1970, 1980, 1990, 2000. Because a crosswalk was not available for 1960 Census tracts, the 1970 Census was used for women born in the 1960's ($n = 98$). The majority of these women (82%) were born between years 1965 and 1969, supporting the use of the 1970 Census.

Census tracts were mapped to earlier censuses and census tract data were standardized using the Longitudinal Tract Database [55–57]. The LTDB uses population and area weighting to account for changes in the geographical boundaries of census tracts over time. The LTDB normalizes the census tract data from previous years to 2010 Census tract boundaries, allowing for comparison of data across censuses. Following the extraction of decennial values, linear interpolation methods were used to estimate annual values from the decennial data. SES-related variables, common to 5 US Censuses (1970, 1980, 1990, 2000, 2010), were extracted, including 1) *neighborhood-level education*: % of individuals with a high school diploma; 2) *neighborhood-level poverty*: % of families below the poverty line; 3) *neighborhood-level unemployment*: % of individuals > 16 years of age in the work force who were unemployed; and 4) *neighborhood-level income*: median family income. Prior to linear interpolation, median family income was adjusted for inflation to reflect 2010 dollars. Using the Consumer Price Index of the US Bureau of Labor Statistics, the adjustment (based on the percent change in price between indicated years) was computed by dividing the annual average Consumer Price Index for All Urban Consumers for 2010 by the annual average for the indicated earlier year.

Ovarian reserve
Antimullerian hormone (AMH). Blood was drawn from each study participant between menstrual cycle days 2 to 4. The concentration of AMH (ng/mL) was assayed using two commercially available enzyme-linked immunosorbent assays (ELISAs) from Beckman Coulter, both of which use a two-site sandwich immunoassay. The majority of the samples (85%) were assayed using the Immunotech assay until this assay was retired. The remainder of the samples were assayed using the second generation assay (Gen II). In a subset of 44 women in whom both assays were performed, regression analyses showed excellent correspondence between the assays ($R^2 = 0.94$), which has also been demonstrated in prior studies [58, 59]. The AMH values

based on the Immunotech assay were adjusted using the equation of the line with Immunotech predicting Gen II. Gen II assay sensitivity was 0.16 ng/mL, the intra-assay coefficient of variation (CV) was 1.4%, and the inter-assay CV was 12.5%.

Antral follicle count (AFC). Transvaginal ultrasound (TVUS) assessment of AFC was performed between menstrual cycle days 2 and 4 by one of two reproductive endocrinologists. The transverse, longitudinal, and anteroposterior diameters of each ovary were measured with electronic calipers using a Shimadzu SDU-450XL machine with a variable 4- to 8-mHz vaginal transducer. Follicles (defined as all echo-free structures in the ovaries) with a mean diameter across two dimensions of 2–10 mm were counted. Each measurement was taken twice and the average was taken. The total number of follicles across both ovaries was summed to calculate AFC. Evaluation of a sub-sample of 50 OVA study participants showed that inter-rater reliability between the two reproductive endocrinologists was excellent ($r = 0.92$) as was test-retest reliability for each reproductive endocrinologist measured over 2 consecutive months (average $r = 0.91$).

Analytical plan

Separate linear regression models were fit, examining each of four maternal neighborhood-level SES variables (education [% of individuals with a HS diploma]; poverty [% of families below the poverty line]; unemployment [% of individuals > 16 years who are unemployed]; and income [median family income]) in relation to each of two dependent measures, marking offspring ovarian reserve—AMH and AFC. In adjusted, multivariate models, all specified predictors were examined simultaneously, including all of the covariates of interest (age, maternal age, race/ethnicity, educational attainment, smoking, BMI, menarcheal age, hormonal contraceptive use, and parity) and each of the maternal neighborhood-level SES variables. The final multivariate models reflect the variables remaining after backward elimination of main effects with $P > .10$. The standardized linear regression parameters of these models are reported. Linear regression assumptions were evaluated by visual inspection and conventions for quantitative guidelines. These efforts revealed minor violations of assumptions (i.e., non-normality of residuals) that were accommodated by applying a square root transform on the positively skewed distributions of AMH and AFC.

The covariates were coded according to the following: Participant age and maternal age (abstracted from participants' birth certificates) was coded in years. Race/ethnicity categories (white, African-American, Latina, Chinese, and Filipina) were dummy coded into four (k-1) variables using white as the reference group. Participant educational

attainment categories (HS degree or less, some college, college degree, graduate degree) were dummy coded into three (k-1) variables using HS degree or less as the reference group. Cigarette smoking was coded (never smoked, current/past smoking) and BMI (kg/m^2) was logarithmically transformed to correct positive skew. Menarcheal age was coded in years, hormonal contraceptive use was coded (no history of use, positive history of use) and parity was coded (no live births, 1+ live births). Maternal neighborhood-level SES variables were examined as continuous variables in their original units.

Results

In Table 1, information pertaining to the sample sociodemographics characteristics, general health, ovarian reserve, reproductive factors, and maternal neighborhood-level SES is reported. The average age of the sample was 34.3 (5.6) and the average age of the participants' mothers at the time of their births (as derived from participant birth certificates) was 26.2 (5.8). The racial/ethnic composition of the sample was 24.9% white, 43.4% African-American, 14% Latina, 13.7% Chinese, and 4.0% Filipina. This distribution differs from the total OVA Study sample ($N = 1019$; 27.4% white, 24.1% African-American, 22.6% Latina, 21.9% Chinese, and 4.0% Filipina) due to the greater number of African-American women (vs. other race/ethnic groups) who were born in the state of California and, therefore, had a birth certificate available for analysis. The sample was well-educated with 58.3% of women holding a college degree or greater, compared to 33% of women at the US population level [60]. 28.9% smoked cigarettes currently or in the past and women on average were overweight (BMI = 29.2 [7.9] kg/m^2). Ovarian reserve indicators showed the average AMH level was 3.2 (2.6) ng/mL and the average number of antral follicles (AFC) was 15.7 (9.5). The majority of women (76%) used a hormonal form of birth control in the past and 40.6% gave birth to at least one child. Finally, examination of the neighborhoods of the participants' mothers at the time of their births (derived from US Census data), showed the percent of individuals with a HS diploma was 66.3% on average, the percent of families living below the poverty line was 11.7% on average, the percent of individuals who were unemployed was 8% on average, and the median family income adjusted to 2010 USD was $46,497 on average.

In Table 2, bivariate correlations of unadjusted associations between maternal neighborhood characteristics and offspring ovarian reserve markers, transformed AMH and AFC, are reported. Overall, bivariate correlations suggest that greater socioeconomic disadvantage in the neighborhoods of women during pregnancy is related to lower ovarian reserve among their adult offspring. Specifically, neighborhood-level education and family income was related positively to AMH ($r = .254$, $P < .001$, $r = .196$, P

Table 1 Sample characteristics ($n = 350$)

	Mean (SD)	Range	n (%)
Socio-demographics:			
Age (years)	34.3 (5.6)	25–45	–
Maternal age (years)	26.2 (5.8)	16–44	
Race/ethnicity:			
White (%)	–	–	87 (24.9)
African-American (%)	–	–	152 (43.4)
Latina (%)	–	–	49 (14.0)
Chinese (%)	–	–	48 (13.7)
Filipina (%)	–	–	14 (4.0)
Education:			
< High school (HS) (%)	–	–	7 (2.0)
HS degree (%)	–	–	38 (10.8)
Some college (%)	–	–	101 (28.9)
College degree (%)	–	–	139 (39.7)
Graduate degree (%)	–	–	65 (18.6)
General Health:			
Smoking (current/past) (%)	–	–	101 (28.9)
Body mass index (BMI) (kg/m^2)	29.2 (7.9)	17.1–58.4	–
Ovarian Reserve:			
Antimullerian hormone (AMH)	3.2 (2.6)	0.2–13.8	–
Antral follicle count (AFC)	15.7 (9.5)	0–49	–
Reproductive Factors:			
Menarcheal age (years)	12.4 (1.7)	8–17	–
History of hormonal contraceptive use (%)	–	–	266 (76.0)
Parity (1+ live births) (%)	–	–	142 (40.6)
Maternal Neighborhood (census-tract level):			
Education: % of individuals with a HS diploma	66.3 (17.1)	20.2–98.3	–
Poverty: % of families below poverty line	11.7 (10.0)	0.6–54.8	–
Unemployment: % of unemployed individuals > 16 years	8.0 (4.3)	1.5–23.3	–
Income: Median family income (adj. to 2010 USDs)	46,497 (17,638)	13,012–110,355	–

Table 2 Correlations between maternal neighborhood characteristics during pregnancy and offspring ovarian reserve in adulthood

	Maternal Neighborhood: Education	Maternal Neighborhood: Poverty	Maternal Neighborhood: Unemployment	Maternal Neighborhood: Income	AMH	AFC
Maternal Neighborhood: Education	–	−.481***	−.589***	.631***	.254***	.173**
Maternal Neighborhood: Poverty		–	.714***	−.545***	−.106†	.045
Maternal Neighborhood: Unemployment			–	−.645***	−.085	.020
Maternal Neighborhood: Income				–	196***	.125*
AMH					–	.726***
AFC						–

†$P < .10$; *$P < .05$; **$P < .01$; ***$P < .001$

< .001, respectively) while greater neighborhood-level poverty was related inversely to AMH ($r = -.106$, $P < .10$). Neighborhood-level education and family income was similarly related positively to AFC ($r = .173$, $P < .001$, $r = .125$, $P < .05$, respectively). As expected, associations between the maternal neighborhood characteristics (education, poverty, unemployment, income) were all significant (all P's < .001) as was the association between AMH and AFC ($r = .726$, $P < .001$).

In Table 3, results of covariate-adjusted linear regression models examining maternal neighborhood characteristics during pregnancy and offspring ovarian reserve in adulthood are reported. In the final models, following the backward elimination of main effects with $P > .10$, associations are evident between maternal neighborhood-level SES and offspring ovarian reserve. Specifically, greater maternal neighborhood education was related to *higher* ovarian reserve as marked by higher levels of offspring AMH (beta = .142, $P < .001$) and AFC (beta = .092, $P < .10$) with models accounting for 19.6% and 21.5% of the variance in AMH and AFC, respectively. Conversely, greater maternal neighborhood poverty was related to *lower* ovarian reserve as marked by lower offspring AMH (beta = -.144, $P < .01$), with the model accounting for 19.5% of the variance in AMH.

To illustrate the significant findings in Table 3, additional linear models were fit replacing the continuous maternal neighborhood SES indicators with coarsened indicators. The effects of the categorical maternal neighborhood SES indicators are represented graphically in Fig. 1, showing ovarian reserve markers (in untransformed units) across categories of maternal neighborhood-level SES, adjusted for all covariates. Across categories of maternal neighborhood education (1 = neighborhoods with < 50% of individuals having earned a HS diploma; 2 = neighborhoods with 50–79% of individuals having earned a HS diploma; and 3 = neighborhoods with > = 80% of individuals having earned a HS diploma), adjusted marginal means for AMH were 2.5 (SE = 0.3) ng/mL, 3.2 (SE = 0.2) ng/mL, and 3.8 (SE = 0.3) ng/mL, respectively (F(2,324) = 3.6, P < .05). Contrasts showed significant differences between education categories 1 and 3 ($P < .01$), and marginal differences between education categories 1 and 2 ($P < .10$), and 2 and 3 ($P < .10$). Adjusted marginal means for AFC levels were 14.3 (SE = 1.2), 15.6 (SE = 0.6), and 17.0 (SE = 1.1), respectively, following a similar, albeit non-significant (F(2,323) = 1.2, $P > .05$), pattern of association. Finally, across categories of maternal neighborhood poverty (1 = neighborhoods with < 5% of families living below the poverty line; 2 = neighborhoods with 5–19% of families living below the poverty line; and 3 = neighborhoods with > = 20% of families living below the poverty line, adjusted marginal means for AMH were 3.7 (SE = 0.3) ng/mL, 3.2 (SE = 0.2) ng/mL, and 2.4 (SE = 0.3) ng/mL, respectively (F(2,324) = 3.4, P < .05). Contrasts

showed significant differences between poverty categories 1 and 3 ($P < .05$) and 2 and 3 ($P < .05$).

Discussion

Building on a robust literature showing lower SES is related to earlier menopausal timing [23–33], the current study focused on adverse prenatal exposures related to maternal SES, hypothesizing that greater maternal socioeconomic disadvantage would be associated with lower ovarian reserve in the adult offspring. Results supported this hypothesis. In a healthy, community-based sub-sample of reproductive age participants in the OVA Study, maternal SES measured indirectly through US Census-derived maternal neighborhood characteristics was related to ovarian reserve in the adult offspring. Specifically, greater maternal neighborhood-level education (% of individuals with a high school diploma) was related to higher offspring ovarian reserve as marked by both AMH and AFC. In addition, greater maternal neighborhood-level poverty (% of families below the poverty line) was related to lower offspring ovarian reserve as marked by AMH. These associations were present independently of offspring SES indexed by educational attainment as well as other potential confounding factors, including maternal age and offspring characteristics (age, race/ethnicity, cigarette smoking, BMI, menarcheal age, history of hormonal contraceptive use, and parity). Because the ovarian follicle pool is established in utero, the current findings are important in suggesting that SES-related adversity exposures during this period may have a detrimental impact on the size or health of the initial follicle endowment, leading to accelerated follicle loss over time.

There are several notable strengths of the current study. First, the current study implemented a novel methodological strategy to characterize SES-related adversity exposures in the prenatal period, a time period that is often neglected in the literature yet is critically important for the initial endowment of the ovarian follicle pool and subsequent trajectories of ovarian follicle loss over time, culminating at menopause. The methodological approach of the current study involved the ascertainment of objective SES-related data derived from US Censuses characterizing the neighborhoods in which the mothers of the OVA Study participants lived. Second, the current study is the first study to our knowledge to examine maternal SES, extending the current literature which has focused almost exclusively on SES in the offspring. The current study is also the first study to our knowledge to examine maternal SES in relation to established biomarkers of ovarian reserve (AMH, AFC), extending the current literature which has focused almost exclusively on menopausal timing. The inclusion of these biomarkers offers a unique opportunity to examine prenatal exposures in relation to variability in ovarian aging among younger women when fertility preservation may still be possible. Although there are prior

Table 3 Final multivariate linear regression models examining maternal neighborhood characteristics during pregnancy and offspring ovarian reserve in adulthood, adjusted for covariates.* Results show variables remaining in the models after backward elimination of main effects with $P > .10$

			DV: AMH	
	Beta	P	b	95% CI for b
1. Predictors:				
Age	−.318	.000	−.040	(−0.052, −0.028)
BMI	−.170	.001	−.472	(−0.748, −0.196)
Maternal Neighborhood:				
Education (% of individuals with a HS diploma)	.142	.006	.588	(0.168, 1.008)
2. Predictors:				
Age	−.382	.000	−.048	(−0.061, −0.035)
BMI	−.157	.003	−.435	(−0.719, −0.152)
Maternal Neighborhood:				
Poverty (% of families below the poverty line)	−.144	.007	−1.033	(−1.778, −0.288)
3. Predictors: Maternal Neighborhood:				
Unemployment (% of unemployed individuals)	–	n.s.	–	–
4. Predictors: Maternal Neighborhood:				
Income (median family income)	–	n.s.	–	–

			DV: AFC	
	Beta	P	b	95% CI for b
1. Predictors:				
Age	−.398	.000	−.086	(−0.107, −0.064)
Hormonal contraceptives	−.119	.017	−.338	(−0.616, −0.061)
Maternal Neighborhood:				
Education (% of individuals with a HS diploma)	.092	.064	.649	(−0.038, 1.337)
2. Predictors: Maternal Neighborhood:				
Poverty (% of families below the poverty line)	–	n.s.	–	–
3. Predictors: Maternal Neighborhood:				
Unemployment (% of unemployed individuals)	–	n.s.	–	–
4. Predictors: Maternal Neighborhood:				
Income (median family income)	–	n.s.	–	–

*Covariates examined simultaneously included age (in years); maternal age (in years); race/ethnicity (using white as the reference group vs. African-American, Latina, Chinese, or Filipina); educational attainment (using HS degree or less as the reference group vs. some college, college degree, or graduate degree); smoking (0 = never smoked, 1 = current/past smoking); BMI (kg/m^2, log transformed); menarcheal age (in years); hormonal contraceptives (0 = no history of use, 1 = positive history of use; and parity (0 = no live births, 1 = 1+ live births)

studies of prenatal adversity exposures, none have considered SES exposures in particular [40–45] and only one examined a biomarker of ovarian reserve [46]. Lastly, the current study drew from a large, well-characterized group of reproductive age participants in the OVA Study. These women were healthy, regularly cycling, and not taking hormonal contraceptives, eliminating numerous potential confounds, including the inclusion of women with polycystic ovarian syndrome (PCOS).

There are several notable weaknesses of the current study. First, maternal neighborhood-level SES is only an indirect marker of individual-level maternal SES. It is possible that high SES mothers may live in lower SES neighborhoods and/or be able to avoid exposures associated with low SES environments. In this way, use of a neighborhood-level marker may not be an adequate representation of an individual mother's experiences. The current study did not have direct measures of maternal SES such as educational

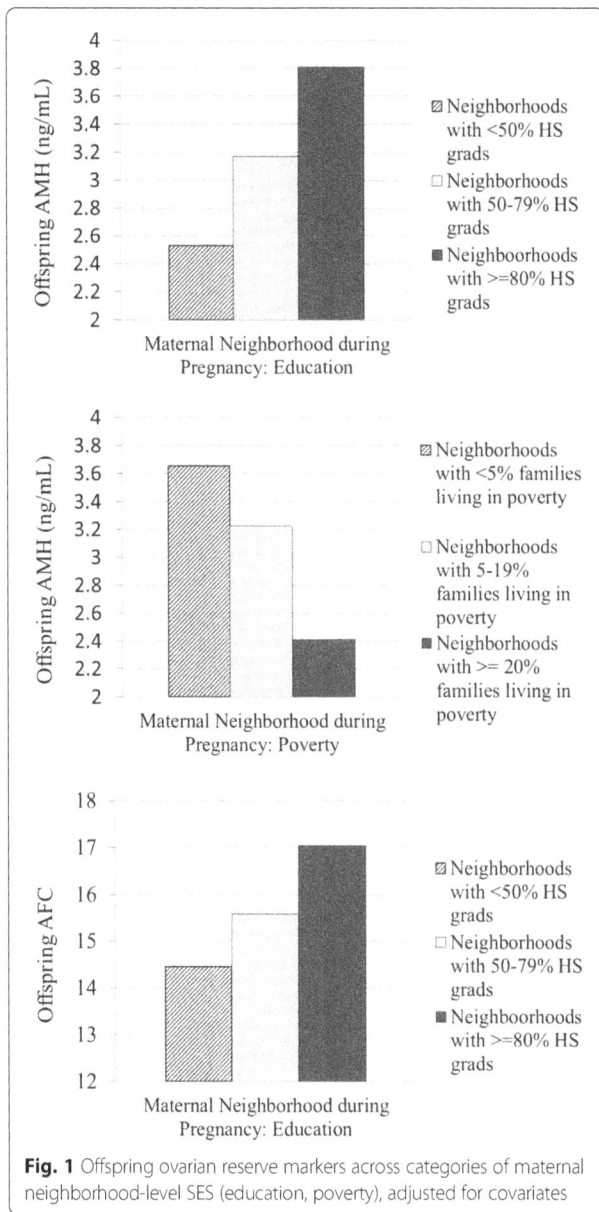

Fig. 1 Offspring ovarian reserve markers across categories of maternal neighborhood-level SES (education, poverty), adjusted for covariates

attainment, income level, or wealth. Second, although the current study attempted to isolate the prenatal period, realistically, it is not possible to discern the impact of exposures related to the prenatal period versus the postnatal period. In fact, it is likely that the neighborhood level SES exposures present prenatally persisted into infancy and childhood may have continued to exert a deleterious influence on the offspring ovarian reserve. In this way, pointing to initial follicle endowment as the specific process that may have been disrupted remains speculative, although it is noteworthy that the effects of maternal neighborhood-level SES on offspring ovarian reserve were independent of offspring SES. Lastly, the current study did not have measures that might help elucidate *why* maternal neighborhood-level SES may impact offspring ovarian

reserve. The current study did not have direct assessments of relevant variables such as maternal health behaviors, nutritional status, and general health as well as potentially correlated exposures such as environmental toxicants known to be endocrine-disrupting.

Future research should improve upon the weaknesses of the current study by focusing on particular maternal and environmental factors that might be driving observed associations between maternal neighborhood-level SES and offspring ovarian reserve. Prior study findings highlight more broadly the impact of early life environments on subsequent reproductive health outcomes. For example, using a novel study design, women who grew up in Sylhet, Bangladesh were shown to have hormonal profiles consistent with lower ovarian reserve and reduced fertility compared to their Bangladeshi counterparts who migrated to Britain as children (versus as adults) as well as to other European-born women who grew up in Britain [61, 62]. This suggests that early life adversity exposures in Bangladeshi neighborhoods, possibly reflecting exposures to nutritional stress, infectious disease, or other yet unidentified stressors, may detrimentally impact adulthood reproductive health outcomes. In animal models, experimental studies have focused on poor maternal nutritional status in particular, showing maternal undernutrition and malnutrition were related to markers of impaired folliculogenesis, lower ovarian reserve, and increased oxidative stress in the adult offspring [63–67]. Consistent with these findings, in a prior study of women, maternal nutritional deprivation during famine was associated with earlier menopausal timing in the offspring [44] as was pre-pregnancy diabetes [43].

In parallel, other studies have investigated the relevance of maternal smoking to offspring reproductive health. In animal models, experimental studies showed that exposure to maternal smoking, similar to study findings regarding maternal nutritional status, was related to negative reproductive health outcomes in the adult offspring, including indicators of sub-fertility, lower ovarian reserve, and increased oxidative stress [68–70]. Consistent with these findings, in a prior study of women, maternal smoking during pregnancy was associated with earlier menopausal timing in the offspring [41]. These authors suggested that maternal smoking might influence the hormonal environment in utero in a way that negatively impacts the formation of the ovarian reserve and subsequent follicle loss. In fact, lower estradiol and estriol levels have been documented in pregnant smokers [71–74]. Because estradiol appears to play a role in the maintenance of the primordial follicle pool [75], lower estradiol levels associated with maternal smoking may allow premature follicle growth, hastening the depletion of the ovarian reserve.

Taken together, mounting epidemiological and experimental evidence suggests that variation in adulthood ovarian function has developmental origins in the intrauterine and early childhood environments, suggesting particular exposures during these sensitive periods may shape trajectories of ovarian aging. Exposures related to maternal nutritional stress and maternal smoking, which are also significantly correlated with lower SES [76–78], are strong candidates for inclusion in future research to address whether maternal neighborhood-level SES in the current study may be marking behavioral, anthropometric, or other health-related characteristics of the mother.

In addition, although less strongly supported, it is possible that maternal neighborhood-level SES may be marking toxicant exposures that cluster in low SES environments [79–81]. A particular group of chemical exposures known to interfere with the actions of hormones termed "endocrine-disrupting chemicals (EDCs)" [82, 83] are common in personal care and household products with recent evidence documenting elevations in particular EDCs (e.g., lead, cadmium, bisphenol A [BPA]) among lower SES individuals [84]. Exposures to EDCs have been related to a host of reproductive health outcomes, including earlier onset puberty, infertility, endometriosis, PCOS, uterine fibroids, and pregnancy complications [85–94]. With respect to ovarian aging outcomes in particular, a recent review [95] summarized relevant human and animal literatures, suggesting environmental toxicants accelerate folliculogenesis and follicular atresia, including in the primordial stage and extending across the spectrum of ovarian follicle development. Notably, in a large representative sample of US women ($n = 31,575$) EDCs (i.e., polychlorinated biphenyl [PCBs], pesticides, furans, and phthalates) were associated with earlier onset menopause up to 3.8 years earlier, following adjustment for covariates [96]. In addition, prospective studies showed higher urinary phthalate and BPA levels were related to decreases in ovarian reserve as marked by lower AFC, although participants were patients seeking infertility treatment [97, 98]. To our knowledge, no studies have examined EDCs in relation to biomarkers of ovarian reserve (AFC, AMH) in healthy, reproductive age women.

Conclusions

In conclusion, results from the current study showed maternal neighborhood-level SES was related to offspring ovarian reserve, independently of a host of confounding variables, including offspring SES. These findings suggest that in the prenatal period, adverse exposures related to increased maternal socioeconomic disadvantage may have a detrimental impact on offspring ovarian aging possibly via disruptions in the initial follicle endowment. Future work, however, is necessary to elucidate the mechanisms that may explain this association, including whether specific maternal (e.g., health behaviors) or environmental (e.g., EDCs) factors that are commonly correlated with

neighborhood-level SES may be driving these associations. Future work should also be guided by a focus on the timing and time course of exposures as well as the dual consideration of both maternal and offspring characteristics. The clinical implications of these results are that risk factors for accelerated ovarian aging in offspring may be identified in mothers prenatally. Insofar as such risk factors are able to be modified prenatally or even before conception, this work offers novel directions for potential interventions to improve the health of mothers and their environments, thereby maximizing the long-term reproductive health of their offspring. Moreover, as evidence mounts that reproductive health and aging are related more broadly to cardiovascular risk [17–21], the implications of this work for the general health and well-being of women are far-reaching.

Abbreviations
AFC: Antral follicle count; AMH: Antimullerian hormone; BMI: Body mass index; BPA: Bisphenol A; EDC: Endocrine-disrupting chemical; ELISA: Enzyme-linked immunosorbent assay; FSH: Follicle stimulating hormone; LTDB: Longitudinal Tract Database; OVA Study: Ovarian Aging Study; PCB: Polychlorinated biphenyl; PCOS: Polycystic ovarian syndrome; SES: Socioeconomic status

Acknowledgements
Not applicable.

Funding
Preparation of this manuscript and the research described here were supported by NIH/NICHD and NIH/NIA (R01 HD044876); NIH/UCSF-CTSI (UL1 RR024131); NIH/NIA (K08 AG03575); NIH/NICHD (R03 HD080893); and University of Washington, Research and Intramural Funding Program (RIFP).

Authors' contributions
MEB (primary author) participated in the conceptualization, data collection, statistical analysis, manuscript drafting, and critical discussion; PE (co-investigator and co-author) participated in the conceptualization, data collection, manuscript drafting, and critical discussion; JV (co-author) participated in the conceptualization, data collection, manuscript drafting and critical discussion; NFW (co-investigator and co-author) participated in the conceptualization, manuscript drafting and critical discussion; KDC (co-investigator and co-author) participated in the conceptualization, manuscript drafting and critical discussion; SEG (co-author) participated in the conceptualization, statistical analysis, manuscript drafting and critical discussion; MIC (senior author) participated in the conceptualization, data collection, manuscript drafting, and critical discussion. All authors read and approved the final manuscript.

Competing interests
The authors declare that they have no competing interests.

Author details
[1]Department of Family and Child Nursing, University of Washington, Box 357262, Seattle, WA 98195, USA. [2]California Department of Public Health, California Environmental Health Tracking Program, Richmond, CA 94804, USA. [3]Department of Biobehavioral Nursing and Health Informatics, University of Washington, Seattle, WA 98195, USA. [4]Department of Sociology, University of Washington, Seattle, WA 98195, USA. [5]Department of Medicine, University of California San Francisco, San Francisco, CA 94143, USA. [6]Department of Obstetrics, Gynecology, & Reproductive Sciences, University of California San Francisco, San Francisco, CA 94143, USA.

References

1. Atsma F, Bartelink M, Grobbee DE, van der Schouw YT. Postmenopausal status and early menopause as independent risk factors for cardiovascular disease: a meta-analysis. Menopause-J N Am Menopause Soc. 2006;13(2):265–79.

2. Cui R, Iso H, Toyoshima H, Date C, Yamamoto A, Kikuchi S, et al. Relationships of age at menarche and menopause, and reproductive year with mortality from cardiovascular disease in Japanese postmenopausal women: the JACC study. J Epidemiol. 2006;16(5):177–84.

3. de Kleijn M, van der Schouw Y, van der Graaf Y. Reproductive history and cardiovascular disease risk in postmenopausal women. A review of the literature. Maturitas. 1999;33:7–36.

4. Fioretti F, Tavani A, Gallus S, Franceschi S, La Vecchia C. Menopause and risk of non-fatal acute myocardial infarction: an Italian case-control study and a review of the literature. Hum Reprod. 2000;15(3):599–603.

5. Jacobsen BK, Knutsen SF, Fraser GE. Age at natural menopause and total mortality and mortality from ischemic heart disease: the Adventist health study. J Clin Epidemiol. 1999;52(4):303–7.

6. Jacobsen BK, Nilssen S, Heuch I, Kvale G. Does age at natural menopause affect mortality from ischemic heart disease? J Clin Epidemiol. 1997;50(4):475–9.

7. Joakimsen O, Bonaa KH, Stensland-Bugge E, Jacobsen BK. Population-based study of age at menopause and ultrasound assessed carotid atherosclerosis - the Tromso study. J Clin Epidemiol. 2000;53(5):525–30.

8. Lisabeth LD, Beiser AS, Brown DL, Murabito JM, Kelly-Hayes M, Wolf PA. Age at natural menopause and risk of ischemic stroke. The Framingham Heart Study Stroke. 2009;40(4):1044–9.

9. Palmer JR, Rosenberg L, Shapiro S. Reproductive factors and risk of myocardial infarction. Am J Epidemiol. 1992;136(4):408–16.

10. Parashar S, Reid KJ, Spertus JA, Shaw LJ, Vaccarino V. Early menopause predicts angina after myocardial infarction. Menopause-J N Am Menopause Soc. 2010;17(5):938–45.

11. Shuster LT, Rhodes DJ, Gostout BS, Grossardt BR, Rocca WA. Premature menopause or early menopause: long-term health consequences. Maturitas. 2010;65(2):161–6.

12. Vander Schouw YT, Vander Graaf Y, Steyerberg EW, MJC E, Banga JD. Age at menopause as a risk factor for cardiovascular mortality. Lancet. 1996;347(9003):714–8.

13. Harlow SD, Gass M, Hall JE, Lobo R, Maki P, Rebar RW, et al. Executive summary of the stages of reproductive aging workshop+10: addressing the unfinished agenda of staging reproductive aging. Menopause-J N Am Menopause Soc. 2012;19(4):387–95.

14. Nelson SM. Biomarkers of ovarian response: current and future applications. Fertil Steril. 2013;99(4):963–9.

15. Iliodromiti S, Anderson RA, Nelson SM. Technical and performance characteristics of anti-Mullerian hormone and antral follicle count as biomarkers of ovarian response. Hum Reprod Update. 2015;21(6):698–710.

16. Hansen KR, Hodnett GM, Knowlton N, Craig LB. Correlation of ovarian reserve tests with histologically determined primordial follicle number. Fertil Steril. 2011;95(1):170–5.

17. Appt SE, Chen HY, Clarkson TB, Kaplan JR. Premenopausal antimullerian hormone concentration is associated with subsequent atherosclerosis. Menopause-J N Am Menopause Soc. 2012;19(12):1353–9.

18. Bleil ME, Gregorich SE, McConnell D, Rosen MP, Cedars MI. Does accelerated reproductive aging underlie premenopausal risk for cardiovascular disease? Menopause. 2013;20(11):1139–46.

19. de Kat AC, Verschuren WM, Eijkemans MJC, Broekmans FJM, van der Schouw YT. Anti-Mullerian hormone trajectories are associated with cardiovascular disease in women results from the Doetinchem cohort study. Circulation. 2017;135(6):556.

20. de Kat AC, Verschuren WMM, Eijkemans MJC, van der Schouw YT, Broekmans FJM. The association of low ovarian reserve with cardiovascular disease risk: a cross-sectional population-based study. Hum Reprod. 2016;31(8):1866–74.

21. Verit FF, Akyol H, Sakar MN. Low antimullerian hormone levels may be associated with cardiovascular risk markers in women with diminished ovarian reserve. Gynecol Endocrinol. 2016;32(4):302–5.

22. Gold EB. The timing of the age at which natural menopause occurs. Obstet Gynecol Clin N Am. 2011;38(3):425.

23. Castelo-Branco C, Bluemel JE, Chedraui P, Calle A, Bocanera R, Depiano E, et al. Age at menopause in Latin America (vol 13, pg 706, 2006). Menopause-J N Am Menopause Soc. 2006;13(5):850.

24. Gold EB, Bromberger J, Crawford S, Samuels S, Greendale GA, Harlow SD, et al. Factors associated with age at natural menopause in a multiethnic sample of midlife women. Am J Epidemiol. 2001;153(9):865–74.

25. Gold EB, Sternfeld B, Kelsey JL, Brown C, Mouton C, Reame N, et al. Relation of demographic and lifestyle factors to symptoms in a multi-racial/ethnic population of women 40-55 years of age. Am J Epidemiol. 2000;152(5):463–73.

26. Lawlor DA, Ebrahim S, Smith GD. The association of socio-economic position across the life course and age at menopause: the British Women's heart and health study. BJOG Int J Obstet Gynaecol. 2003;110(12):1078–87.

27. Luoto R, Kaprio J, Uutela A. Age at natural menopause and sociodemographic status in Finland. Am J Epidemiol. 1994;139(1):64–76.

28. Magursky V, Mesko M, Sokolik L. Age at menopause and onset of climacteric in women of Martin-District, Czechoslovakia - statistical survey and some biological and social correlations. Int J Fertil. 1975;20(1):17–23.

29. Rodstrom K, Bengtsson C, Milsom I, Lissner L, Sundh V, Bjourkelund C. Evidence for a secular trend in menopausal age: a population study of women in Gothenburg. Menopause-J N Am Menopause Soc. 2003;10(6):538–43.

30. Santoro N, Brockwell S, Johnston J, Crawford SL, Gold EB, Harlow SD, et al. Helping midlife women predict the onset of the final menses: SWAN, the study of Women's health across the nation. Menopause-J N Am Menopause Soc. 2007;14(3):415–24.

31. Stanford JL, Hartge P, Brinton LA, Hoover RN, Brookmeyer R. Factors influencing the age at natural menopause. J Chronic Dis. 1987;40(11):995–1002.

32. Torgerson DJ, Avenell A, Russell IT, Reid DM. Factors associated with onset of menopause in women aged 45-49. Maturitas. 1994;19(2):83–92.

33. Wise LA, Krieger N, Zierler S, Harlow BL. Lifetime socioeconomic position in relation to onset of perimenopause. J Epidemiol Community Health. 2002;56(11):851–60.

34. Brevini TA, Zanetto SB, Cillo F. Effects of endocrine disruptors on developmental and reproductive functions. Current Drug Targets - Immune Endocrine & Metabolic Disorders. 2005;5(1):1–10.

35. Buck Louis GMSundaram R. Exposome: time for transformative research. Stat Med. 2012;31(22):2569–75.

36. Cohen Hubal EA, Moya J, Selevan SG. A lifestage approach to assessing children's exposure. Birth defects research Part B, Developmental and reproductive toxicology. 2008;83(6):522–9.

37. Heimler I, Trewin AL, Chaffin CL, Rawlins RG, Hutz RJ. Modulation of ovarian follicle maturation and effects on apoptotic cell death in Holtzman rats exposed to 2,3,7,8-tetrachlorodibenzo-p-dioxin (TCDD) in utero and lactationally. Reprod Toxicol. 1998;12(1):69–73.

38. Lee CK, Kang HS, Kim JR, Lee BJ, Lee JT, Kim JH, et al. Effects of aroclor 1254 on the expression of the RAPJ gene and reproductive function in rats. Reproduction, Fertility, and Development. 2007;19(4):539–47.

39. Lemasters GK, Perreault SD, Hales BF, Hatch M, Hirshfield AN, Hughes CL, et al. Workshop to identify critical windows of exposure for children's health: reproductive health in children and adolescents work group summary. Environ Health Perspect. 2000;108(3):505–9.

40. Treloar SA, Sadrzadeh S, Do KA, Martin NG, Lambalk CB. Birth weight and age at menopause in Australian female twin pairs: exploration of the fetal origin hypothesis. Hum Reprod. 2000;15(1):55–9.

41. Strohsnitter WC, Hatch EE, Hyer M, Troisi R, Kaufman RH, Robboy SJ, et al. The association between in utero cigarette smoke exposure and age at menopause. Am J Epidemiol. 2008;167(6):727–33.

42. Tom SE, Cooper R, Kuh D, Guralnik JM, Hardy R, Power C. Fetal environment and early age at natural menopause in a British birth cohort study. Hum Reprod. 2010;25(3):791–8.

43. Steiner AZ, D'Aloisio AA, DeRoo LA, Sandler DP, Baird DD. Association of intrauterine and early-life exposures with age at menopause in the sister study. Am J Epidemiol. 2010;172(2):140–8.

44. Yarde F, Broekmans FJM, van der Pal-de Bruin KM, Schonbeck Y, te Velde ER, Stein AD, et al. Prenatal famine, birthweight, reproductive performance and age at menopause: the Dutch hunger winter families study. Hum Reprod. 2013;28(12):3328–36.

45. Ruth KS, Perry JRB, Henley WE, Melzer D, Weedon MN, Murray A. Events in early life are associated with female reproductive ageing: a UK biobank study. Sci Rep. 2016;6:9.

46. Fraser A, McNally W, Sattar N, Anderson EL, Lashen H, Fleming R, et al. Prenatal exposures and anti-mullerian hormone in female adolescents. Am J Epidemiol. 2013;178(9):1414–23.

47. AJW MGEAH. Initial and cyclic recruitment of ovarian follicles. Endocr Rev. 2000;21(2):200–14.

48. Hansen KR, Knowlton NS, Thyer AC, Charleston JS, Soules MR, Klein NA. A new model of reproductive aging: the decline in ovarian non-growing follicle number from birth to menopause. Hum Reprod. 2008;23(3):699–708.

49. te Velde ERPearson PL. The variability of female reproductive ageing. Hum Reprod Update. 2002;8(2):141–54.

50. te Velde ER, Scheffer GJ, Dorland M, Broekmans FJ, Fauser BC. Developmental and endocrine aspects of normal ovarian aging. Mol Cell Endocrinol. 1998;145(1–2):67–73.

51. Bleil ME, Gregorich SE, Adler NE, Sternfeld B, Rosen MP, Cedars MI. Race/ ethnic disparities in reproductive age: an examination of ovarian reserve estimates across four race/ethnic groups of healthy, regularly cycling women. Fertil Steril. 2014;101(1):199–207.

52. Rosen MP, Johnstone E, McCulloch CE, Schuh-Huerta SM, Sternfeld B, Reijo-Pera RA, et al. A characterization of the relationship of ovarian reserve markers with age. Fertil Steril. 2012;97(1):238–43.

53. Schuh-Huerta SM, Johnson NA, Rosen MP, Sternfeld B, Cedars MI, Pera RAR. Genetic variants and environmental factors associated with hormonal markers of ovarian reserve in Caucasian and African American women. Hum Reprod. 2012;27(2):594–608.

54. Gordon N. How does the adult Kaiser Permanente membership in northern California compare with the larger community? Oakland, CA: Kaiser Permanente Division of Research; 2006.

55. Logan JR, Xu ZW, Stults BJ. Interpolating US decennial census tract data from as early as 1970 to 2010: a longitudinal tract database. Prof Geogr. 2014;66(3):412–20.

56. Logan JR, Stults BJ, Xu ZW. Validating population estimates for harmonized census tract data, 2000-2010. Ann Am Assoc Geogr. 2016;106(5):1013–29.

57. Diversity and Disparities, Longitudinal Tract Database (LTDB). Accessed 1 June 2017; Available from: https://s4.ad.brown.edu/Projects/Diversity/Researcher/LTDB.htm.

58. Majumder K, Gelbaya TA, Laing I, Nardo LG. The use of anti-Mullerian hormone and antral follicle count to predict the potential of oocytes and embryos. Eur J Obstet Gynecol Reprod Biol. 2010;150(2):166–70.

59. Yates A, Rustamov O, Roberts S, Lim H, Pemberton P, Smith A, et al. Anti-Mullerian hormone-tailored stimulation protocols improve outcomes whilst reducing adverse effects and costs of IVF. Hum Reprod. 2011;26(9):2353–62.

60. Current Population Survey (CPS), US Census Bureau, 2015. Accessed 1 Sept 2017; Available from: https://www.census.gov/programs-surveys/cps.html.

61. Nunez-de la Mora A, Chatterton RT, Choudhury OA, Napolitano DA, Bentley GR. Childhood conditions influence adult progesterone levels. PLoS Med. 2007;4(5):813–21.

62. Begum K, Muttukrishna S, Sievert LL, Sharmeen T, Murphy L, Chowdhury O, et al. Ethnicity or environment: effects of migration on ovarian reserve among Bangladeshi women in the United Kingdom. Fertil Steril. 2016;105(3):744.

63. Bernal AB, Vickers MH, Hampton MB, Poynton RA, Sloboda DM. Maternal undernutrition significantly impacts ovarian follicle number and increases ovarian oxidative stress in adult rat offspring. PLoS One. 2010;5(12):12.

64. Sloboda DM, Howie GJ, Pleasants A, Gluckman PD, Vickers MH. Pre- and postnatal nutritional histories influence reproductive maturation and ovarian function in the rat. PLoS One. 2009;4(8):8.

65. Connor KL, Vickers MH, Beltrand J, Meaney MJ, Sloboda DM. Nature, nurture or nutrition? Impact of maternal nutrition on maternal care, offspring development and reproductive function. J Physiol-London. 2012;590(9):2167–80.

66. Rae MT, Palassio S, Kyle CE, Brooks AN, Lea RG, Miller DW, et al. Effect of maternal undernutrition during pregnancy on early ovarian development and subsequent follicular development in sheep fetuses. Reproduction (Cambridge, Eng). 2001;122(6):915–22.

67. Faria TD, Brasil FD, Sampaio FJB, Ramos CD. Maternal malnutrition during lactation affects folliculogenesis, gonadotropins, and leptin receptors in adult rats. Nutrition. 2010;26(10):1000–7.

68. Kilic S, Yuksel B, Lortlar N, Sertyel S, Aksu T, Batioglu S. Environmental tobacco smoke exposure during intrauterine period promotes granulosa cell apoptosis: a prospective, randomized study. J Matern-Fetal Neonatal Med. 2012;25(10):1904–8.

69. Camlin NJ, Sobinoff AP, Sutherland JM, Beckett EL, Jarnicki AG, Vanders RL, et al. Maternal smoke exposure impairs the long-term fertility of female offspring in a murine model. Biol Reprod. 2016;94(2):12.

70. Camlin NJ, Jarnicki AG, Vanders RL, Walters KA, Hansbro PM, McLaughlin EA, et al. Grandmaternal smoke exposure reduces female fertility in a murine model, with great-grandmaternal smoke exposure unlikely to have an effect. Hum Reprod. 2017;32(6):1270–81.

71. Palomaki GE, Knight GJ, Haddow JE, Canick JA, Wald NJ, Kennard A. Cigarette smoking and levels of maternal serum alpha-fetoprotein, unconjugated estriol, and HCG- impact on down-syndrome screening. Obstet Gynecol. 1993;81(5):675–8.

72. Petridou E, Panagiotopoulou K, Katsouyanni K, Spanos E, Trichopoulos D. Tobacco smoking, pregnancy estrogens, and birth weight. Epidemiology. 1990;1(3):247–50.

73. Bernstein L, Pike MC, Lobo RA, Depue RH, Ross RK, Henderson BE. Cigarette smoking in pregnancy results in marked decrease in maternal HCG and estradiol levels. Br J Obstet Gynaecol. 1989;96(1):92–6.

74. Kaijser M, Granath F, Jacobsen G, Cnattingius S, Ekbom A. Maternal pregnancy estriol levels in relation to anamnestic and fetal anthropometric data. Epidemiology. 2000;11(3):315–9.

75. Kezele PSkinner MK. Regulation of ovarian primordial follicle assembly and development by estrogen and progesterone: endocrine model of follicle assembly. Endocrinology. 2003;144(8):3329–37.

76. Black C, Moon G, Baird J. Dietary inequalities: what is the evidence for the effect of the neighbourhood food environment? Health Place. 2014;27:229–42.

77. Darmon NDrewnowski A. Does social class predict diet quality? Am J Clin Nutr. 2008;87(5):1107–17.

78. Leventhal AM. The sociopharmacology of tobacco addiction: implications for understanding health disparities. Nicotine Tob Res. 2016;18(2):110–21.

79. Brown P. Race, class, and environmental health: a review and systematization of the literature. Environ Res. 1995;69(1):15–30.

80. Brulle RJ, Pellow DN. Environmental justice: human health and environmental inequalities. Annu Rev Public Health. 2006;27:103–24.

81. Evans GW, Kantrowitz E. Socioeconomic status and health: the potential role of environmental risk exposure. Annu Rev Public Health. 2002;23:303–31.

82. Diamanti-Kandarakis E, Bourguignon JP, Giudice LC, Hauser R, Prins GS, Soto AM, et al. Endocrine-disrupting chemicals: an Endocrine Society scientific statement. Endocr Rev. 2009;30(4):293–342.

83. Zoeller RT, Brown TR, Doan LL, Gore AC, Skakkebaek NE, Soto AM, et al. Endocrine-disrupting chemicals and public health protection: a statement of principles from the Endocrine Society. Endocrinology. 2012;153(9):4097–110.

84. Tyrrell J, Melzer D, Henley W, Galloway TS, Osborne NJ. Associations between socioeconomic status and environmental toxicant concentrations in adults in the USA: NHANES 2001-2010. Environ Int. 2013;59:328–35.

85. Buck Louis GM, Sundaram R, Schisterman EF, Sweeney AM, Lynch CD, Gore-Langton RE, et al. Persistent environmental pollutants and couple fecundity: the LIFE study. Environ Health Perspect. 2013;121(2):231–6.

86. Buttke DE, Sircar K, Martin C. Exposures to endocrine-disrupting chemicals and age of menarche in adolescent girls in NHANES (2003-2008). Environ Health Perspect. 2012;120(11):1613–8.

87. Cobellis L, Latini G, De Felice C, Razzi S, Paris I, Ruggieri F, et al. High plasma concentrations of di-(2-ethylhexyl)-phthalate in women with endometriosis. Hum Reprod. 2003;18(7):1512–5.

88. Gerhard I, Daniel V, Link S, Monga B, Runnebaum B. Chlorinated hydrocarbons in women with repeated miscarriages. Environ Health Perspect. 1998;106(10):675–81.

89. Greenlee AR, Arbuckle TE, Chyou PH. Risk factors for female infertility in an agricultural region. Epidemiology. 2003;14(4):429–36.

90. Hoover RN, Hyer M, Pfeiffer RM, Adam E, Bond B, Cheville AL, et al. Adverse health outcomes in women exposed in utero to diethylstilbestrol. N Engl J Med. 2011;365(14):1304–14.

91. Korrick SA, Chen C, Damokosh AI, Ni J, Liu X, Cho SI, et al. Association of DDT with spontaneous abortion: a case-control study. Ann Epidemiol. 2001;11(7):491–6.
92. Mayani A, Barel S, Soback S, Almagor M. Dioxin concentrations in women with endometriosis. Hum Reprod. 1997;12(2):373–5.
93. McLachlan JA, Simpson E, Martin M. Endocrine disrupters and female reproductive health. Best Pract Res Clin Endocrinol Metab. 2006;20(1):63–75.
94. Takeuchi T, Tsutsumi O, Ikezuki Y, Takai Y, Taketani Y. Positive relationship between androgen and the endocrine disruptor, bisphenol a, in normal women and women with ovarian dysfunction. Endocr J. 2004;51(2):165–9.
95. Vabre P, Gatimel N, Moreau J, Gayrard V, Picard-Hagen N, Parinaud J, et al. Environmental pollutants, a possible etiology for premature ovarian insufficiency: a narrative review of animal and human data. Environ Health. 2017;16:18.
96. Grindler NM, Allsworth JE, Macones GA, Kannan K, Roehl KA, Cooper AR. Persistent organic pollutants and early menopause in US women. PLoS One. 2015;10(1):12.
97. Messerlian C, Souter I, Gaskins AJ, Williams PL, Ford JB, Chiu YH, et al. Urinary phthalate metabolites and ovarian reserve among women seeking infertility care. Hum Reprod. 2016;31(1):75–83.
98. Souter I, Smith KW, Dimitriadis I, Ehrlich S, Williams PL, Calafat AM, et al. The association of bisphenol-a urinary concentrations with antral follicle counts and other measures of ovarian reserve in women undergoing infertility treatments. Reprod Toxicol. 2013;42:224–31.

16

Anti-Müllerian hormone and its relationships with subclinical cardiovascular disease and renal disease in a longitudinal cohort study of women with type 1 diabetes

Catherine Kim[1]* ⓘ, Yuanyuan Pan[2], Barbara H. Braffett[2], Valerie L. Arends[3], Michael W. Steffes[3], Hunter Wessells[4], Aruna V. Sarma[5] and for the DCCT/EDIC Research Group

Abstract

Background: Reproductive age may be a risk factor for vascular disease. Anti-Müllerian hormone (AMH) is produced by viable ovarian follicles and reflects reproductive age. We examined whether AMH concentrations were associated with markers of subclinical cardiovascular disease (CVD) and kidney disease among women with type 1 diabetes.

Methods: We performed a cross-sectional analysis of the Epidemiology of Diabetes Interventions and Complications Study. Participants included women with type 1 diabetes and ≥ 1 AMH measurement ($n = 390$). In multivariable regression models which adjusted for repeated measures, we examined the associations between AMH with CVD risk factors, estimated glomerular filtration rate, and albumin excretion ratio. We also examined whether initial AMH concentrations were associated with the presence of any coronary artery calcification (CAC) or carotid intima media thickness (cIMT).

Results: After adjustment for age, AMH was not associated with waist circumference, blood pressure, lipid profiles, or renal function. Higher initial AMH concentrations had borderline but non-significant associations with the presence of CAC after adjustment for age (odds ratio [OR] 1.08, 95% confidence interval [CI] 1.00, 1.16) which were minimally altered by addition of other CVD risk factors, although women in the 3rd quartile of AMH had lower odds of CAC than women in the lowest quartile (OR 0.40, 95% CI 0.17, 0.94). After adjustment for age, higher AMH was associated with statistically significant but only slightly higher cIMT (0.005 mm, $p = 0.0087$) which was minimally altered by addition of other CVD risk factors.

Conclusions: Among midlife women with type 1 diabetes, AMH has slight but significant associations with subclinical measures of atherosclerosis. Future studies should examine whether these associations are clinically significant.

Trial registration: NCT00360815 and NCT00360893 Study Start Date April 1994.

Keywords: Ovarian reserve, Anti-Müllerian hormone, Coronary artery calcification, Type 1 diabetes

---

* Correspondence: cathkim@umich.edu
[1]Departments of Medicine, Obstetrics & Gynecology, and Epidemiology, University of Michigan, 2800 Plymouth Road, Building 16, Room 430W, Ann Arbor, MI 48109-2800, USA
Full list of author information is available at the end of the article

Background

Reproductive age, traditionally categorized as reproductive stage (i.e. premenopausal or postmenopausal) [1], may be a risk factor for chronic diseases including cardiovascular disease (CVD) and kidney disease apart from chronologic age. For example, an early age (less than 40 years) of menopause may increase risk of both coronary disease and stroke [2], and early age at menopause is also associated with end stage renal disease among women with type 1 diabetes [3]. Presumably, such associations are mediated through ovarian hormone effects on the vascular endothelium, or conversely through the impact of chronic conditions on ovarian function [4], although the key hormones and exact mechanisms of action are not known. A serum marker of reproductive age is anti-Müllerian hormone (AMH), a dimeric glycoprotein that is produced solely by functioning ovarian follicles [5]. AMH is a member of the transforming growth factor-beta superfamily, which encompass a broad group of receptors with endothelial activity [6], and hypothetically could affect vascular disease via these receptors. In addition, AMH has relatively minimal variations within the menstrual cycle and has recently been incorporated into the STRAW (Stages of Reproductive Aging Workshop) staging system for reproductive aging [1]. As women approach menopause, concentrations of AMH decline to undetectable values [7]. Thus, AMH has been increasingly used to predict ovarian reserve in healthy populations as well as in women experiencing assisted reproductive technology [8–11].

Cross-sectional studies suggest that lower AMH concentrations are independently associated with hypertensive disorders of pregnancy [4] as well as higher blood pressure [12, 13] and less favorable lipid concentrations [13, 14]. We have previously reported that AMH was not associated with hemoglobin A1c in the EDIC cohort [15]. Reports examining AMH and subclinical atherosclerosis are few and conflict [6, 13, 16, 17]. To our knowledge, no reports in women have examined whether AMH is associated with markers of renal function.

Women with type 1 diabetes have an increased risk of CVD and kidney disease compared to women without diabetes [18]. Whether reproductive age independently increases risk for CVD in this high-risk population is not known. The Diabetes Control and Complications Trial (DCCT) was a randomized trial that enrolled participants with type 1 diabetes in order to compare the impact of intensive vs. conventional diabetes therapy upon microvascular complications [19]. During the follow-up Epidemiology of Diabetes Interventions and Complications (EDIC) study, coronary artery calcification (CAC) and serial measures of common cIMT were assessed, as well as AMH and serial measures of CVD risk factors. Thus, we were able to examine whether AMH was associated with CVD risk factor profile and measures of subclinical atherosclerosis among women with type 1 diabetes. In addition, estimated glomerular filtration rate (eGFR) and albumin excretion ratio (AER) were evaluated serially throughout DCCT and EDIC, and we were able to examine whether AMH was associated with these markers of renal disease. As previous reports have noted a U-shaped relationship between AMH and CVD risk factors [13], our hypotheses were that extremes of AMH are associated with CVD risk factor profile and measures of subclinical atherosclerosis and renal disease among women with type 1 diabetes.

Methods

The DCCT and EDIC studies have been described in detail (14). Briefly, the DCCT was a multicenter, randomized clinical trial designed to compare the impact of intensive and conventional diabetes treatment on the development and progression of early microvascular complications of type 1 diabetes [20]. From 1983 to 1989, 1441 patients (including 680 women) were enrolled at 29 centers. The intensive treatment regimen was designed to achieve glycemic control as close to the non-diabetic range as possible using ≥3 daily insulin injections or an insulin pump. Conventional treatment consisted of 1–2 daily insulin injections without stipulated target glucose concentrations. The DCCT included a primary prevention cohort and a secondary intervention cohort. The primary prevention cohort consisted of 726 subjects with no retinopathy, urinary albumin excretion rate < 40 mg/24 h, and diabetes duration of 1–5 years at DCCT baseline. The secondary intervention cohort consisted of 715 subjects who had non-proliferative retinopathy, urinary albumin excretion rate ≤ 200 mg/24 h, and diabetes duration of 1–15 years. Individuals were excluded if they had hypertension (defined by systolic blood pressure [SBP] levels ≥140 or diastolic blood pressure [DBP] levels ≥90 mmHg), were taking any blood pressure or lipid-lowering medications, or had a history of symptomatic ischemic heart disease or symptomatic peripheral neuropathy. Of the 680 women in the original DCCT cohort, 657 were postpubertal and premenopausal at DCCT baseline.

In 1994, 615 women from the original DCCT cohort enrolled in the Epidemiology of Diabetes Interventions and Complications (EDIC) study, designed to follow participants for long-term micro and macrovascular complications. During EDIC, a standardized annual history and physical examination included a standardized interview regarding menstrual patterns or discontinuation of menses, gynecologic surgeries, and use of exogenous sex hormones [21]. This report focuses upon the relationship between AMH, CVD risk factors, and markers of subclinical atherosclerosis during EDIC for women who had not undergone hysterectomy or oophorectomy by EDIC year 17 and also had initial serum AMH measures assessed during EDIC years 1–4, prior to CAC measures at EDIC year 8 (n = 349) and cIMT measures at EDIC year 6 (n = 390) (Fig. 1). Since AMH is made only by ovulating ovaries, it is undetectable after menopause, and previous reports noted that AMH levels were undetectable at 6 years prior to menopause [22]. We desired to limit the number of undetectable values, and so we measured AMH only prior to menopause. We also desired to have at least 2 values per woman, as AMH declines linearly prior to menopause. Therefore, for women who were naturally menopausal at EDIC year 17, AMH was assessed as close to EDIC baseline as possible and also assessed 7 years prior to their final menstrual period (n = 148). In a subset of these women who had reached natural menopause by EDIC year 17 (n = 50), AMH was measured every other year prior to

menopause to ensure that the declines in AMH were linear over time. For women who were still premenopausal at EDIC year 17, AMH was assessed as close to EDIC baseline as possible and also assessed at EDIC year 10. The median number of AMH measurements per woman was 2, with an interquartile ratio of 1–4, at an average of 6.3 years apart.

Clinical and biochemical endpoints were obtained annually by history, physical exam, and laboratory testing [23]. Body mass index (BMI), waist circumference, insulin dosage, SBP and DBP, and hemoglobin A1c (HbA1c) were assessed at randomization and quarterly during DCCT and annually in EDIC [24]. Lipid profiles and urinary albumin excretion rates (AER)/glomerular filtration rates (GFR) were obtained on alternate years. Total cholesterol, triglyceride, and high-density lipoprotein cholesterol (HDL) concentrations were determined by

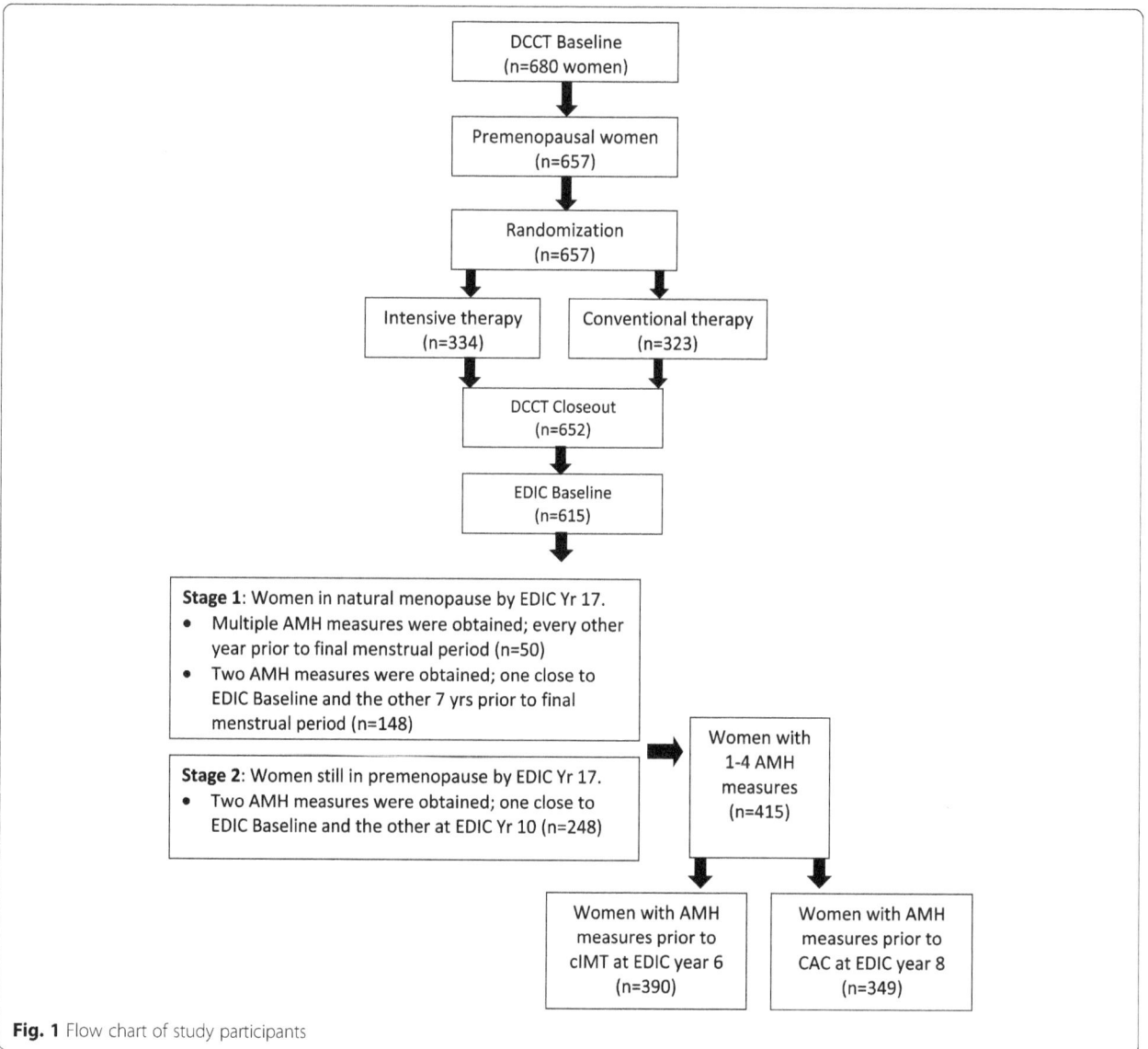

Fig. 1 Flow chart of study participants

enzymatic methods, and low-density lipoprotein choles-terol (LDL) was calculated using the Friedewald equa-tion [25]. Medication use was assessed at each exam by EDIC staff. Cigarette use was also self-reported and smoking was defined as reporting any cigarette use currently.

AMH assays were performed on previously stored samples by the EDIC Central Biochemistry Laboratory in Minneapolis, MN using ELISA (Beckman Coulter DSL, Webster, TX second generation kit) with a quanti-fication limit of 0.08 ng/ml [26], lower than reported for earlier generation assays [27]. Inter-assay coefficients of variation (CV) provided by the manufacturer were 8.0% at 0.15 ng/ml, 4.8% at 0.85 ng/ml and 6.7% at 4.28 ng/ml (mean = 6.5%); intra-assay CV is 4.6% at 0.14 ng/ml, 2.4% at 0.84 ng/ml and 3.3% at 4.41 ng/ml (mean = 4.0%). In the EDIC Central Biochemistry Laboratory, coeffi-cients of variation were 8.1% at a mean concentration of 3.3 ng/ml and 4.2% at a mean concentration of 8.3 ng/ml. For values less than the 0.08 ng/ml limit of quanti-fication but above the lower limit of detection, SoftMax Pro software (Sunnyvale, CA) was used to plot values, fit a cubic regression curve, and create splines which were then used to estimate AMH concentrations.

Carotid ultrasonography was performed at approxi-mately 1, 6, and 12 years after the initiation of the EDIC study [28]. Carotid IMT (mm) was assessed in a central unit (Tufts University, Boston, MA) by a single reader. Computed tomography of the heart was performed once during approximately the 8th EDIC year of follow-up [28]. At that visit, participants were scanned twice over calibra-tion phantoms of known calcium concentration with scans read centrally by readers who were masked to sub-ject identity and previous treatment assignment. The aver-age coronary artery CAC Agatston score from the 2 scans was used in the analysis. Presence of CAC was defined as an Agatston score > 6.25 mm^3, which represents a value that is <1% likely to be attributable to interscan variability.

Statistical analysis
We compared the distribution of CVD risk factors at EDIC baseline by quartile of the initial measure of AMH for each woman using analysis of variance for continu-ous variables and the chi square test for categorical vari-ables. Next, we examined whether AMH concentrations were associated with concurrent CVD risk factor values before and after adjustment for age. General linear mixed models accounted for multiple AMH measures and CVD risk factor measurements within each woman using PROC MIXED. Models examining blood pressure and renal function were additionally adjusted for anti-hypertensive medication use (angiotensin converting en-zyme inhibitors, angiotensin receptor blockers, beta blockers) at the time of blood pressure measurement;

other models examined lipid concentrations adjusted for lipid-lowering medication at the time of measurement. AMH was also modelled as a quadratic term, but this did not change the significance of the associations, so models are presented that assume a linear relationship between AMH and CVD risk factors.

We examined the relationship between continuous mea-sures of AMH and presence of CAC using logistic regres-sion models. Models used the initial AMH level during EDIC years 1–4 the primary independent variable and CAC >0 at EDIC year 8 as the dependent variable, un-adjusted and adjusted for concurrent CVD risk factors measured during the same year as the initial AMH value. Due to prior studies suggesting non-linear relationships between AMH and CVD risk factors as well as non-linear relationships between AMH and CAC in unadjusted com-parisons, we performed a sensitivity analysis that exam-ined AMH in quartiles rather than as a continuous variable. Similarly, we examined the relationship between continuous measures of AMH and cIMT using linear re-gression models with the initial AMH level during EDIC years 1–4 as the primary independent variable and con-tinuous cIMT measure as the dependent variable, un-adjusted and adjusted for concurrent CVD risk factors measured during the same year as the initial AMH value. As these models examined only a single measure of AMH, adjustment for repeated measurements within women were not performed. All analyses were performed using SAS version 9.2 (SAS Institute, Cary, NC).

Results
Characteristics of women at EDIC baseline by quartile of AMH value at their initial AMH measurement are shown in Table 1. Women in the lowest quartile of AMH were the oldest and women in the highest quartile of AMH were the youngest. Women in the lowest quar-tile of AMH had higher BMI, waist circumference, SBP, total cholesterol, LDL, and triglyceride concentrations and had lower eGFR than women in other quartiles. Duration of diabetes, cigarette use, OCP use, BMI, waist circumference, DBP, and HDL did not vary significantly by AMH quartile. Hypertension, use of hypertensive medications, and use of lipid-lowering medications was uncommon. The women in the lowest AMH quartile had the highest prevalence of CAC at year 8 (Table 2), followed by women in the highest AMH quartile, women in quartile 2, and then women in quartile 3. Al-though there was no relationship between quartile in AMH and cIMT at year 1, women in the lowest quartile of AMH had the highest cIMT at years 6 and year 12 followed by women in quartiles 2, 3, and 4.

Table 3 shows the associations between continuous measures AMH and concurrent individual CVD risk fac-tors before and after adjustment for age, medication use,

Table 1 Participant characteristics at EDIC baseline by quartile of women's initial AMH measurement (*n* = 390 women)

Range of AMH (ng/dl)	Quartile 1 <0.96 *n* = 99	Quartile 2 0.96–2.70 *n* = 97	Quartile 3 2.70–4.61 *n* = 98	Quartile 4 >4.61 *n* = 97	*p*-value
Age (years)	40.6 ± 6.2	34.6 ± 6.5	32.6 ± 6.0	31.0 ± 5.6	<0.0001
Diabetes duration (years)	14.4 ± 5.0	13.9 ± 5.2	14.4 ± 5.5	13.8 ± 5.4	0.78
Current smoking (%)	26.6%	20.4%	14.7%	15.1%	0.13
Current oral contraceptive use (%)	9.6%	18.3%	17.9%	11.8%	0.23
Body mass index (kg/m^2)	26.8 ± 4.7	25.1 ± 3.8	25.8 ± 3.9	25.7 ± 3.8	0.05
Waist circumference (cm)	80.9 ± 11.2	77.2 ± 7.6	77.4 ± 8.6	78.7 ± 8.8	0.02
Systolic blood pressure (mm Hg)	118.4 ± 13.0	113.2 ± 10.8	112.4 ± 11.2	111.7 ± 12.1	0.0005
Diastolic blood pressure (mm Hg)	73.9 ± 8.9	72.8 ± 9.0	71.5 ± 8.4	72.0 ± 9.9	0.27
Hypertension[a]	10.6%	7.5%	10.5%	14.0%	0.57
Total cholesterol (mg/dl)	200.5 ± 37.6	174.4 ± 31.0	179.3 ± 30.7	189.1 ± 33.1	<0.0001
Low-density lipoprotein cholesterol (mg/dl)	123.5 ± 34.8	101.8 ± 26.2	106.1 ± 26.8	113.1 ± 26.7	<0.0001
High-density lipoprotein cholesterol (mg/dl)	59.6 ± 14.5	59.6 ± 13.6	59.7 ± 13.8	59.8 ± 14.7	0.99
Triglycerides (mg/dl)	86.5 ± 45.0	65.1 ± 28.1	66.9 ± 30.5	80.6 ± 43.4	0.0001
Lipid medication use (%)	1.1%	2.2%	0%	0%	0.29
Log albumin excretion ratio (mg/day)	2.3 ± 1.0	2.5 ± 1.1	2.2 ± 1.0	2.6 ± 1.1	0.02
Estimated glomerular filtration rate (mL/min/1.73 m^2)	106.2 ± 11.9	114.4 ± 16.2	113.3 ± 12.5	116.7 ± 13.3	<0.0001

[a]Hypertension defined as systolic blood pressure ≥ 140 OR diastolic blood pressure ≥ 90 OR anti-hypertensive medication use
Means ± standard deviations or percentages shown

and multiple AMH and risk factor observations per woman. Such analyses account for the fact that when there are multiple observations per woman, the resulting values are correlated i.e. cluster. In these adjusted analyses, AMH values were not associated with any CVD risk factors or measures of renal function. When AMH was modeled as a quadratic term, these associations did not change.

There were 349 women who had AMH measurements during years 1–4 and CAC measurements at EDIC year 8. Table 4 shows the odds of having any CAC by AMH, before and after adjustment for age and other CVD risk factors. After adjustment for age, AMH had non-significant borderline associations with any CAC which was not altered after adjustment for covariates. In a sensitivity analysis, and due to the U-shaped relationship with prevalence of CAC in unadjusted analyses, we also examined the relationship between AMH in quartiles and the presence of any CAC. Compared to women in the lowest quartile of AMH, women in the 3rd or

Table 2 Presence of coronary artery calcification (CAC) and diameter of common carotid intima media thickness (cIMT) by baseline quartile of women's initial AMH measurement

	Quartile 1	Quartile 2	Quartile 3	Quartile 4	*p*-value
CAC > 0 (%)[a]	33.7%	17.2%	11.1%	20.5%	0.002
CIMT year 1 (mm)[b]					
Mean ± SD	0.620 ± 0.095	0.584 ± 0.059	0.595 ± 0.075	0.595 ± 0.075	
Median	0.613	0.576	0.579	0.601	
Range	(0.449–0.841)	(0.474–0.755)	(0.466–0.791)	(0.441–0.750)	0.22
CIMT year 6 (mm)[c]					
Mean ± SD	0.642 ± 0.104	0.609 ± 0.087	0.595 ± 0.086	0.596 ± 0.088	
Median	0.618	0.595	0.588	0.589	
Range	(0.451–1.10)	(0.432–0.927)	(0.429–0.824)	(0.413–0.928)	0.002

[a]Women who had AMH measures years 1–4 and CAC measurements at year 8 (*n* = 349)
[b]Women who had initial AMH measurements at EDIC year 1 and cIMT at year 1 (*n* = 172)
[c]Women who had initial AMH measurements at EDIC years 1–4 and cIMT measurements at EDIC year 6 (*n* = 390)
Means ± standard deviations or percentages shown

Table 3 Associations between AMH (ng/dl) and levels of concurrent cardiovascular disease risk factors and renal function (n = 390 women with n = 781 observations)

	Unadjusted	Adjusted for age and medication use[a]
Systolic blood pressure (mm Hg)	−0.32 (−0.60, −0.03)	0.005 (−0.29, 0.30)
Diastolic blood pressure (mm Hg)	−0.01 (−0.21, 0.18)	0.11 (−0.10, 0.31)
Total cholesterol (mg/dl)	−0.21 (−0.95, 0.53)	−0.02 (−0.81, 0.77)
Low-density lipoprotein cholesterol (mg/dL)	0.02 (−0.63, 0.66)	0.02 (−0.66, 0.71)
High-density lipoprotein cholesterol (mg/dL)	−0.14 (−0.44, 0.16)	−0.05 (−0.37, 0.28)
Triglycerides (mg/dL)	−0.25 (−1.22, 0.73)	−0.10 (−1.16, 0.85)
Log albumin excretion ratio (mg/day)	0.02 (−0.003, 0.04)	0.01 (−0.01, 0.04)
Estimated glomerular filtration rate (mL/min/1.73 m^2)	0.57 (0.25, 0.88)	0.02 (−0.29, 0.34)
Waist circumference (cm)	−0.11 (−0.34, 0.12)	−0.05 (−0.29, 0.20)

[a]Antihypertensive medication use for systolic and diastolic blood pressure, log AER, eGFR, and lipid-lowering medication use for total cholesterol, LDL, HDL, and triglycerides. Age was the only adjustment made in the waist circumference model
Beta-coefficients and 95% confidence intervals shown from repeated measures regression models. Each beta-coefficient is per 1 ng/dl increment in AMH

highest quartile of AMH had a slightly lower odds of any CAC after adjustment for age (odds ratio 0.40, 95% confidence interval [CI] 0.17, 0.94) which was similar in models which adjusted for both age and systolic blood pressure (OR 0.40, 95% CI 0.17, 0.94) and age and hemoglobin A1c (OR 0.40, 0.17, 0.94) although attenuated in models that examined age, total cholesterol, and high-density cholesterol (OR 0.46, 95% CI 0.19, 1.13). These results did not differ when treatment group was added as a covariate (data not shown).

The association between AMH and cIMT at years 1 and 6 are shown in Table 5. For cIMT measured at year 1, AMH was not associated with cIMT at year 1 before or after adjustment for age. For cIMT measured at year 6, AMH was associated with statistically significant although only very slightly higher cIMT which was not altered after adjustment for CVD risk factors. In a sensitivity analysis, when we examined AMH in quartiles, there was no association between quartile of AMH and degree of cIMT at year 1 or degree of cIMT at year 6. Quartile of AMH was not associated with change in cIMT between EDIC years 1 to 6 (results not shown), nor was quartile of AMH associated with change in cIMT between EDIC years 6 to 12 (results not shown).

Discussion

Women with type 1 diabetes have a higher prevalence of reproductive disorders compared to women without diabetes, including irregular menses [29], subfertility [30], and possibly polycystic ovary syndrome [31]. In addition, women with type 1 diabetes are at greater risk for CVD

and renal disease than women without diabetes [18]. Thus, among women with type 1 diabetes, it plausible that reproductive dysfunction could play a role in risk of CVD and/or renal disease. AMH is increasingly used in the diagnosis and management of reproductive disorders and for reproductive staging [9]. In this cohort of women with type 1 diabetes, AMH was not associated with CVD risk factors after adjustment of age. After adjustment for age, there were associations between AMH and CAC as well as between AMH and cIMT, although the associations, when present, were slight and of unclear clinical significance. AMH was associated with significantly although minimally higher cIMT. Women who had intermediate AMH concentrations, i.e. AMH concentrations that were neither in the lowest nor the highest quartile, had the lowest odds of CAC compared to women in the lowest quartile of AMH.

Previous studies have suggested that AMH, a proxy for reproductive age, might correlate with CVD risk factors independent of chronologic age. Only one report has examined women with type 1 diabetes. In another cohort of 150 premenopausal women with type 1 diabetes, higher concentrations of AMH were associated with lower levels of SBP before and after adjustment for age [13]. There was a U-shaped relationship between AMH and HDL, where extremes of HDL were associated with low AMH concentrations. As with the current report as well as our previous report examining HbA1c and AMH [15], there was no significant correlation between AMH and DBP, AMH and LDL, or between AMH and other diabetes characteristics including

Table 4 Association between initial measurement of AMH (ng/dl) during years 1–4 and CAC at year 8 before and after adjustment for concurrent CVD risk factors (n = 349 women)

	Unadjusted	Adjusted for age	Adjusted for age and SBP	Adjusted for age, total cholesterol, and HDL	Adjusted for age and A1c
AMH	1.01 (0.94–1.08)	1.08 (1.00–1.16)	1.08 (1.00–1.16)	1.08 (1.00–1.17)	1.08 (1.00–1.16)

Odds ratios and 95% confidence intervals shown

Table 5 Associations between initial AMH (ng/dl) during years 1–4 and cIMT (mm) before and after adjustment for concurrent CVD risk factors

	Unadjusted	Adjusted for age	Adjusted for age and SBP	Adjusted for age, total cholesterol, and HDL	Adjusted for age and A1c
Models for year 1 cIMT[a]					
AMH	0.00009 ± 0.002	0.002 ± 0.002	0.002 ± 0.002	0.002 ± 0.002	0.002 ± 0.002
p-value	0.95	0.11	0.10	0.22	0.13
Models for year 6 cIMT[b]					
AMH	0.00008 ± 0.002	0.005 ± 0.002	0.005 ± 0.002	0.004 ± 0.002	0.004 ± 0.002
p-value	0.66	0.0087	0.008	0.019	0.014

[a]Women who had AMH measurement at year 1 and cIMT measurements at EDIC year 1 (n = 172)
[b]Women who had AMH measurement at year 1 and cIMT measurements at EDIC year 6 (n = 390)
Least square means and standard errors shown

diabetes duration, HbA1c, or BMI after adjustment for age. We may not have found an association between AMH and SBP due to differences between the study populations. Although both studies performed AMH and CVD risk factor measurements at similar ages, EDIC did not exclude women with histories of irregular menses, and it is possible that the relationship between AMH and SBP differs among regularly cycling women. We also adjusted for the use of anti-hypertensive medications, although this should have accentuated any existing associations between AMH and blood pressure. We were also able to examine multiple AMH measurements and CVD risk factor measurements within each woman over time in a larger population.

Studies of AMH and CVD risk factors in populations without diabetes conflict, although the associations between AMH and CVD risk factors, when documented, have been modest. Reports in populations without diabetes have noted that AMH concentrations were not cross-sectionally associated with blood pressure or lipid profiles after adjustment for age and BMI [12, 32]. Tehrani et al. reported that women in the lowest quartile of AMH eventually had slightly greater increases in total cholesterol and LDL over a decade compared to women in other quartiles [14]. However, adjustment for medication use was not noted, and the increases were slight, the equivalent of 0.39 mg/dl per year, and adjustment for age was performed by transforming actual AMH levels into age-specific AMH levels, which might have minimized the impact of age-adjustment. AMH was not associated with progression in other risk factors; to our knowledge, previous reports have not examined whether AMH is associated with renal function.

Whether AMH could subsequently increase risk of atherosclerosis via CVD risk factors or through an independent pathway has not been well-studied. One report in macaques (n = 66) suggested that AMH was associated with atherosclerotic plaque size [16]. Macaques in the lowest tertile of AMH had greater plaque area than macaques in the highest tertile. Similarly, Looby et al. [17] noted that in a cohort consisting of HIV positive

and negative women, postmenopausal women had higher prevalence of coronary plaque vs. perimenopausal women vs. premenopausal women. AMH concentrations were undetectable in the first two groups and detectable in the last group. Other adjustments were not performed, so the association may have been due to other factors characterizing the menopausal transition. Our report suggests that if AMH and odds of CAC are associated, the relationship is not linear. Women in the highest quartile of AMH may have similar risk of CAC compared to women in the lowest quartile of AMH. While explanations are speculative, it is possible that elevated values of AMH correspond with other disorders, such as polycystic ovary syndrome, which increase the risk of CVD, and women with low values of AMH have minimal ovarian reserve, which may also increase the risk of CVD. Although mechanisms are speculative, AMH has been linked with molecules with endothelial activity, including vascular endothelial growth factor (VEGF) [33]. VEGF regulates angiogenesis, and extremes of VEGF confer decreased CVD risk [34]. Administration of VEGF has been demonstrated to stimulate AMH receptor 2 expression, which in turn can increase AMH binding in animal models [33]. Thus, AMH may be a marker for angiogenesis dysregulation. Alternatively, higher concentrations of inflammatory and endothelial dysfunction markers among lymphoma patients including interleukin 6 are significantly correlated with decreased AMH concentrations [35] as well as CVD risk [36], suggesting that AMH may also be linked with CVD through this pathway.

The two studies examining the relationship between AMH and cIMT conflict. Among women with type 1 diabetes, AMH and cIMT and between AMH and other measures of vascular flow were not related [13]. In a population of women without diabetes [6], Figueroa-Vega et al. lower AMH concentrations were strongly associated with thicker cIMT in 60 postmenopausal women. In that report, we note that the majority of postmenopausal women in this report had detectable and even elevated concentrations of AMH exceeding 5 ng/dl, despite having undergone natural menopause an average of 5 years before enrollment and use of an AMH assay with a high detection limit (0.375 ng/ml), contrary to previous reports suggesting that AMH declines to undetectable concentrations before the final menstrual period [7, 8, 14, 37, 38]. We found that that higher concentrations of AMH were associated with slightly thicker cIMT even after adjustment for covariates, although the magnitude of the association was so slight as to render clinical significance questionable.

Strengths of this report include its well-phenotyped population of women with type 1 diabetes, enabling examination of AMH with CVD risk factors as well as CAC, cIMT, and renal function. We were able to assess whether AMH was assessed with progression in cIMT as well as single measures of cIMT. As our report included women with type 1 diabetes, our results may not extend to women without diabetes, who are at lower CVD risk. We have previously reported that type 1 diabetes is associated with lower AMH concentrations [39], and thus diabetes may have modified the relationship between AMH and CVD risk factor severity and between AMH and atherosclerosis. Women in EDIC represent a cohort of a randomized trial population and experienced excellent glycemic control, and thus may not represent a more generalized population of persons with type 1 diabetes. It is possible that ovarian reserve may have stronger associations with subclinical atherosclerosis in a population with a higher severity of disease; despite their increased CVD risk from type 1 diabetes, women were in their forties at the time of their CAC and cIMT assessment, and the burden of disease was low. Similarly, end-stage renal disease was uncommon in the EDIC cohort [40], and it is possible that the relationship between AMH and renal disease would have been more pronounced in a population with a higher incidence of disease. Finally, we note that due to our sampling strategy of AMH measures prior to menopause, our power was limited to detect relationships between lower concentrations of AMH with greater burden of subclinical atherosclerosis or adverse risk factors.

Conclusions

Among women with type 1 diabetes, AMH has minimal associations with CVD risk factors apart from chronologic age, but AMH may have a non-linear relationship with CAC and associations with cIMT. Future investigations should replicate these findings between AMH, particular in larger populations without diabetes. The clinical significance of these associations is not known and should be corroborated with investigations of outcomes. The role of reproductive stage in CVD risk has been controversial [41]. Reproductive stage is also strongly associated with other end-organ complications,

including bone disease [42] and urologic conditions such vaginal atrophy [43], and investigation of the role of ovarian reserve in these complications should also be conducted. Future investigations should also explore whether the reproductive abnormalities experienced by women with type 1 diabetes are CVD risk factors apart from ovarian markers such as AMH.

Abbreviations

AER: Albumin excretion ratio; AMH: Anti-Müllerian hormone; BMI: Body mass index; CAC: Coronary artery calcification; CIMT: Carotid intima media thickness; CVD: Cardiovascular disease; DBP: Diastolic blood pressure; DCCT: Diabetes Control and Complications Trial; EDIC: Epidemiology of Diabetes Interventions and Complications; eGFR: Estimated glomerular filtration rate; HDL: High-density lipoprotein cholesterol; LDL: Low-density lipoprotein cholesterol; SBP: Systolic blood pressure

Acknowledgments

Not applicable.

Funding

The DCCT/EDIC has been supported by U01 Cooperative Agreement grants (1982–93, 2011–2016), and contracts (1982–2011) with the Division of Diabetes Endocrinology and Metabolic Diseases of the National Institute of Diabetes and Digestive and Kidney Disease (current grant numbers U01 DK094176 and U01 DK094157), and through support by the National Eye Institute, the National Institute of Neurologic Disorders and Stroke, the Genetic Clinical Research Centers Program (1993–2007), and Clinical Translational Science Center Program (2006-present), Bethesda, Maryland, USA. Additional support for this work was provided by DP3 DK098129. A complete list of participants in the DCCT/EDIC Research Group is presented in the Supplementary Material published online for the article in *N Engl J Med* 2015;372:1722–33. Industry contributors have had no role in the DCCT/EDIC study but have provided free or discounted supplies or equipment to support participants' adherence to the study: Abbott Diabetes Care (Alameda, CA), Animas (Westchester, PA), Bayer Diabetes Care (North America Headquarters, Tarrytown, NY), Becton Dickinson (Franklin Lakes, NJ), Eli Lilly (Indianapolis, IN), Extend Nutrition (St. Louis, MO), Insulet Corporation (Bedford, MA), Lifescan (Milpitas, CA), Medtronic Diabetes (Minneapolis, MN), Nipro Home Diagnostics (Ft. Lauderdale, FL), Nova Diabetes Care (Billerica, MA), Omron (Shelton, CT), Perrigo Diabetes Care (Allegan, MI), Roche Diabetes Care (Indianapolis, IN), and Sanofi-Aventis (Bridgewater NJ).

Authors' contributions

CK interpreted the data regarding AMH distributions and associations with CVD and CVD risk factors and wrote the manuscript. BB and YP performed the analysis, interpreted the data, and revised the manuscript. AS and HW revised the manuscript, interpreted the data, and performed data collection. VA and MS performed the AMH and other assays, interpreted the data, and reviewed the manuscript. All authors read and approved the final manuscript.

Competing interests

The authors declare that they have no competing interests.

Author details

[1]Departments of Medicine, Obstetrics & Gynecology, and Epidemiology, University of Michigan, 2800 Plymouth Road, Building 16, Room 430W, Ann Arbor, MI 48109-2800, USA. [2]The Biostatistics Center, George Washington University, Rockville, MD, USA. [3]Department of Laboratory Medicine and Pathology, University of Minnesota, Minneapolis, MN, USA. [4]Department of Urology, University of Washington, Seattle, WA, USA. [5]Department of Urology, University of Michigan, Ann Arbor, MI, USA.

References

1. Harlow S, Gass M, Hall J, Lobo R, Maki P, Rebar R, et al. Executive summary of the stages of reproductive aging workshop + 10; addressing the unfinished agenda of staging reproductive aging. J Clin Endocrinol Metab. 2012;97(4):1159–68.
2. Wellons M, Ouyang P, Schreiner P, Herrington D, Vaidya D. Early menopause predicts future coronary heart disease and stroke: the multi-ethnic study of atherosclerosis (MESA). Menopause. 2012;19(10):1081–7.
3. Sjoberg L, Pitkaniemi J, Harjutsalo V, Haapala L, Tiitinen A, Tuomilehto J, et al. Menopause in women with type 1 diabetes. Menopause. 2011;18(2):158–63.
4. de Kat A, Broekmans F, Laven J, van der Schouw Y. Anti-Mullerian hormone as a marker of ovarian reserve in relation to cardiometabolic health: a narrative review. Maturitas. 2015;80:251–7.
5. Aksglaede L, Sorensen K, Boas M, Mouritsen A, Hagen C, Jensen R, et al. Changes in anti-Mullerian hormone (AMH) throughout the lifespan: a population-based study of 1027 healthy males from birth (cord blood) to the age of 69 years. J Clin Endocrinol Metab. 2010;95:5357–64.
6. Figueroa-Vega N, Moreno-Frias C, Malacara J. Alterations in adhesion molecules, pro-inflammatory cytokines and cell-derived microparticles contribute to intima-media thickness and symptoms in postmenopausal women. PLoS One. 2015;10(5):e0120990.
7. Dolleman M, Depmann M, Eijkemans M, Heimensem J, Broer S, van der STroom E, et al. Antimullerian hormone is a more accurate predictor of individual time to menopause than mother's age at menopause. Hum Reprod. 2014;29(3):584–91.
8. Broer S, Eijkemans M, Scheffer G, van Rooij I, de Vet A, Themmen A, et al. Anti-mullerian hormone predicts menopause: a long-term follow-up study in normoovulatory women. J Clin Endocrinol Metab. 2011;96(8):2532–9.
9. Dewailly D, Andersen C, Balen A, Broekmans F, Dilaver N, Fanchin R, et al. The physiology and clinical utility of anti-Mullerian hormone in women. Hum Reprod. 2013;20(3):370–85.
10. Tehrani F, Solaymani-Dodaran M, Tohidi M, Goharai M, Azizi F. Modeling age at menopause using serum concentration of anti-Mullerian hormone. J Clin Endocrinol Metab. 2013;98:729–35.
11. Nair S, Slaughter J, Terry J, Appiah D, Ebong I, Wang E, et al. Anti-mullerian hormone (AMH) is associated with natural menopause in a population-based sample: the CARDIA Women's study. Maturitas. 2015;81:493–8.
12. Bleil M, Gregorich S, McConnell D, Rosen M, Cedars M. Does accelerated reproductive aging underlie premenopausal risk for cardiovascular disease. Menopause. 2013;20(11):1139–46.
13. Yarde F, Spiering W, Franx A, Visseren F, Eijkemans M, de Valk H, et al. Association between vascular health and ovarian ageing in type 1 diabetes mellitus. Hum Reprod. 2016;31(6):1354–62.
14. Tehrani F, Erfani H, Cheraghi L, Tohidi M, Azizi F. Lipid profiles and ovarian reserve status: a longitudinal study. Hum Reprod. 2014;29(11):2522–9.
15. Kim C, Dunn R, Braffett B, Cleary P, Arends V, Steffes M et al. Ovarian reserve in women with type 1 diabetes in the DCCT/EDIC Study. Diabet Med. 2015;33(5):691–2.
16. Appt S, Chen H, Clarkson T, Kaplan J. Premenopausal antimullerian hormone concentration is associated with subsequent atherosclerosis. Menopause. 2012;19(12):1353–9.
17. Looby S, Fitch K, Srinivasa S, Lo J, Rafferty D, Martin A, et al. Reduced ovarian reserve relates to monocyte activation and subclinical coronary artherosclerotic plaque in women with HIV. AIDS. 2016;30:383–93.
18. Orchard T, Dorman J, Maser R, Becker D, Drash A, Ellis D, et al. Prevalence of complications in IDDM by sex and duration. Pittsburgh epidemiology of diabetes complications study II. Diabetes. 1990;39(9):1116–24.
19. DCCT/EDIC Research Group, Nathan D, Zinman B, Cleary P, Backlund J, Genuth S, et al. Modern-day clinical course of type 1 diabetes mellitus after 30 years' duration: the diabetes control and complications trial/epidemiology of diabetes interventions and complications and Pittsburgh epidemiology of diabetes complications experience (1983-2005). Arch Intern Med. 2009;169(14):1307–16.
20. Diabetes Control and Complications Trial/Epidemiology of Diabetes Interventions and Complications Research Group. Retinopathy and nephropathy in patients with type 1 diabetes four years after a trial of intensive therapy. The Diabetes Control and Complications Trial/Epidemiology of Diabetes Interventions and Complications Research Group. N Engl J Med. 2000;342(6):381–9.
21. Kim C, Cleary P, Cowie C, Braffett B, Dunn R, Larkin M, et al. Effect of glycemic treatment and microvascular complications on menopause in women with type 1 diabetes in the diabetes control and complications trial/epidemiology of diabetes interventions and complications (DCCT/EDIC) cohort. Diabetes Care. 2014;37(3):701–8.
22. Sowers M, Eyvazzadeh A, McConnell D, Yosef M, Jannausch M, Zhang D, et al. Anti-mullerian hormone and inhibin B in the definition of ovarian aging and the menopause transition. J Clin Endocrinol Metab. 2008;93(9):3478–83.
23. Epidemiology of Diabetes Interventions and Complications (EDIC) Group. Design, implementation, and preliminary results of a long-term follow-up of the diabetes control and complications trial cohort. Diabetes Care. 1999;22:99–111.
24. Steffes M, Cleary P, Goldstein D, Little R, Wiedmeyer HM, Rohlfing C, et al. Hemoglobin A1c measurements over nearly two decades: sustaining comparable values throughout the diabetes control and complications trial and the epidemiology of diabetes interventions and complications study. Clin Chem. 2005;51(4):753–8.
25. Friedewald W, Levy R, Fredrickson D. Estimation of low-density lipoprotein cholesterol in plasma without use of the preparative ultracentrifuge. Clin Chem. 1972;18:499–502.
26. Kumar A, Kalra B, Patel A, McDavid L, Roudebush W. Development of a second generation anti-Müllerian hormone (AMH) ELISA. J Immunol Methods. 2010;362:51–9.
27. Broer S, Broekmans F, Laven J, Fauser B. Anti-Mullerian hormone: ovarian reserve testing and its potential clinical implications. Hum Reprod Update. 2014;20(5):688–701.
28. Purnell J, Zinman B, Brunzell J. The effect of excess weight gain with intensive diabetes mellitus treatment on cardiovascular disease risk factors and atherosclerosis in type 1 diabetes mellitus: results from the diabetes control and complications trial/epidemiology of diabetes interventions and complications study (DCCT/EDIC). Circulation. 2013;127:180–7.
29. Strotmeyer E, Steenkiste A, Foley T Jr, Berga S, Dorman J. Menstrual cycle differences between women with type 1 diabetes and women without diabetes. Diabetes Care. 2003;26:1016–21.
30. Jonasson J, Brismar K, Sparen P, Lambe M, Myren O, Ostenson C, et al. Fertility in women with type 1 diabetes: a population-based cohort study in Sweden. Diabetes Care. 2007;30:2271–6.
31. Escobar-Morreale H, Roldan-Martin M. Type 1 diabetes and polycystic ovary syndrome: systematic review and meta-analysis. Diabetes Care. 2016;39:639–48.
32. Cui L, Qin Y, Gao X, Lu J, Geng L, Ding L, et al. Anti-Mullerian hormone: correlation with age and androgenic and metabolic factors in women from birth to postmenopause. Fertil Steril. 2016;105(2):481–5.
33. Fang Y, Lu X, Liu L, Lin X, Sun M, Fu J, et al. Vascular endothelial growth factor induces anti-Mullerian hormone receptor 2 overexpression in ovarian granulosa cells of in vitro fertilization/intracytoplasmic sperm injection patients. Mol Med Rep. 2016;13(6):5157–62.
34. Kaess B, Preis S, Beiser A, Sawyer D, Chen T, Seshadri S, et al. Circulating vascular endothelial growth factor and the risk of cardiovascular events. Heart. 2015;102(23):1898–901.
35. Paradisi R, Vicenti R, Macciocca M, Seracchioli R, Rossi S, Fabbri R. High cytokine expression and reduced ovarian reserve in patients with Hodkin lymphoma or non-Hodgkin lymphoma. Fertil Steril. 2016;106(5):1176–82.
36. Looker H, Colombo M, Agakov F, Zeller T, Groop L, Thorand B, et al. Protein biomarkers for the prediction of cardiovascular disease in type 2 diabetes. Diabetologia. 2015;57(2):1363–71.

37. Sowers M, McConnell D, Yosef M, Jannausch M, Harlow S, Randolph J Jr. Relating smoking, obesity, insulin resistance, and ovarian biomarker changes to the final menstrual period. Ann N Y Acad Sci. 2010;1204:95–103.

38. Freeman E, Sammel M, Lin H, Gracia C. Anti-mullerian hormone as a predictor of time to menopause in late reprodutive age women. J Clin Endocrinol Metab. 2012;97(5):1673–80.

39. Kim C, Pan H, Braffett B, Cleary P, Arends V, Steffes M, et al. AMH in women with and without type 1 diabetes in the EDIC and MBHMS cohorts. Fertil Steril. 2016;106(6):1446–52.

40. DCCT/EDIC Research Group, de Boer I, Sun W, Cleary P, Lachin J, Molitch M, et al. Intensive diabetes therapy and glomerular filtration rate in type 1 diabetes. N Engl J Med. 2011;365(25):2366–76.

41. Kim C, Cushman M, Khodneva Y, Lisabeth L, Judd S, Kleindorfer D, et al. Risk of incident coronary heart disease events in men compared to women by menopause type and race. J Am Heart Assoc. 2015;4(7):piie001881.

42. Cauley J. Bone health after menopause. Curr Opinn Endocrinol Diabetes Obes. 2015;22(6):490–4.

43. Palacios S, Meija A, Neyro J. Treatment of the genitourinary syndrome of menopause. Climacteric. 2015;1:23–9.

17

The challenges of midlife women: themes from the Seattle midlife Women's health study

Annette Joan Thomas[1][*] [ID], Ellen Sullivan Mitchell[2] and Nancy Fugate Woods[3]

Abstract

Background: Midlife, the period of the lifespan between younger and older adulthood, has been described as a period of transition in women's lives. Investigators studying midlife have focused on women 40 to 65 years of age, who typically experience multiple social, psychological and biological challenges, among them the menopausal transition. Investigators have reported a diverse array of stressful events, for example, health concerns, family problems, work-related issues, deaths, frustrated goal attainment, and financial worries; however, none have identified which life events midlife women experience as the most salient. The purpose of this study was to understand the meaning behind the experiences that midlife women identify as the most challenging.

Methods: Participants were enrolled in The Seattle Midlife Women's Health Study, a longitudinal study spanning up to 23 years. Summative content analysis, incorporating manifest and latent analysis approaches, was used to identify life experiences that women described as the most challenging looking back over 15 years of being in the study. Eighty-one women responded to the question, "Since you have been in our study (since 1990 or 1991), what has been the most challenging part of life for you?"

Results: Women identified the most challenging aspects of midlife as changing family relationships, re-balancing work/personal life, re-discovering self, securing enough resources, and coping with multiple co-occurring stressors. Within these themes the most frequently reported challenges were: multiple co-occurring stressors, divorce/breaking up with a partner, health problems of self, and death of parents. Few women mentioned menopause as the most challenging aspect of their lives.

Conclusion: Women found themselves searching for balance in the midst of multiple co-occurring stressors while coping with losses and transitions, for some in a context of limited resources. Menopause was infrequently mentioned. Future research to identify the challenges experienced by more diverse populations of women and further understanding of the dynamics among multiple co-occurring stressors is needed to provide individualized health care appropriately to midlife women.

Keywords: Midlife women, Challenges, Multiple co-occurring stressors, Divorce, Health concerns, Deaths of parents, Parenting

* Correspondence: thomaann@seattleu.edu
[1]College of Nursing, Seattle University, Seattle, Washington, USA
Full list of author information is available at the end of the article

Background

Midlife, the period of the lifespan between younger and older adulthood, has been described as a period of transition in women's lives. Investigators studying midlife have focused on women 40 to 65 years of age, who typically experience multiple social, psychological and biological transitions. Among these are the biological transition of menopause, developmental transitions related to the aging/emerging self, and situational transitions such as divorce, taking on caregiving responsibilities for parents, or launching children [1].

In an investigation of the meaning of midlife, Woods and Mitchell [2] found that participants in the Seattle Midlife Women's Health Study described experiencing a diverse array of stressful events, for example, health problems, family problems, work-related issues, deaths, frustrated goal attainment, and financial concerns [2]. Women reported health problems they were experiencing as well as those their parents experienced with similar frequency. Deaths were also a common experience for these women. Family challenges included challenges with adolescent children, domestic violence, divorce or separation from a spouse, and the ending of relationships. Work problems included difficulty finding work, workplace conflicts, and downsizing of workplaces. These midlife women also reported frustrated goal attainment, such as being unable to complete an academic program or lack of personal time while working. In addition, they experienced financial stresses such as inability to pay college tuition for a child or afford essentials. SMWHS participants also rated their perceived stress levels in a health diary throughout their participation the study [3]. Greater perceived stress levels were significantly related to employment, history of sexual abuse, depressed mood, negative appraisal of aging changes, and poorer perceived health. Although symptoms such as hot flashes, sleep disruption, difficulty concentrating, and depressed mood were associated with greater perceived stress, the menopausal transition, itself, was unrelated to perceived stress. Improvement in role burden, social support, and income adequacy were associated with significantly lower perceived stress levels. Although SMWHS participants reported stressful experiences during midlife and rated their stress levels in a variety of dimensions of their lives over an extended period of time, it was not clear which stressors were most salient to them.

One approach to understanding experiences midlife women find most salient is inquiring about challenges they face. "Challenges" refer to experiences that require great physical or mental effort and determination that test one's strength, skill, or ability. In comparison, a stressor is a stimulus or threat that places real or perceived demands on the body, emotions, mind, or spirit of an individual. The word challenge, used in this study, is a word embroidered with strength and courage, allowing for the possibility that all challenges may not be perceived as stressful or appraised as negative. Due to the design of the original survey instrument, the words "challenge" and "stressor" as well as "challenging" and "stressful" were interchangeable in this report. In recent studies, women have reported challenges due to racism such as derogatory remarks, discriminatory actions such as sexual harassment [4] as well as menopausal symptoms, such as forgetfulness or difficulty concentrating (cognitive function), mood disturbances, and sleeping problems [3].

A commonly reported challenge of midlife is managing multiple responsibilities attributable to women's multiple roles. During midlife many women have been married or partnered, have already had children (some are young, others are leaving for college or jobs), have jobs of their own, manage their household with or without any additional help, and care for their aging parents. Kenny [5] studied stressors reported by 299 women aged 18–66 years and found that midlife women had more stressors than younger or older women and that midlife women identified roles involving family, work, and eldercare as sources of stress [5], but did not identify which of these sources of stress was the most salient.

During midlife, some women experience severing a relationship with a long-term partner. In addition to being emotionally wounded, women may experience a substantially reduced household income. Women in midlife tend to experience higher rates of loneliness and distress post-divorce than do younger divorced women [6].

Women in midlife begin to experience health problems of their own, such as cardiac problems [7] and sleeping difficulties [8]. Evidence from recent studies suggests that some of these health problems are related to women's stressful experiences. Investigators for the Study of Women's Health Across the Nation (SWAN) sleep study, examined very stressful life events using an 18-item version of the Psychiatric Epidemiology Research Interview Life Events Scale (PERI), which evaluated eight areas: school, work, romantic relationships, children, family, criminal and legal matters, finances and health. Women who had high chronic stress levels had lower subjective sleep quality, more waking after sleep onset (WASO) and were more likely to report insomnia compared to women who had low to moderate chronic stress profiles [8].

Allostatic load has been proposed as the accumulation of stress over time that affects health leading to preclinical signs of disease [9]. Allostasis refers to the ability to achieve stability and to maintain homeostasis during changing conditions through physiological or behavioral means and is adaptive in the short-term [10] but can revert to chronic stress in the long-term (allostatic load). Some events in daily life can generate chronic stress resulting in "wear and tear" on a woman's body, resulting in allostatic load [11]. Physiologic responses to stress are mediated by epinephrine and/or cortisol, which in turn elevate heart rate and blood pressure. Constant elevation of these responses over time can result in atherosclerosis increasing the risk for myocardial infarction and stroke [10]. Thus, health problems and allostatic load may be a result of chronic exposure to stressors or challenges.

Some of the questions that remain unanswered about midlife women's experiences of stress include: *Which life events do midlife women experience as the most stressful? Which of these life events are the most challenging to midlife women?*

Although studies of midlife women have documented multiple sources of stress, the impact of stressful life events and perceived stress on symptoms, subclinical changes, and diagnosed disease such as cardiovascular disease, to date there are no studies that reveal the most salient challenges for midlife women. The purpose of this study was to identify the experiences that midlife women found most challenging as they reflected on their experiences over more than a decade of their lives.

Methods
Study design and population
Data reported here were collected as part of a longitudinal study, the Seattle Midlife Women's Health Study (SMWHS). Women entered the study between 1990 and the early part of 1992 when most were in the early stages of the menopausal transition (MT) or not yet in the transition. All households within census tracts with a wide income range and mixed ethnicity were contacted by telephone for interested and eligible women. Women who were eligible were between 35 and 55 years of age, had at least one menstrual period within the last year, had a uterus and at least one ovary, were not pregnant, and could read and understand English. Out of 11,222 telephone contacts, 820 women were eligible, and 508 women entered the study [12].

The University of Washington Institutional Review Board approved each phase of the Seattle Midlife Women's Health Study (SMWHS) and approved informed consent forms. Each participant signed informed consent forms before entering the study.

Women completed an initial in-person interview administered by a trained registered nurse interviewer. A subset of the 508 women kept a health diary and from late 1996 to 2005 provided urine samples. All women were mailed a yearly Health Questionnaire and kept a menstrual calendar.

Sample
Eligible participants for this study ($N = 81$) provided data from the 2006 Health Questionnaire answering specifically the following question: "Since you have been in our study, what has been the most challenging part of life for you?" A total of 83 women responded to the 2006 Health Questionnaire. Two women did not answer this specific question leaving 81 women's answers for analysis. Women not eligible for this study did not answer the 2006 Health Questionnaire.

At enrollment in the parent study, women who were eligible for inclusion were midlife women with a mean age of 39.3 years (SD 3.0 years) and in the current study were approximately 53–54 years, an education of 16.6 years (SD 2.7 years), and mean family income of $38,320 (SD $14,782). Most (86%) were employed. Eligible women described themselves as African American (3.6%), Asian/Pacific Islander (8.3%), or White (88.1%). Women eligible for this study identified themselves as never married or never partnered (6%), married or partnered (76.2%), divorced or separated (16.7%) and widowed (1.2%). Most (67%) of the eligible women were parents.

As seen in Table 1, women with data included in the current analyses compared to those who were ineligible were similar with respect to family income, employment status, and marital status. They differed significantly by age, years of education, and race/ethnicity; women in the current study were younger, had more years of education, fewer were African American and more were White women, and fewer women were parents.

Analysis
Summative Content Analysis approach as described by Hsieh and Shannon [13] was used to identify life experiences that midlife women described as challenges looking back over 15 years when they participated in the SMWHS. Summative content analysis is a method that researchers use to interpret the content of data through coding in order to identify themes about the study participants' life experiences. Consistent with the approach, content analysis of data in this study started with identifying and quantifying key words or phrases in the text with the purpose of understanding the contextual use of the words or phrases. Some of the key words and categories that were identified prior to analysis were derived from the categories of the Life Event Questionnaire [14] while others were newly identified from the text. Potter and Levine-Donnerstein [15] refer to this first level of analysis as manifest content analysis whereby the appearance of the particular word or content is analyzed rather than the meaning derived. Each response was read over initially for a first impression. Subsequent readings included circling of key words or phrases in the women's answers in order to develop a

Table 1 Sample Characteristics at Start of Study (1990–1991) for the Eligible and Ineligible Women in the Challenges of Midlife Women from the SMWHS

Characteristic	Eligible N = 81	Ineligible N = 427	p value[a]
	Mean (SD)	Mean (SD)	
Age (years)	39.3 (3.0)	42.2 (4.7)	<.0001
Years of Education	16.6 (2.7)	15.5 (2.9)	<.0017
Gross Family Income	38, 320 (14,782)	35, 460 (15,258)	= .1210
Characteristic	% (N)	% (N)	p value[b]
Currently Employed	86%	86.3%	= .9428
Race/Ethnicity % (N)			
African American	3.6% (3)	13% (55)	= .0152
Asian/Pacific Islander	8.3% (7)	8.5% (36)	= .9528
White	88.1% (74)	74.8% (317)	= .0093
Other (Latina/Hispanic, Mixed/NativeAmerican)		3.8%	= .0749
Marital status % (N)			
Never married/partnered	6% (5)	7.1(30)	= .7211
Married/partnered	76.2% (64)	67.0% (284)	= .1028
Divorced/separated	16.7% (14)	24.1% (102)	= .1469
Widowed	1.2% (1)	1.9% (8)	= .6634
Ever a parent?			
Yes	60.7%	72.9%	0.0268
No	26.2%	27.1%	0.8673

[a]independent t-test
[b]Chi-square test

coding scheme. The women's responses were divided into five themes with categories listed under each main theme. The responses were listed under the appropriate category and ranged from one sub-category to five sub-categories, meaning that the women identified from one to five types of challenges. Disagreements about coding the challenges were discussed among the investigators (AJT, NFW) until a resolution was found.

In this study, counting of key words and phrases enabled the authors to identify patterns in the data and to contextualize the codes, which subsequently led the authors to discover meanings, a process which Morse and Field [16] refer to as latent content analysis, an aspect of the summative content analysis approach. Credibility or internal consistency of findings was assured by aligning the textual evidence with interpretation of data by the authors, all of whom are content experts [17].

Results
The midlife women's challenges revealed one overarching theme, "Searching for balance in the midst of multiple co-occurring stressors while coping with losses and transitions, for some in a context of limited resources" and five themes: 1) Changing Family relationships, 2) Re-balancing Work and Personal Life, 3) Rediscovering

Self, 4) Securing Enough Resources, and 5) Coping with Multiple Co-Occurring Stressors. Each theme was further divided into categories. If a response contained more than one challenge, the challenges were each counted individually as well as placed into the Multiple Co-Occurring Stressor category. For example, if a response conveyed parenting a teenager, husband's health, and a parent's death, there would be three separate types of challenges as well as the Multiple Co-Occurring Stressor challenge.

Searching for balance in the midst of multiple co-occurring stressors while coping with losses and transitions, for some in a context of limited resources
Data analysis revealed an overarching theme, "Searching for balance in the midst of multiple co-occurring stressors while coping with losses and transitions, for some in a context of limited resources," that encapsulated the experiences of all study participants and permeated the themes and sub-themes that emerged from the data. Women reported challenges related to changing family relationships, including those with several generations of family members, e.g. children and parents, while also striving to rebalance their work and personal life. In addition, they struggled with rediscovering

themselves, in the context of changing relationships. Securing sufficient financial resources posed challenges for many. A noteworthy set of challenges is related to coping with multiple co-occurring stressors. Each of these is discussed in greater detail below.

Changing family relationships

The theme of *Changing Family Relationships* refers to the changing relationships that women had with different family members: husband/partner, children, aging parents, siblings, and in-laws.

Changing relationships with partner

A number of women described changes in their long-term relationship with their partners as a primary life stressor. These changes ranged from a declining partner's health and necessity to provide caregiving, to separation or divorce after many years together, to the untimely death of a partner. Some women, especially those who reported divorce/breaking up with partner, reported more than one challenge. For example, one woman explained that an all-encompassing life challenge was a combination of events she summed up as "my divorce, my children leaving home and my parents dying all in the same 2-year period." Like others, another woman wrote, "The death of my brother in [year] and my divorce the same year" presented the most challenge. A partner's declining health was another new life challenge for many study participants. Women disclosed having to deal with their partners' declining health, including heart attacks, depression, disability, surgery, high blood pressure, reluctance to be more active, and alcoholism as a challenge. Like others, one study participant explained, "The most challenging has been watching my husband sink more and more into alcoholism and not being able to stop him." Another woman shared, "The challenges have changed from year to year- [year] I had an ectopic pregnancy- and infertility before/after- 0 kids. [years]- Graduate school and full-time work was challenging. [year]- currently, my husband's health problems and disability are most challenging."

For other midlife women the most challenging experiences were around the transition from an old to a new partner relationship. Similar to others, for one woman the life-midlife turmoil included "Losses and transitions –death of both parents, divorce from long term partner, beginning a new life with a new partner and his child."

Changing relationships with children

For many women in the study, changes in relationships included challenges with parenting that ranged from foster-parenting, parenting step-children, leaving children, children moving back in, to children moving out (Empty Nest), death of a child, or dealing with infertility.

For some of the women many of these issues were intertwined. For most women in the study, problems with parenting teenage children presented a new challenge. For others, step-parenting or foster parenting was most difficult. One woman explained, "Foster-parenting teens, most often teens who have been victims of abuse." Another one reflected parenting step-children was a new life challenge for her. She explained, "Dealing with being a blended family. Trying to parent stepchildren who would rather not have me around…" was quite difficult. For others, dealing with more than simply parenting teens added to the complexity of the parenting experience. Like many other women, one study participant listed multiple challenges, "My current job, my daughter from age 15-18, my mother's death, my husband's unemployment."

Children leaving home (e.g., for college) and children moving back home were also challenging for some women. One woman explained, "Family life – Change from having little children to them all growing up and leaving – changing relationship with husband because of that and personal changes" was strenuous. A woman whose child came back home said, "getting older, stiffer, clumsier. Seeing my finances shift, caring for 2 elderly parents and having a grown child move home w/ no finances" was wearisome. One woman in the study shared, "My son dying in [year] from suicide" was her greatest midlife challenge.

For childless women in the study, a midlife challenge represented a realization that biological parenthood will never be part of their life experience. One woman reflected, "The challenges have changed from year to year – [year] I had an ectopic pregnancy – and infertility before/after resulting in 0 kids. [years]– Graduate school and full-time work was challenging. Currently my husband's health problems and disability is the greatest challenge." Another woman indicated, "accepting that I would never be a biological parent, never have my 'own' kids, and possibly never become 'important' to my two step-children (now grown and living away). Everyone else's pregnancies, baby showers, and 'kid talk' is also a challenge."

Changing relationships with aging parents

Caregiving for parents, death of parents, parents' health problems, and relationships with parents encompassed the women sharing about their relationships with aging parents. Like others, one woman shared, "Caregiving for parents and losses are challenging – Losing father [year], father-in-law [year], mother-in-law [year], and only having my mother still living." For some study participants, death of a parent was the most challenging part of their midlife experience. Others described, "Losing my Dad to brain cancer," and "Experiencing my parents' death" as the most challenging part of midlife. One woman remembered, "Within four months, my mother had a severe stroke, my father died and a month later (to the day) my mother passed away." For other study participants who still had their parents, "parents getting old" and "Dad's health" were cited as the most challenging.

Changing sibling relationships

The issues surrounding women's changing relationships with siblings consisted of three key narratives: death of a sibling, relationship problems with siblings, and seeking harmonious sibling relationships. Women recounted, "the death of my brother in [year] and my divorce the same year" and "Dealing with not getting along with my older sister" as some examples of the most challenging part of midlife.

Changing relationships with in-laws

With aging in-laws, for some women in the study challenges came from having to move in together. One woman reported, "Moving in and living with all of my In-Laws" was the most challenging thing she had to do.

Re-balancing work and personal life

For many women in the current study, stressful job/career, unemployment, balancing multiple roles, job change/ career change, job loss/ unemployment, finding a job with health benefits, and facing retirement necessitated re-balancing work and personal life. Only three out of 81 women in the study cited their job as the most challenging part of midlife. For the majority of women, feeling overworked, and having to balance multiple roles was difficult. Like others, one woman explained: "Balancing all aspects of my life - as a mother, as a wife, as a teacher and as a woman and as the major head of the household (cooking, cleaning, etc.) currently is the greatest challenge of my life." For others, the greatest challenges came from "Getting into a more interesting career," dealing with personal health issues such as a breast cancer diagnosis, going through a divorce, or losing a partner, losing a job and seeking new employment with benefits. One woman elaborated,

"Finding and sustaining suitable employment with health care benefits. Having intermittent medical coverage caused me to postpone a surgery (hyperparathyroid) for 3 years" as the most significant issue she had to deal with in midlife.

Re-discovering self

Re-discovering self was important to many women in the current study. Health problems, existential issues, self-esteem/ self-acceptance, returning to school, the menopausal transition, and personal changes were the five sub-themes related to the self. Many women commented about health problems they had. Health problems included heart surgery, arthritis, physical disability due to arthritic pains, chronic pain, breast cancer, motor vehicle accident resulting in the diminished use of the woman's right hand, blot clot in the leg, and as one woman summarized: "getting older, stiffer, clumsier."

Women focused on making meaning of or appraising various aspects of their lives. Some of the women focused on accepting not being able to achieve their goals in life, realizing that the number of active years is limited, others on seeking new relationships. A number of women remarked about the newly found comfort with whom they were and self-acceptance. Similar to others, one study participant concluded, "Becoming more comfortable with myself. Accepting myself & having better self-esteem…" was most challenging. In order to re-discover oneself, some women returned to graduate school or decided to finish the university degree they once started. Surprisingly, only four out of 81 women in the current study commented on their menopausal transition symptoms as being the most challenging aspect of midlife, which included hot flashes, mood swings, difficulty remembering things, and excessive uterine bleeding.

Securing enough resources

Generating enough resources was an all-encompassing task for many study participants. The women found financial challenges, partner's unemployment, and lack of health insurance as very stressful life issues.

Some women revealed financial challenges such as supporting children in private schools with a partner's sporadic job situation, financing college, and becoming financially secure as stressful. Many of them described how they coped with such situations in life. For example, one woman enumerated, "I have to work 2 jobs and long hours to support my children, but never seem to get ahead…" Another woman explained, "having to close a business, including laying off people, not paying business debts, selling off furniture, etc., and then having to sell our home to pay off a bank loan" as most challenging. For some women the difficult financial decisions were related to their partner's unemployment. One example was "…Constant threat of strikes or job lay off for my husband and eventually job loss was difficult."

Lack of health insurance was also a great concern to women. One woman related that "Finding and sustaining suitable employment with health care benefits" and "Having intermittent medical coverage" were the greatest challenges for her.

Coping with multiple co-occurring stressors

As stated in the preceding paragraphs many women in the current study had to deal with multiple life stressors in their midlife years, many of them occurring at or around the same time. The majority of women identified multiple co-occurring stressors as they described their most challenging experiences. One woman commented, "Dealing with stress – job stress, health stress, social stress, family stress, etc. For a time, it seemed to snow-ball with no end in site." Some women explained that being overworked and balancing multiple roles were the most challenging part of midlife. Two examples were, "Fulfilling obligations of work and family" and "Balan-cing all aspects of my life - as a mother, as a wife, as a teacher and as a woman and as the major head of the household (cooking, cleaning, etc.)."

Discussion

Seattle Midlife Women's Health Study participants found themselves searching for balance in the midst of multiple co-occurring stressors while coping with losses and transitions, for some in a context of limited re-sources. Themes of challenges for this group of midlife women included 1) changing family relationships, 2) re-balancing work and personal life, 3) re-discovering self, 4) securing enough resources, and 5) coping with multiple co-occurring stressors.

Research about self-in-relation to others [18] provides a useful framework for understanding the salience of these categories of challenging experiences. Taking care of fam-ily members with whom women have affiliations or con-nections is central to the lives of many women. Women's affiliations are organized around being able to make and maintain relationships with others. Taking care of others (partners, children, parents) is one way of describing how women's connections are formed. For many women, the threat of terminating a connection is viewed not only as a loss of connection, but as a total loss of self. Losses were exemplified in this study as many women identified di-vorce and losing their parents as the most challenging as-pect of midlife in *Changing family relationships.* In an ethnographic qualitative research study from Australia [19], Dare and colleagues found that while many midlife women cope with the menopausal transition and their children leaving the house, the aging and death of their parents [20] and the effect of divorce [6] present more ser-ious long-term challenges to these women.

In addition to relational issues, the workplace con-tinues to provide many challenges for women. Overwork is a common experience, detailed well in Hochshild's "Second Shift" [21]. The combination of responsibilities women assume beyond their employment remain daunt-ing for U.S. women, with many not having access to help with child care and household maintenance. Indeed, Hochshild's observations were that women worked the equivalent of a 'second shift' after they returned home after employment. Thus, launching children may be emancipatory for both the late adolescent and young adult children as well as their midlife mother.

Recent study of women's multiple roles, including work-family conflicts, has largely focused on younger, re-productive age women with preschool or school-aged chil-dren. Recognition of the continuity of the challenge of balancing competing demands of work and family for midlife women, and the addition of caring responsibilities for their parents, points to increased complexity of achiev-ing balance and leading to the use of the term "sandwich generation" [22] to describe the compression of midlife women's lives by their children's and parents' needs.

In addition to rebalancing work and personal life, women faced challenges of re-discovering themselves in the context of their changing relationships. Miller and Stiver [18], proposed that a woman's sense of self and self-worth is often grounded in her ability to make and maintain relationships, and that these connections, not separations, can lead to strong, healthy development. In-dividual development, seen in the category of *Re-disco-vering Self,* proceeds by means of connection. Women connect with other women by finding relationships that foster mutual growth or mutuality. Mutuality benefits both people to grow and develop in and as a result of the relationship. This mutuality may manifest itself in a woman with breast cancer connecting with a breast can-cer support group or with others who have a different health problem. Women may develop further by ques-tioning their existence, their purpose, or raising other existential questions that surface in midlife and relating these questions to someone with whom they share mu-tuality. According to Miller and Stiver [18], the inclin-ation toward connection that women feel in themselves is a strength. Any matter in question in relation to the self may enable women to develop themselves further by sharing with another person; this forwardness of mutual-ity increases the strength of the relationship.

Women's descriptions of challenges related to re-discovering themselves reflected their interest in the next stage of their lives. Current literature about women's experiences of aging emphasize the "third chapter:" Sarah Lawrence-Lightfoot coined this term to designate the years when one is neither old nor young, a period that can be transformative in women's lives. In her case studies of adults, Lawrence-Lightfoot explores themes of engage-ment over retreat, labor over leisure, and reinvention over retirement, emphasizing the importance of active engage-ment, purposefulness, and new learning as themes in the stories that people write about in the third chapter of their lives [23]. Mary Catherine Bateson [24] also examines the middle years, revising Erik Erickson's model of human de-velopment to include a second stage of adulthood in which the challenges include engagement over withdrawal. Her discussion of lifelong learning as part of human devel-opmental processes emphasizes the achievement of wis-dom and humility as one confronts the challenges of aging. Both Lawrence-Lightfoot [23] and Bateson [24] invite consideration of midlife as a period during which it is possible to actively compose a life story or narratives into which we can live as we age.

Often before a woman has the opportunity for self-introspection, she may find that dealing with concerns about material resources, such as financial worries, employment and health insurance take precedence. Although the majority of women in this study were not living in poverty, women experience disproportionately lower incomes than men. For the fourth quarter of 2017, the Bureau of Labor Statistics reported weekly median earnings for women who were full-time wage or salary workers as $771.00, which was 82% of the $944.00 median weekly earnings for men [25]. During midlife, both men and women reach their peak earning capacity. Women who leave the labor force to raise their children or those women who have been laid off, struggle with access to benefits from employment, such as healthcare and often lag behind in their cumulative retirement benefits in comparison to men. A woman's exposure to securing enough resources is also impacted by her partner's employment status. For example, when a woman's partner faces unemployment, the family experiences the consequences, especially if the employment benefits, such as health insurance, are from the partner's employer. If a woman's income is the primary household income, job loss can also result in loss of healthcare if the healthcare benefits are from her employer.

The most commonly experienced challenges for midlife women across all themes were identified as *Coping with Multiple Co-occurring Stressors*. Midlife women reported multiple co-occurring stressors when asked what was the most challenging for them during the past 15 years. Midlife is marked by women who are overworked with multiple roles and responsibilities. Lanza di Scalea et al. [26] investigated role stress, role reward, and mental health in a cross-sectional sample of 2549 women, who were 45–55 years with roles such as being employed, married, a mother, and/or a caregiver, revealing 34% of the sample were involved in 2 roles and 50% of the sample were involved in 3 roles [26]. The roles reported [26] were similar to those reported in this study as challenges in a woman's job, being married/partnered, being a parent, and taking care of elderly parents.

Only four women (4/81 = 5%) in the SMWHS sample reported the menopausal transition as being part of the most challenging aspects of midlife, identifying hot flashes, mood swings, difficulty remembering, and excessive uterine bleeding. Thus, their challenges were not with experiencing the menopausal transition itself, but, experiencing symptoms. This finding is surprising given that 85% of midlife women report one or more symptoms, such as hot flashes, depressed mood, and/or sleep disturbances [27]. In

the Penn Ovarian Aging Study, 26 % of women disclosed moderate to severe hot flashes and 9 % revealed having daily hot flashes [28]. Also, The Study of Women's Health Across the Nation (SWAN) identified 60–80% of women experience hot flashes at some point during the menopausal transition [29]. Despite the prevalence of symptoms, it is possible that the stressful nature of the menopausal transition has been over-emphasized [30].

This study has several limitations. First, the sample size consisted of responses from only 81 women, most of whom were White, employed, and married or partnered. The average age was 39 years at enrollment (approximately 53–54 years at the time of the current study) with an average of 17 years of education and 61% were parents. The participants included in this component of the SMWHS differed from those in the parent study who, at enrollment, were older, made less money, were more ethnically diverse, were less likely to be married, and more likely to be parents. Additionally, the women's answers to the Health Questionnaire usually included only 2–3 sentences, and their responses to a written questionnaire vs interview made further clarification of their responses impossible. Future investigations should include more ethnic diversity. Geronimus and colleagues [31] studied weathering on Black and White adults aged 18 to 64 years using logistic regression and odds ratios and found that Black women have a larger allostatic load compared to either Black men or White women and that marked differences were between non-poor Black women and non-poor White women suggesting that race is a key component in the impact of chronic stress on health [31].

The current investigation had several strengths. This study is the first to examine midlife women's descriptions of their challenges over an extended reference period of 15 years while participating in the Seattle Midlife Women's Health Study. Results of this study included the most commonly reported challenges over the past 15 years of midlife explained by the women themselves. These findings are important as they reveal the challenges most salient to midlife women and may also help providers to identify women at high risk for allostatic overload (e.g., sustained high blood pressure, sustained high levels of cortisol as a result of chronic high levels of stress), which may lead to heart disease, stroke, or sleeping problems. Further, providers will find these results informative in order to individualize care, so that they can determine resources and interventions to help this specific age group of women who perform so many roles with all their associated responsibilities.

Conclusion
The over-arching theme of searching for balance in the midst of multiple co-occurring stressors, while coping with losses and transitions, for some in a context of

limited resources, spanned five categories. The most frequently reported challenges identified were multiple co-occurring stressors. Further study of multiple co-occurring stressors is warranted. Perhaps a single stressor, e.g., divorce, precipitates several related stressors. For example, loss of life partner precipitates loss of income, loss of children and separation from a relational network of mutual friends of the couple. Also, experience of a single stressor, such as development of a chronic illness, may precede other stressors such as job loss, a need to relocate living arrangements and the financial stressors of paying for medications. Inquiring about a focal stressor and its consequences may help women elaborate a series of stressors that more fully illuminates midlife women's experiences.

Acknowledgements
We acknowledge all the women who participated in the SMWHS. Only the authors of this paper contributed to this manuscript.

Authors' contributions
AJT conducted the literature review, analyzed the data and had primary responsibility for writing the manuscript. NFW contributed to the design and literature review, analyzed the data and edited the manuscript. ESM edited the manuscript. ESM and NFW were PIs of the Seattle Midlife Women's Health Study and collected all data. All authors read and approved the final manuscript.

Author's information
Annette Joan Thomas, College of Nursing, Seattle University,
Ellen Sullivan Mitchell, Department of Family and Child Nursing, University of Washington School of Nursing,
Nancy Fugate Woods, Department of Biobehavioral Nursing and Health Informatics, University of Washington School of Nursing,

Competing interests
NFW is guest editor of this journal. Peer review and all decisions made regarding this manuscript were made by an associate editor at a different institution. AJT and ESM have no competing interests.

Author details
[1]College of Nursing, Seattle University, Seattle, Washington, USA. [2]Family and Child Nursing, University of Washington, Seattle, Washington, USA. [3]Biobehavioral Nursing and Health Informatics, University of Washington, Seattle, Wahsington, USA.

References
1. Smith-DiJulio K, Woods N, Mitchell E. Well-being during the menopausal transition and early postmenopause: a longitudinal analysis. Menopause. 2008;15(6):1095–102.
2. Woods NF, Mitchell ES. Women's images of midlife: observations from the Seattle midlife Women's health study. Health Care Women Int. 1997;18:439–53.
3. Woods NF, Mitchell ES, Percival DB, Smith-DeJulio K. Is the menopausal transition stressful? Observations of perceived stress from the Seattle midlife Women's health study. Menopause. 2009;16(1):90–7.
4. Woods-Giscombé CL, Lobel M. Race and gender matter: a multidimensional approach to conceptualizing and measuring stress in African American women. Cult Divers Ethn Minor Psychol. 2008;14(3):173–82.
5. Kenny J. Women's inner balance: a comparison of stressors, personality traits and health problems by age groups. J Adv Nurs. 2000;31:639–50.
6. Sakraida TJ. Common themes in the divorce transition experience of midlife women. J Divorce and Remarriage. 2005;43(1,2):69–88.
7. Stevens S, Thomas SP. Recovery of midlife women from myocardial infarction. Health Care for Women Int. 2012;33(12):1096–113.
8. Hall MH, Casement MD, Troxel WM, et al. Chronic stress is prospectively associated with sleep in midlife women: the SWAN sleep study. Sleep. 2014; 10(38):1645–55.
9. McEwen BS, Wingfield JC. The concept of allostasis in biology and biomedicine. Horm Behav. 2003;43(1):2–15.
10. McEwen BS. Physiology and neurobiology of stress and adaptation: central role of the brain. Physiol Rev. 2007;87:873–904.
11. McEwen BS. Protective and damaging effects of stress mediators. N Engl J Med. 1998;338:171–9.
12. Mitchell ES, Woods NF. Symptom experiences of midlife women: observations from the Seattle midlife women's health study. Maturitas. 1996; 25:1–10.
13. Hsieh H-F, Shannon S. Three approaches to qualitative content analysis. Qual Health Res. 2005;15(9):1277–88.
14. Norbeck JS. Modification of life event questionnaires with female respondents. Res Nurs Health. 1984;7(1):61–71.
15. Potter WJ, Levine-Donnerstein D. Rethinking validity and reliability in content analysis. J Appl Commun Res. 1999;27:258–84.
16. Morse JM, Field PA. Qualitative research methods for health professionals. 2nd ed. Thousand Oaks, CA: Sage; 1995.
17. Weber RP. Content analysis. Beverly Hills, CA: Sage; 1990.
18. Miller JB, Stiver IP. The healing connection: how women form connections in therapy and in life. Boston: Beacon Press; 1997.
19. Dare JS. Transitions in midlife: contemporary experiences. Health Care for Women Int. 2011;32:111–33.
20. Perrig-Chiello P, Hopflinger F. Aging parents and their middle-aged children: demographic and psychosocial challenges. European J Aging. 2005;2:183–91.
21. Hochshild AR, Machung A. The second shift: working parents and revolution at home. New York: Avon Books; 1989.
22. Raphael D, Schlesinger B. Caring for elderly parents and adult children being at home: interactions of the sandwich generation family. Soc Work Res and Abstr. 1993;29(1):1–10.
23. Lawrence-Lighfoot S. The third chapter: passion, risk, and adventure in the 25 years after 50. New York: Sarah Crichton Books; 2009.
24. Bateson MC. Composing a further life: the age of active wisdom. New York: Vintage Books; 2010.
25. Bureau of Labor Statistics, U.S. Department of Labor, The Economics Daily, Median weekly earnings 767 for women, 937 for men, in third quarter 2017 on the Internet athttps://www.bls.gov/opub/ted/2017/median-weekly-earnings-767-for-women-937-for-men-in-third-quarter-2017.htm. Accessed 29 Mar 2018.
26. Lanza di Scalea T, Matthews KA, Avis NE, et al. Role stress, role reward, and mental health in a multiethnic sample of midlife women: results from the study of women's health across the nation (SWAN). J Women's Health. 2012;21(5):481–9.
27. Woods NF, Mitchell ES. Symptoms during the perimenopause: prevalence, severity, trajectory and significance in women's lives. Proceeding of the NIH State-of-the-Science Conference on management of menopause-related symptoms. Am J Med. 2005;118(Suppl 2):14–24.

28. Freeman EW, Grisso JA, Berlin J, et al. Symptom reports from a cohort of African American and white women in the late reproductive years. Menopause. 2001;8(1):33–42.
29. Gold E, Colvin A, Avis N, et al. Longitudinal analysis of vasomotor symptoms and race/ethnicity across the menopausal transition: study of women's health across the nation (SWAN). Am J Public Health. 2006;96(7):1226–35.
30. Judd FK, Hickey M, Bryant C. Depression and midlife: are we overpathologising the menopause? J Affect Disord. 2012;136:199–211.
31. Geronimus AT, Hicken M, Keene D, Bound J. "Weathering" and age patterns of allostatic load scores among blacks and whites in the United States. Am J Pub Health. 2006;96(5):826–33.

18

Undesirable stressful life events, impact, and correlates during midlife: observations from the Seattle midlife women's health study

Annette Joan Thomas[1][*] [iD], Ellen Sullivan Mitchell[2] and Nancy Fugate Woods[3]

Abstract

Purpose: To examine the undesirable stressful life events midlife women experience, including: 1) which life events midlife women reported most frequently; 2) which life events women rated as most undesirable; and 3) whether age, years of education, income, employment, race/ethnicity, marital status, being a parent, and the menopausal transition stage were associated with the impact scores of the life event categories.

Background: In addition to the menopausal transition, midlife is a time of increased responsibilities for women related to multiple roles such as taking care of children, caring for elderly parents, managing households, and working outside the home. These multiple roles put midlife women at risk for increased stress with little time for themselves in order to relieve stress.

Methods: The sample used in this study is part of a larger longitudinal study, The Seattle Midlife Women's Health Study. Women ($N = 380$ for Occasion 1) completed the 77-item Life Events Scale on four occasions during the course of the SMWHS: Occasion 1 (1990), Occasion 2 (1992), Occasion 3 (1997), and Occasion 4 (2000). In addition to descriptive analyses of frequency of life events and the undesirable impact of life events, demographic correlates (age, education, income, employment, being a parent as well as marital status, race/ethnicity, and menopausal transition stages) were examined in relation to the stressful life event scores.

Results: Highest scores of undesirable life events were for categories of both Financial and Family/Friends over 3 of the 4 occasions. Health and Crime/Legal scores were among the highest for 2 occasions. Impact of the undesirable stressful life events was greatest for categories of Family/Friends; Personal/Social; Work; and, Health. Age, income, marital status, being a parent, and menopausal transition stage were each associated with specific categories of the stressful event impact scores.

Conclusion: Most commonly reported undesirable life events were not those women described as having the greatest impact. Impact of life event stress reflected women's social roles and connections as seen in the categories with the highest impact scores: Family/Close Friends, Personal/Social, and Work. Menopausal transition stages were related only to undesirable health events.

Keywords: Stressful life events, Menopausal transition, Midlife women

* Correspondence: thomaann@seattleu.edu
[1]College of Nursing, Seattle University, Seattle, USA
Full list of author information is available at the end of the article

Introduction

Although stressful life events have been the focus of research for a variety of populations, there has been relatively little attention paid to understanding the stressful aspects of midlife women's lives. Many of the studies that have investigated stress in midlife women have used measurements of perceived stress, scales rated at different time points, descriptions, or health-related quality of life; few have used life event scales.

One approach to studying perceived stress among midlife women has been to ask women to rate their stress levels over a period of time, such as the past 24 h, and to relate their ratings to events in their lives, for example progression through the menopausal transition stages. Woods and colleagues [1] examined the relationship of menopausal transition (MT)-related factors (MT stage, urinary estrone glucuronide, follicle-stimulating hormone, aging), psychosocial factors (income adequacy, role burden, social support, parenting, employment, history of sexual abuse, depressed mood) and symptoms (hot flashes, depressed mood, lower sexual desire, difficulty getting to sleep, night-time awakening, early morning awakening, forgetfulness, difficulty concentrating) on perceived stress recorded by Seattle Midlife Women's Health Study (SMWHS) participants in a daily health diary. They found that perceived stress ratings were unrelated to the menopausal transition stage, but significantly associated with symptoms. Decrease in role burden, social support, and income adequacy was associated with significantly lower levels of perceived stress. Using multivariate models, Freeman and colleagues [2] examined perceived stress on symptoms women experienced during the menopausal transition and found that perceived stress was strongly correlated with symptom severity in the Penn Ovarian Aging Study. Women who reported high stress scores were 40% more likely to report irritability, anxiety, mood swings, concentration difficulties, and headache compared to those women who reported low stress scores [2].

Another approach has been to examine women's own descriptions of their stressful experiences as they relate to midlife and menopause [3–5]. Woods and Mitchell [3] found that one of the stressful aspects of women's anticipation of menopause was described as uncertainty about what to expect [5]. Thomas [4] recently reported results of content analysis of women's descriptions of their most challenging experiences during 15 years of participation in the Seattle Midlife Women's Health Study, revealing that in addition to challenges involving divorce/breaking up with a partner, death of a parent, and health concerns of their own, a common feature for midlife women was experiencing multiple co-occurring stressors. However, when women looked back over the time period during which they experienced the menopausal transition, menopause did not figure prominently in their most challenging experiences [4].

Other approaches have included researching the impact of stress on modifiable lifestyle factors. To illustrate, in a cross-sectional study from Australia, Seib and colleagues [6] used structural equation modeling to investigate the impact of stress on lifestyle and quality of life using the Life Stressor Checklist-revised (LSC-R; to determine high magnitude stressors) and found that women who reported high magnitude stressors also reported high BMI and more chronic illness. Also, duration of exposure to life stressors was associated with higher depressive symptom scores and sleep disturbance scores [6].

Few studies investigating stress in midlife women utilized life event scales; and, most of these investigations have involved cross-sectional data. For example, in a cross-sectional study from Iran involving women 35 to 55 years, Horri et al. [7] investigated the relationship between education and metabolic syndrome using the stressful life events (SLE) scale and found that the prevalence of metabolic syndrome in women with eight or more SLEs was higher compared to those women who reported fewer than eight SLEs. Furthermore, poorly educated women reported a greater number of SLEs. In a case-control study from New England, Rosman et al. [8] used the Psychiatric Epidemiology Research Interview (PERI) scale to determine the cumulative impact of stressful life events in women on the development of Takotsubo Cardiomyopathy (TC: defined as acute stress-induced cardiomyopathy, a temporary condition where the left ventricle changes shape and the heart becomes suddenly weakened mimicking symptoms of a heart attack) versus women who have had myocardial infarctions (MI) and healthy controls (HC) and found that the death of a relative/close friend and illness/injury to a relative/close friend were more prevalent in women who had TC than those that had a MI or HC. In addition, the onset of TC was associated with multiple SLEs during the 6 months prior to hospitalization suggesting that grief and cumulative stress may play a major role in the onset of Takotsubo Cardiomyopathy [8].

Asking women about their experiences of what researchers have determined are major stressful events, such as a death or an experience of personal injury, is an alternative way to study the stressful aspects of women's lives. Investigators for the Study of Women and Health Across the Nation (SWAN) explored women's ratings of life events that were upsetting using the Psychiatric Epidemiology Research Interview (PERI) Life Events Scale, which involved events related to school, work, romantic relations, children, family, crime and legal matters, finances, and health. Hall and colleagues [9] used PERI scores over 9 years to characterize women's experiences as low, medium, and high levels of chronic stress and related these to sleep [9]. Although SWAN participants rated the degree to which these events were upsetting, researchers have not yet examined the type of stressful events most prevalent in this population.

To date, few studies have focused on the nature of stressful life events midlife women experience, how they view these events, e.g., as undesirable or desirable, and their impact over time as women age. Most early work on stressful life events focused on experiences of men: the original life events scale was developed and used with male naval shipyard personnel [10]. Consequently, experiences that women would rate as stressful were not reflected in any of the earlier stressful life events scales. Norbeck [11] is one of the few investigators to have studied stressful life events among women, having focused on a population of single and married adult women of childbearing age, interviewing them about major events or disruptions that occurred in their lives during the past year and during their preschool child's first year of life. Norbeck [11] identified stressful events related to contraception, parenting, single-parenting, custody issues, being the victim of assaultive acts, and having difficulty obtaining employment as salient concerns of these women and subsequently created the Life Events Questionnaire (LEQ), a 77-item self-rated scale to assess women's experiences of life events and their impact, described in greater detail in the methods section. Midlife women have unique concerns, which may or may not differ from those they had during their childbearing years. To date, there have been limited reports of life events experienced by midlife women and how they are appraised and none that characterize how women's experiences change over time during the menopausal transition. Stressful life events may be related to women's roles and demographic characteristics that reflect social advantage, but to date these have not been studied.

The Seattle Midlife Women's Health Study (SMWHS) provides a unique data source that allows for characterizing the patterns of stressful life events examined on four occasions over a ten-year period. These data allow exploration of whether certain types of stressful life events, for example, those related to finances, change over time.

The overall goal of this study was to describe the stressful life events midlife women experience as undesirable and their impact or rating of the event as they progressed through the menopausal transition during the 10 years they were in the SMWHS. The specific aims were to determine 1) which life events midlife women reported most frequently; 2) which events women rated as most undesirable; and 3) whether age, years of education, income, employment, race/ethnicity, marital status, being a parent, and the menopausal transition stages were associated with the impact scores of the life event categories.

Methods
Study design and population
Data reported here were from the Seattle Midlife Women's Health Study (SMWHS), an observational,

longitudinal study of approximately 23 years, from 1990 to 2013 [12]. Women entered the study between 1990 and the early part of 1992 when most were in the early stages of the menopausal transition (MT) or not yet in the transition. All households within census tracts with a wide income range and mixed ethnicity were contacted by telephone for interested and eligible women. Women who were eligible were between 35 and 55 years of age, had at least one menstrual period within the last year, had a uterus and at least one ovary, were not pregnant, and could read and understand English. Out of 11,222 telephone contacts, 820 women were eligible, and 508 women entered the study [12].

Women completed an initial in-person interview administered by a trained registered nurse interviewer. A subset of the 508 women kept a health diary and from late 1996 through 2005 provided urine samples. All women were mailed a yearly Health Questionnaire and kept a menstrual calendar.

Sample
Participants in the current study provided at least one and up to four Life Event Scale (LES) questionnaires beginning in 1990 and who were in either the late reproductive (LR), early transition (ET), late transition (LT) or early post-menopause (PM) sometime during the course of the study. When women started the study, they were on average 42 years, well-educated (16 years of education), earning a gross family income of $35, 740 (SD $15, 440), most were employed (86%), and married (71%). Women identified themselves as African American (12%), Asian/Pacific Islander (9%), White (76%), Latina (1%), and Mixed/Native American (3%). Seventy-five percent of the women were parents (See Table 1).

The Life Event Scale (LES) was administered on four occasions: Occasion 1(1990), Occasion 2 (1993), Occasion 3 (1997), and Occasion 4 (2000). Attrition rates for the initial LES during Occasion 1 (1990) included 67 women who were unable to be contacted, five women who became ineligible, and 64 who left the study for personal reasons resulting in 380 women. For the 2nd occasion (1992), thirty-six women were unable to be contacted, a total of 18 women became ineligible, and 32 women left for personal reasons resulting in 233 women. During the third occasion, 18 women were unable to be contacted, ten became ineligible, and 15 who left for personal reasons generating 220 participants. For the fourth and final occasion (2000), nineteen women were unable to be contacted, 138 women became ineligible, and 34 left for personal reasons leaving 191 women.

As seen in Table 1, the mean age of the sample increased at each testing occasion ($F = 169$, $df = 3$, $p < .001$) from 42 years to 50 years, on average, as expected for a longitudinal study. The number of years of education of

Table 1 Demographic Characteristics of Participants Providing Data for the Life Events Scale for Four Occasions

Characteristic	Occasion 1 N = 380	Occasion 2 N = 233	Occasion 3 N = 220	Occasion 4 N = 191
	Mean (SD)	Mean (SD)	Mean (SD)	Mean (SD)
Age	42 (5)	44 (5)	47 (4)	50 (4)
Years of Education	16 (3)	16 (3)	16 (3)	16 (3)
Gross Family Income	35,740 (15,440)	No Data	40,920 (15,042)	43,580 (14,478)
Currently Employed	86%	97%	89%	90%
Race/Ethnicity				
African American	12%	8%	7%	7%
Asian/Pacific Islander	9%	9%	9%	9%
White	76%	81%	84%	84%
Latina	1%	1.5%	1%	0
Mixed/Native Amer	3%	1.5%	0	0
Marital Status				
Never married/ partnered	6%	6%	6%	4%
Married/ partnered	71%	65%	68%	65%
Divorced/ separated	22%	28%	25%	30%
Widowed	2%	1%	2%	1%
If a parent?				
Yes	75%	67%	70%	68%
No	25%	33%	30%	32%
Menopausal Transition				
Stage (MTS), % (N)				
Late Reproduction (LR)	70% (N = 142)	58% (100)	43% (66)	38% (47)
Early Transition (ET)	22% (45)	33% (57)	37% (57)	25% (31)
Late Transition (LT)	5% (11)	5% (8)	13% (20)	22% (27)
Post Menopause (PM)	2% (4)	4% (7)	7% (10)	16% (20)

the women remained the same over time. The participants who remained in the study earned higher incomes over time, possibly reflecting that those with lower incomes tended to leave the study ($F = 18.602$, $df = 2$, $p < .001$). At least 86% of the women were employed as indicated by a higher percentage reporting employment on each occasion and the possibility that those who weren't employed were more likely to leave the study (Pearson's Chi Square = 18.864, $df = 3$, $p < .001$). Ethnic composition of the sample also changed over time (Chi Square = 18.907, $df = 9$, $p = .026$) resulting in a higher proportion of White women

remaining enrolled with fewer African American, Latina and Mixed/Native American women completing the study. There were no significant differences between occasions for marital status (Pearson's Chi Square = 7.221, $df = 9$, $p = .614$) although there is a slight decrease in the percentage of married women, suggesting that these women divorced or dropped out of the study and there is a slight increase in the percentage of divorced women over the course of the study. There was a slight decrease, although not statistically significant, in the number of parents who remained in the study (Pearson's Chi Square = 5.161, $df = 3$, $p = .160$). As expected, there were significant differences among the women in menopausal transition stages across all occasions (Chi square = 81.440, $df = 9$, $p < .001$) with women progressing from the late reproductive (LR) to early (ET) and late (LT) transition and to post-menopause over time.

Measures

The measures used in this analysis included the Life Events Scale and Menstrual Calendars to determine menopausal transition stage. Demographic characteristics included age, years of education, income, employment, race/ethnicity, marital status, and being a parent.

The life events scale

The Life Events Scale (LES) is an adaptation of Norbeck's Life Events Questionnaire (LEQ) [11] created for use with midlife women by the investigators of The Seattle Midlife Women's Health Study (SMWHS). An enumeration of each item is given in the Appendix. The LES is a 77-item, self-rated scale that assesses whether or not a stressful event happened over the past year and how stressful the event was. The LES was given four times during the course of the SMWHS: Occasion 1 (1990), Occasion 2 (1992), Occasion 3 (1997), and Occasion 4 (2000). The LES has the same nine sections or categories as the LEQ: Health, Work, Residence, Love & Marriage, Family & Close Friends, Parenting, Personal & Social, Financial, and Crime & Legal Matters.

The LES differs from the LEQ in the wording of the questions seen in the categories of Work; Family and Close Friends; and, Personal and Social. The following items were changed to reflect relevance to midlife. In the Work category, one item, "job changed," was added. For Family and Close Friends, "death of parents" and "birth of a grandchild" were added; and "acquired or lost a pet" was omitted. The questions were adapted in item 5a (see items listed in Appendix) to include "grandchild" and in item 5g to include "other family members (than a parent)." In the Personal and Social category, one item was added, "lost a friend for other reasons." In summary, after the adaptations for midlife women, both the LEQ and the LES totaled 77 items.

Women were asked to indicate whether or not a life event had occurred over the past year (yes/no); to evaluate if the event was undesirable, neutral or desirable; and, to rate the impact of the event as 1) no effect, 2) small effect, 3) moderate effect, or 4) great effect. For this investigation, undesirable mean total scores and undesirable total impact scores were reported for all 9 sections of the LES as well as the totals for the individual undesirable items under each section over 4 separate occasions spanning 10 years.

Menopausal transition stages

Menopausal Transition Stages (MTS) were labeled according to the stages of reproductive aging developed by Mitchell, Woods, and Mariella [13]: Late reproductive stage (LR), early menopausal transition (ET), late menopausal transition (LT), or post-menopause (PM), and match those labels recommended at the Stages of Reproductive Aging Workshop (STRAW) [14], and STRAW + 10 [15–17]. The data were obtained from menstrual calendars and coded as LR, ET, LT, or PM based on criteria developed by the Seattle Midlife Women's Health Study (SMWHS) [13] and validated by Harlow and colleagues [17, 18]. The late reproductive (LR) stage includes the time in midlife before the onset of persistent menstrual cycle irregularity when cycles are regular; Early transition (ET) stage is defined as persistent irregularity of more than 6 days of absolute difference between the start of any two consecutive menstrual cycles during the year, with no skipped periods; Late transition (LT) is defined as persistent skipping of one or more menstrual periods. A skipped period was defined as 60 or more consecutive days of amenorrhea during the calendar year [18]. Persistence indicated the irregular cycle or skipped period took place one or more times in the ensuing 12 months. The final menstrual period (FMP) was identified retrospectively after 1 year of amenorrhea. The first day of the FMP was used to determine age of onset of the FMP. Early post menopause (PM) was the time frame within 5 years after the FMP.

Demographic characteristics

Age was measured in years, as was education. Income from all sources was measured as gross family monthly pay in dollars. Current employment (part time or full time) was assessed using employed or not employed. Ethnicity was self-reported as African American, Asian/Pacific Islander, White, Latina, or Mixed/Native American. Marital status was self-reported as never married/never partnered, married/partnered, divorced/separated, or widowed. Parental status was assessed by asking women whether or not they were parents, including parenting adopted and foster children (See Table 1).

Data analysis Descriptive statistics (mean, standard deviation) were used to describe the individual items of the Life Event Scale (LES), scale scores, estimates of undesirable impact of the LES and demographic variables by occasion when the questionnaires were administered. To assess the relationship between demographic factors (age, years of education, gross family income, employment, race/ethnicity, marital status, being a parent) and life event stress, Pearson's r was used for continuous variables and analysis of variance was used for categorical variables (menopausal transition stage, race/ethnicity). Descriptive statistics, Pearson's r, and analyses of variance were performed using SPSS v23.

Results

Frequency of undesirable events

The total scores (number of items reported, standard deviation, N, adjusted means) of undesirable events for each category of the Life Event Scale rated over the past year are presented in Table 2. The total scores were calculated to identify which categories had the highest number of undesirable events. Adjusted mean total scores represent the simple average number of items for each of the subscales, e.g., health, work, etc., calculated by dividing the total number of items selected by the total number of items in each subscale to enable comparison across subscales, e.g., health vs. work.

Overall categories with the highest adjusted total scores for undesirable events were: Financial; Love and Marriage; and, Family and Close Friends. The categories with the highest adjusted total scores varied over the years of the study. For Occasion 1, the largest adjusted mean total number of stressful events by category were: Financial (.10), Family and close Friends (.09), Health (.08), and Parenting (.08). For Occasion 2, the largest adjusted mean total number of stressful events were in the categories of Love and Marriage (.11), Financial (.06), and Crime/Legal (.06). For Occasion 3, Family and Friends (.06) and Financial (.06) categories followed by Health, Personal/Social, Crime/Legal Matters (.05 each) were the largest adjusted mean total number of stressful events and for Occasion 4, the largest adjusted mean total number of events were in the categories of Family and Friends (.06), Health, Personal/Social, Financial, and Crime/Legal Matters (.05 each).

To summarize, over the four occasions, the adjusted mean total for the Financial category was among the highest, followed by Family and Friends for three of the four occasions. Health/Parenting and Crime/legal categories had the highest adjusted total means for Occasions 1 and 2, respectively. Thus, some categories of the most frequently experienced life events changed over the occasions of the study.

Table 2 Number of all *Undesirable* Events by LES Categories[a] by Occasion (Mean N of Items Reported (SD), Adjusted Mean)

Category (Number of Items)	Occasion N = 381	Occasion N = 235	Occasion 3 N = 221	Occasion 4 N = 192
Health (9)	.73 (.99) .08	.48 (.79) .05	.42 (.73) .05	.42 (.76) .05
Work (15)	.64 (1.00) .04	.69 (1.00) .05	.48 (.92) .03	.54 (.95) .04
Residence (4)	.18 (.46) .05	.09 (.31) .02	.05 (.22) .01	.07 (.31) .02
Love & Marriage (13)	.71 (1.20) .05	.50 (.98) .11[b]	.38 (.86) .03	.31 (.70) .02
Family & Close Friends (8)	.72 (.82) .09	.69 (.81) .04	.49 (.71) .06[b]	.51 (.72) .06[b]
Personal & Social (12)	.75 (1.03) .06	.60 (.81) .05	.56 (.84) .05	.58 (.88) .05
Financial (5)	.48 (.72) .10[b]	.29 (.55) .06	.32 (.66) .06[b]	.25 (.49) .05
Crime & Legal Matters (6)	.42 (.65) .07	.37 (.63) .06	.29 (.59) .05	.30 (.59) .05
Parenting (5)	.40 (.69) .08	.26 (.54) .05	.18 (.50) .04	.15 (.44) .04
Total Number of Undesirable Events	5.02 (3.82)	3.98 (2.71)	3.18 (2.97)	3.13 (3.01)

[a] Adjusted mean total scores represent the simple average number of items for each of the subscales, calculated by dividing the total number of items selected per category by the number of items in each category to enable comparison across categories
[b] Represents the highest category per Occasion

Mean impact scores of undesirable events

Over all occasions, the highest rated undesirable impact scores by category included Family and Close Friends. Personal/Social, Health and Work categories also had high impact scores. As seen in Table 3, the LES categories with the highest mean impact scores for undesirable events for Occasion 1 included Family & Close Friends (1.75), followed by Personal/Social (1.49) and Health (1.41). The categories of Family/Close Friends (1.65), Work (1.29), and Personal/Social (1.28) had the highest impact scores for Occasion 2. Similarly, the categories of Family/ Close Friends (1.32), Personal/ Social (1.12) and Work (.96) had the highest mean impact scores for Occasion 3. For the last Occasion, the highest impact scores were Family/ Close Friends (1.36), Personal/Social (1.21), and Work (1.03). Both Occasion 3 and 4 followed the same order of highest impact scores. Of note is that the lowest undesirable impact scores for each occasion were for the Residence category.

Individual items of each category

Analysis of individual items (see Appendix) provided further clarification of which specific items of the categories of life events were most commonly rated and viewed as having the most undesirable impact. The impact scores were rated as 1) no impact, 2) small impact, 3) moderate impact or 4) great impact. An average impact score was calculated by dividing the total of impact ratings by the number of women who reported the items to give the average impact score. The percentage calculated was the total number of women who reported the event, divided by the number of women for that particular occasion.

The most frequently reported individual items in the Health category included a major change in eating habits or major dental work. The most frequently reported Work items were having changed work hours or conditions, changed responsibilities at work, and having troubles at work with an employer or co-worker. Although

Residence was the category with the lowest score totals for undesirable events (see Tables 2 and 3), the most frequently reported individual item was having had a major change in living conditions, such as a home improvement or a decline in home or neighborhood. There were two most frequently reported items in the Love and Marriage category: having had a change in closeness with a husband or life partner and having had a change in a husband or partner's work outside the home. The most frequently reported Family and Close Friends items included having gained a new family member; experiencing a major change in the health or behavior of a family member or close friend; and, experiencing the death of a family member or close friend. The most frequently reported Personal and Social events included having had a vacation; had a trip, not a vacation; and, made a new friend. Most frequently reported Financial concerns involved having had a major change in financial status, improved or worsened, followed by taking on a moderate purchase, such as a car or major appliance. Crime and Legal Matters events were less frequently reported and included being involved in a minor violation of the law, getting traffic tickets or arrested for disturbing the peace, being robbed, or being involved in a car accident. The most frequently reported Parenting events included conflicts with a husband or partner about parenting and a change in childcare arrangements.

Associations of undesirable impact scores with demographic characteristics

Table 4 includes the correlations among the undesirable impact scores of the LES with baseline measures (Occasion 1) of demographic characteristics. Age was significantly correlated with undesirable impact scores for health ($r = 0.103$, $p = .046$): older women had higher undesirable impact scores for health-related events. Women with higher income reported lower undesirable

Table 3 Mean Impact Scores of *Undesirable* Events by LES Categories by Occasion [Mean impact score (SD)]

Category (No. items)	Occasion 1 N = 381	Occasion 2 N = 235	Occasion 3 N = 221	Occasion 4 N = 192
Health (9)	1.41 (1.63)	1.05 (1.49)	.92 (1.45)	.88 (1.43)
Work (15)	1.31 (1.66)	1.29 (1.58)	.96 (1.50)	1.03 (1.50)
Residence (4)	.50 (1.23)	.28 (.91)	.16 (.70)	.21 (.86)
Love & Marriage (13)	1.30 (1.67)	.96 (1.52)	.75 (1.41)	.69 (1.37)
Family & Friends (8)	1.75 (1.76)[a]	1.65 (1.73)[a]	1.32 (1.72)[a]	1.36 (1.74)[a]
Personal & Social (12)	1.49 (1.64)	1.28 (1.52)	1.12 (1.49)	1.21 (1.56)
Financial (5)	1.20 (1.66)	.77 (1.38)	.77 (1.44)	.70 (1.36)
Crime & Legal Matters (6)	.96 (1.41)	.86 (1.41)	.66 (1.27)	.63 (1.21)
Parenting (5)	.90 (1.45)	.59 (1.20)	.42 (1.08)	.36 (1.00)

An average impact score was calculated by dividing the total of impact ratings by the number of women who reported the items to give the average impact score
[a] Depicts the highest impact score per occasion

impact scores for: health events ($r = -.133$, $p = .010$), events concerning residence ($r = -.115$, $p = .025$), love and marriage events ($r = -.133$, $p = .010$) and financial matters ($r = -.192$, $p < .001$). Being a parent was associated with reporting a higher undesirable impact of financial events ($r = .102$, $p = .046$) as well as parenting life event stress, as expected ($r = .259$, $p < .001$). Years of education and employment status were not significantly correlated with any of the undesirable impact scores for the LES categories.

Marital status, race/ethnicity, and menopausal transition stages were also examined for their association with undesirable total impact scores for LES categories using analysis of variance. For the first occasion, marital status was associated significantly with greater undesirable impact scores for Health ($F = 3.109$; 3, 376 df; $p = .026$), Love and Marriage ($F = 6.979$; 3, 376 df; $p < .001$), and Personal and Social events ($F = 3.920$; 3, 376 df; $p < .001$). Post Hoc analysis identified a significant negative mean difference between Married/Partnered and Divorced women indicating that being married was associated with less impact of

stressful health events than being divorced. Being married also was associated with a lesser impact of stressful events in Love and Marriage compared to women who were never married and to women who were divorced. Married women reported less impact of Personal and Social stressful life events than did women who were divorced.

For the second occasion, undesirable impact scores of Love and Marriage ($F = 7.430$; 3, 229 df; $p < .001$) as well as Personal and Social events ($F = 2.770$; 3, 229 df; $p = .042$) were associated with marital status. Married women reported significantly more of an impact of undesirable stressful life events in Love and Marriage than divorced women, while divorced women reported a greater impact of stressful life events in Love and Marriage than women who had never been married. Married women reported a greater impact of undesirable stressful life events in the Personal and Social category than women who were widowed. Marital status was not associated with the LES undesirable mean total impact scores for the third occasion.

Table 4 Correlation Matrix of Impact Scores of Undesirable Events at Baseline (Occasion 1) and Demographic Categories (Pearson's *r*, *p* value, and N for each)

LES subscale/ correlate	Health	Work	Residence	Love and Marriage	Family and Close Friends	Personal and Social	Financial	Crime and Legal Matters	Parenting
Age	0.103* .046 (380)	−.058 .258 (380)	.004 .943 (380)	.003 .946 (380)	.033 .515 (380)	.060 .244 (380)	−.064 .217 (379)	.074 .151 (380)	−.063 .224 (380)
Years of Education	−.072 .163 (380)	.086 .095 (380)	−.027 .602 (380)	.007 .889 (380)	−.063 .222 (380)	−.010 .854 (380)	−.023 .655 (379)	.066 .200 (380)	−.013 .795 (380)
Income	−.133** .010 (375)	−.027 .608 (375)	−.115* .025 (375)	−.133** .010 (375)	−.097 .060 (375)	−.087 .094 (375)	−.192** .000 (374)	−.035 .500 (375)	−.082 .115 (375)
Employment	−.081 .114 (380)	.044 .391 (380)	−.041 .421 (380)	−.087 .089 (380)	.017 .746 (380)	−.066 .196 (380)	−.050 .336 (379)	−.041 .430 (380)	−.028 .583 (380)
If a parent	.046 .368 (380)	−.041 .420 (380)	.018 .727 (380)	−.010 .841 (380)	.009 .859 (380)	.014 .786 (380)	.102* .046 (379)	−.031 .542 (380)	.259** .000 (380)

r = Pearson's Correlation
p is significant if *: α < .05 or **: α < .001
N = Number of women

For Occasion 4, four categories were associated with marital status: Work ($F = 4.231$; 3, 187 df; $p = .006$), Residence ($F = 3.209$; 3, 187 df; $p = .024$), Personal/Social ($F = 3.417$; 3, 187 df; $p = .019$), and Financial/Legal Matters ($F = 2.971$; 3, 187 df; $p = .033$). Women who were never married rated the impact of Work stress and Personal and Social stress significantly higher than married women. Married women rated impact scores significantly higher than divorced women for Work, Residence, Personal and Social, and Financial stress. Married women also reported significantly higher impact scores of Financial stress than women who were widowed.

Ethnicity was significantly associated with the undesirable impact scores for the Financial category, but only for Occasion 2 (F = 3.879; 4, 228 df; $p = .005$) and Occasion 3 (F = 7.772; 3, 216 df; $p < .001$). For Occasion 2, there were significant differences between Hispanic/Latina women and all other ethnicities suggesting that Hispanic/Latina women rated the impact of Financial stress higher than women who were Asian/Pacific Islander, African American, White and Mixed/Native American; however, only three women identified themselves as Hispanic/Latina. Post hoc analyses were not performed for Occasion 3 because at least one group had fewer than two cases. One woman identified herself as Hispanic/Latina for the third occasion and no women identified themselves as Mixed/Native American.

Menopausal transition stages were significantly associated with undesirable mean impact scores only for Health and only for Occasion 1 ($F = 3.700$; 3, 198 df; $p = .013$), but not significant for all other occasions. Significant mean differences from the Post Hoc analysis tests from the analysis of variance for the LES category impact scores for undesirable stressful life events and the menopausal transition stages (LR = Late Reproductive, ET = Early Transition, LT = Late Transition, PM = Post-menopausal) were evident for Occasion 1. Scores for the LR, ET, and LT stages each significantly and negatively differed from the PM stage ($p < .001$, .001, and .008) in the Health category, meaning that the mean impact scores of undesirable Health events decrease as women transition through the menopausal stages; however, there were only four women in the post-menopausal stage during the first occasion.

Discussion

The overall goal of this study was to describe the undesirable life events midlife women experience, women's ratings of the impact of these life events, and factors associated with the experience of stressful life events by category. Over 10 years of follow-up, participants in the Seattle Midlife Women's Health Study reported the highest adjusted mean total score of undesirable life events in the Financial category, followed by Family and Close Friends for three of

the four occasions. Health and Crime/Legal categories were among the highest adjusted mean total scores for two occasions. In contrast, the highest mean *impact* scores for undesirable life events over all four occasions were in the category of Family and Close Friends. Thus, the most commonly reported undesirable life events (financial) may not have been those women described as having the greatest impact (family and close friends).

Women's assessment of the impact of life events reflected their social roles and connections as shaping the kinds of stressful life events they experienced and their impact, as seen in the categories with the highest impact scores of Family/Close Friends, Personal/Social, and Work. Indeed, investigators have recently identified the importance of women's roles and relationships in relation to the types of stressors they experience. Woods-Giscombé et al. [19] differentiated self-stress and network-stress among African American women aged 21 to 78 years. Self-stress referred to stressful events happening to oneself whereas network-stress referred to stressful events happening to family, friends and loved ones, which could indirectly affect the woman herself. African American women reported significantly more network-stress than self-stress [19]. Certainly, Family and Close Friends as well as Personal and Social life events could reflect network-stress as described by Woods-Giscombé et al. [19]. Midlife women's social roles and connections thus may place them at risk for a greater number of stressors altogether as indicated by events related to their networks as well as those that they experience directly. These findings also support the utility of the concept of self in relation, as described by Jean Baker-Miller, whose conception of women's development emphasizes the importance of life experienced in a relational network [20]. Understanding the life experiences women rate as undesirable and high impact requires viewing their experiences from their individual perspectives as they reflect their place in a relational network.

In addition to describing the number and impact of life events in the various categories, the undesirable impact of life events was correlated with several demographic factors. Mean impact scores for undesirable stressful life events were associated with age, not surprising given that one of the categories with the largest number of undesirable stressful life events during Occasion 1 was Health. In fact, women reported a major change in eating habits (29%), a major change in recreation (25%), a major change in sleeping habits (23%), and a major personal illness or injury (22%), all with a moderate to great impact score (See Appendix). Undesirable impact scores for Health, Residence, Love/Marriage, and Financial life events were also correlated with family income, reflecting the effects of social disadvantage on the experience and impact of stressful events. Although education was not correlated with undesirable mean impact scores, the current results are similar to what others have found. Prior studies have examined how social structure is linked to health in midlife and younger women 25–64 years of age. McDonough et al. [21] found that chronic stressors (social life, financial, relationship, child, environment, and family health stress) were significantly and positively related to women's levels of distress and that health status improved as education and household income increased. Furthermore, in the current study, married women reported lower impacts of Health stress than did women who were divorced, results supported by McDonough et al. [21] who revealed that married women reported the best health results while formerly married women reported the worst. Newton et al. [22] investigated midlife women aged 51 to 60 years and found that married women experienced fewer functional limitations and fewer risks of chronic diseases (hypertension, diabetes, heart attacks, chronic heart failure, coronary heart disease, angina, stroke and rheumatoid arthritis) compared to women who were divorced/separated, widowed and never married.

Family income was also associated with the undesirable impact of life events in the Financial category. Women with lower family incomes may have been less able to bear the costs of purchasing and maintaining a residence, and may have had difficulty paying for food, bills or rent. In addition, lower income may place a strain on Love and Marriage; one of the most frequently reported Love and Marriage items was a change in husband or partner's work outside the home (26%) see Appendix.

Being a parent was associated with more Financial stress, such as paying for a child's food and clothing, as well as Parenting stress. Women most frequently reported having a change in childcare arrangements (23%) and conflicts with their husband or partner about parenting (31%) see Appendix.

Strengths and limitations

One of the strengths of this study was that chronic life event stress was investigated in midlife women repeatedly over a decade. Life event stress may reflect the impact of the chronic activation (stress arousal) of the hypothalamic-pituitary-adrenal (HPA) axis. Future investigations may consider how, and if, desirable or positive life events buffer the effects of negative or undesirable stressful life events on HPA axis responses, such as cortisol levels.

Among the limitations of this study was the declining number of participants over time reflecting the attrition that occurs during longitudinal studies and women becoming ineligible due to having completed early post-menopause as well as other causes such as use of

hormone therapy. Also, exploring the influence of factors beyond the demographic variables was beyond the scope of this paper. For example, depressed mood is an important factor that both influences one's perception of life event stress and may be a consequence of a stressful life event. In the current study, 202 of the 380 women who completed the Occasion1 LES, completed a Center for Epidemiologic Studies Depression Scale (CESD) resulting in a mean sum score of 11.4, median score of 10.4, and a SD 7.3. These results indicate that the women who completed the CESD in the current study had a depression score less than 16; the literature suggests a sum score of 16 or more as an indicator of depression. In the longitudinal Study of Women's Health Across the Nation (SWAN), women who experienced more upsetting life events were more likely to experience depressed mood [23, 24]. Future studies of stressful life events of midlife women should include factors such as depression in order to determine whether women with depressed mood identify more stressful life events and rate them as having a greater undesirable impact in addition to determining whether the LES scores predict depressed mood. Also, future studies of patterns of change or continuity over time in life event stress would be insightful for clinicians to help midlife women manage their life event stress.

Conclusion

Midlife women experience a variety of stressful life events with a range of undesirable impact of these events. The types of events and their impact were related to women's roles as well as to factors that afforded them social advantage, such as income. In addition, there were uniform patterns of decline over time of the impact of undesirable life events suggesting that adaptation may occur over time as well as the possible loss of participants experiencing the most stressful events.

Two important messages from these results follow. First, practitioners will benefit from knowing the type of stressful life events occurring for women, especially those related to their roles and social advantage during midlife, a time of many different responsibilities. Second, many women have multiple co-occurring stressors, potentially related to an initiating event, such as divorce. Divorce may propagate additional stressful events, such as loss of income and/or insurance, the need to increase hours worked, difficulty with childcare arrangements, as well as loss of a partner. Undesirable stressful life events that continue over time may place women at risk for development of pathologies such as hypertension, diabetes, heart disease, arthritis, and obesity. More research is needed to understand the potential consequences of this snowballing effect that often happens in midlife women's lives.

Appendix

Table 5 Number of Women (And Percent of Total for each Occasion) Reporting Individual LES Items and Undesirable (U) Impact Scores (Mean, SD) for each Occasion

Item	Occasion 1 (% of total)	U	Occasion 2	U	Occasion 3	U	Occasion 4	U
1. Health subscale	N = 381		N = 235		N = 221		N = 192	
A. *major* personal illness or injury	83 (22%)	3.33 (.83)	36 (15%)	3.5 (.72)	43 (20%)	3.5 (.76)	31 (16%)	3.25 (.74)
B. *major* change in eating habits	111 (29%)	4.0 (.00)	56 (24%)	3.0 (1.00)	46 (21%)	4.00 (ND)	38 (20%)	4.00 (ND)
C. *major* change in sleeping habits	89 (23%)	3.8 (.45)	32 (14%)	3.4 (.55)	45 (20%)	3.0 (ND)	32 (17%)	2.0 (ND)
D. *major* change in usual type and/or amount of recreation	94 (25%)	4.0 (0.00)	56 (24%)	3.5 (.71)	42 (19%)	3.5 (.71)	29 (15%)	3.0 (ND)
E. *major* dental work	65 (17%)	3.0 (ND)	72 (31%)	4.0 (ND)	24 (11%)	3.0 (ND)	17 (9%)	4.0 (ND)
F. *major* difficulty with birth control pills or devices	12 (3%)	4.0 (ND)	3 (1%)	4.0 (ND)	5 (2%)	2.0 (ND)	4 (2%)	3.0 (ND)
g. Pregnancy	21 (6%)	4.0 (ND)	7 (3%)	ND	2 (1%)	ND	0 (0%)	ND
h. miscarriage or abortion	8 (2%)	3.0 (ND)	4 (2%)	4.0 (ND)	0(0%)	ND	0(0%)	ND
i. started menopause	47 (12%)	3.0 (ND)	26 (11%)	4.0 (ND)	31 (14%)	4.0 (ND)	35 (18%)	4.0 (ND)
2. Work								
a. had difficulty finding a job	36 (9%)	4.0 (ND)	27 (12%)	4.0 (ND)	13 (6%)	3.0 (ND)	8 (4%)	4.0 (ND)
b. begun work outside the home	62 (16%)	4.0 (ND)	15 (6%)	3.0 (ND)	15 (7%)	4.0 (ND)	8 (4%)	4.0 (ND)
c. changed job setting, but continued the same kind of work	97 (26%)	4.0 (ND)	47 (20%)	2.0 (ND)	37 (17%)	3.0 (ND)	43 (22%)	3.0 (ND)
d. changed to a new type of work	72 (19%)	4.0 (ND)	35 (15%)	4.0 (ND)	32 (15%)	4.0 (ND)	27 (14%)	4.0 (ND)
e. changed work hours or conditions	161 (42%)	3.5 (.71)	91 (39%)	3.0 (ND)	78 (35%)	4.0 (0.00)	63 (33%)	2.0 (ND)
f. changed responsibilities at work.	138 (36%)	4.0 (ND)	96 (41%)	4.0 (ND)	67 (30%)	4.0 (ND)	53 (28%)	4.0 (ND)
g. had troubles at work with employer or co-workers	128 (34%)	3.5 (.58)	69 (29%)	4.0 (ND)	61 (28%)	4.0 (ND)	40 (21%)	3.0 (ND)
h. had a major business readjustment	46 (12%)	4.0 (ND)	27 (12%)	4.0 (ND)	24 (11%)	4.0 (ND)	14 (7%)	4.0 (ND)
i. been fired or laid off from work	26 (7%)	4.0 (ND)	20 (9%)	4.0	8 (4%)	4.0	10 (5%)	4.0 (ND)
j. retired from work	5 (1%)	4.0 (ND)	3 (1%)	ND	0	ND	3 (2%)	ND
k. started courses by mail or studying at home to help with work	41 (11%)	4.0 (ND)	13 (6%)	ND (ND)	14 (6%)	3.0 (ND)	6 (3%)	3.0 (ND)
l. begun or ended school, college, or training program	65 (17%)	3.0 (ND)	32 (14%)	4.0 (ND)	19 (9%)	ND	12 (6%)	4.0 (ND)
m. changed career goal or academic major	54 (14%)	4.0 (ND)	19 (8%)	ND	25 (11%)	3.0 (ND)	12 (6%)	4.0 (ND)
n. changed school, college or training program	10 (3%)	ND	6 (3%)	2.0 (ND)	4 (2%)	4.0 (ND)	3 (2%)	4.0 (ND)
o. had problems in school, college or training program	9 (2%)	4.0 (ND)	10 (4%)	4.0 (ND)	3 (1%)	2.0 (ND)	1 (< 1%)	3.0 (ND)
3. Residence								
a. had difficulty finding a home	18 (5%)	3.58 (.67)	3 (1%)	2.5 (.71)	3 (1%)	3.0 (ND)	3 (2%)	3.67 (.58)
b. changed residences within the same town or city	39 (10%)	3.13 (1.13)	14 (6%)	4.0 (0.00)	6 (3%)	ND	9 (5%)	4.0 (ND)
c. moved to a different town, city, state, or country	15 (4%)	2.67 (1.21)	14 (6%)	4.0 (0.00)	6 (3%)	ND	4 (2%)	ND
d. had a major change in living conditions (home improvements or a decline in home or neighborhood)	121 (32%)	3.26 (.85)	55 (23%)	2.94 (.77)	44 (20%)	3.10 (.88)	34 (18%)	3.67 (.50)
4. Love and Marriage								
a. begun a new, close personal, romantic relationship	40 (11%)	3.33 (.58)	23 (10%)	3.50 (.71)	22 (10%)	4.0 (ND)	17 (9%)	4.0 (ND)

Table 5 Number of Women (And Percent of Total for each Occasion) Reporting Individual LES Items and Undesirable (U) Impact Scores (Mean, SD) for each Occasion *(Continued)*

Item	Occasion 1 (% of total)	U	Occasion 2	U	Occasion 3	U	Occasion 4	U
b. become engaged	20 (5%)	ND	7 (3%)	ND	4 (2%)	ND	4 (2%)	4.0 (ND)
c. had girlfriend or boyfriend problems (not just friends)(not husband/partner)	48 (13%)	3.43 (.69)	28 (12%)	3.55 (.67)	19 (9%)	3.13 (.83)	12 (6%)	3.33 (.87)
d. broken up with a boyfriend (or girlfriend) or broken an engagement	46 (12%)	3.52 (.80)	20 (9%)	3.58 (.52)	16 (7%)	3.18 (.87)	5 (3%)	4.0 (0.00)
e. gotten married or begun to live with someone (roommate OK)	37 (10%)	3.5 (.58)	15 (6%)	ND	11 (5%)	3.5 (.58)	12 (6%)	ND
f. had change in closeness with husband or life partner	140 (37%)	3.36 (.73)	63 (27%)	3.27 (.83)	42 (19%)	3.28 (.90)	37 (19%)	3.13 (.89)
g. experienced infidelity, (cheating on husband/partner)(either party)	33 (9%)	3.48 (.73)	16 (7%)	3.55 (.69)	12 (5%)	3.83 (.41)	8 (4%)	3.2 (1.30)
h. had trouble with in-laws	36 (9%)	3.07 (.73)	11 (5%)	2.6 (.84)	14 (6%)	2.73 (.91)	8 (4%)	3.25 (.89)
i. separated from husband or life partner due to conflict	29 (7%)	3.67 (.77)	10 (4%)	3.50 (.84)	11 (5%)	4.0 (0.00)	8 (4%)	4.0 (0.00)
j. separated from husband or life partner due to work, travel, school, etc.	36 (9%)	3.17 (.99)	15 (6%)	3.0 (0.00)	10 (5%)	3.25 (.96)	4 (2%)	3.33 (1.16)
k. had a reconciliation with spouse or partner	25 (7%)	ND	10 (4%)	3.50 (.71)	11 (5%)	ND	4 (2%)	ND
l. had a legal divorce	12 (3%)	4.0 (0.00)	3 (1%)	ND	2 (< 1%)	ND	3 (2%)	4.0 (0.00)
m. had a change in husband's or partner's work outside the home (beginning work, ceasing work, changing jobs, retirement, etc.)	100 (26%)	3.48 (.72)	43 (18%)	3.35 (.70)	36 (16%)	3.46 (.69)	35 (18%)	3.00 (.54)
5. Family and Close Friends								
a. gained a new family member (through birth, adoption, relative moving in, includes extended family)	109 (29%)	2.8 (1.03)	51 (22%)	3.67 (.52)	40 (18%)	3.00 (.82)	47 (25%)	3.0 (1.00)
b. had a child or family member leave home (due to marriage, to attend college, or for some other reason)	59 (16%)	3.48 (.81)	27 (12%)	3.9 (.32)	37 (17%)	3.63 (.74)	28 (15%)	3.75 (.50)
c. had a major change in the health or behavior of a family member or close friend (illness, accidents, drug or disciplinary problems, etc.)	165 (43%)	3.41 (.75)	100 (43%)	3.28 (.80)	75 (34%)	3.42 (.72)	79 (41%)	3.55 (.59)
d. had the death of a husband or partner	4 (1%)	4.0 (0.00)	1 (< 1%)	4.0 (ND)	1 (< 1%)	4.0 (ND)	2 (1%)	2.0 (ND)
e. had the death of a child	1 (< 1%)	4.0 (ND)	1 (< 1%)	ND	0	ND	1 (< 1%)	ND
f. had the death of a parent	36 (9%)	3.92 (.27)	19 (8%)	3.79 (.43)	13 (6%)	3.4 (.70)	8 (4%)	3.67 (.82)
g. had the death of another family member or close friend	103 (27%)	3.30 (.78)	60 (26%)	3.22 (.76)	44 (20%)	3.2 (.76)	35 (18%)	3.29 (.64)
h. had a change in the marital status of your parents	8 (2%)	3.5 (.58)	5 (2%)	3.5 (.71)	4 (2%)	4.0 (0.00)	1 (< 1%)	ND
6. Personal and Social								
a. major personal achievement	139 (37%)	3.0 (1.41)	70 (30%)	ND	52 (24%)	4.0 (ND)	48 (25%)	3.0 (1.41)
b. had a major decision regarding the immediate future	154 (40%)	3.62 (.51)	70 (30%)	3.56 (.88)	67 (30%)	3.40 (.89)	55 (29%)	3.88 (.35)
c.								
d. had a change in political beliefs	8 (2%)	3.50 (.71)	5 (2%)	ND	5 (2%)	ND	3 (2%)	ND
e. had a change in religious beliefs	20 (5%)	3.50 (.71)	10 (4%)	ND	15 (7%)	ND	4 (2%)	ND

Table 5 Number of Women (And Percent of Total for each Occasion) Reporting Individual LES Items and Undesirable (U) Impact Scores (Mean, SD) for each Occasion *(Continued)*

Item	Occasion 1 (% of total)	U	Occasion 2	U	Occasion 3	U	Occasion 4	U
f. had a loss or damage of personal property	75 (20%)	3.12 (.83)	41 (17%)	2.97 (.81)	49 (22%)	2.81 (.83)	24 (13%)	3.00 (.79)
g. had a vacation	231 (61%)	3.55 (.69)	151 (64%)	3.00 (ND)	163 (74%)	3.00 (1.00)	125 (65%)	4.00 (0.00)
h. had a trip; not a vacation	171 (45%)	3.15 (.99)	98 (42%)	2.72 (.91)	107 (48%)	3.11 (.93)	96 (50%)	3.00 (.82)
i. had a change in family get-togethers	91 (24%)	3.17 (.80)	60 (26%)	2.80 (.78)	75 (34%)	3.04 (.77)	54 (28%)	3.09 (.81)
j. had a change in social activities (clubs, movies, visiting)	102 (27%)	2.76 (.74)	66 (28%)	2.84 (.60)	56 (25%)	2.78 (.81)	43 (22%)	3.07 (.73)
k. made a new friend	231 (61%)	2.25 (.50)	123 (52%)	4.0 (ND)	100 (45%)	ND	95 (50%)	3.50 (.71)
l. broken up with a friend due to conflict	66 (17%)	3.18 (.83)	30 (13%)	2.93 (.70)	28 (13%)	3.20 (.78)	21 (11%)	3.33 (.72)
m. lost a friend for other reasons (death, moving)	72 (19%)	3.30 (.79)	47 (20%)	2.94 (.69)	25 (11%)	2.80 (.86)	35 (18%)	2.75 (.85)
7. Financial								
a. had a major change in financial status (improved or worsened)	168 (44%)	3.53 (.68)	92 (39%)	3.33 (.76)	79 (36%)	3.58 (.50)	69 (36%)	3.20 (.76)
b. taken on a moderate purchase such as a car, major appliance, etc.	157 (41%)	2.79 (.98)	85 (36%)	2.92 (.90)	70 (32%)	3.0 (.93)	59 (31%)	2.75 (.96)
c. taken on a major purchase or a mortgage loan, such as a home, business, property, etc.	67 (18%)	3.29 (.83)	40 (17%)	2.50 (.71)	39 (18%)	3.0 (.78)	30 (16%)	3.40 (.55)
d. experienced a foreclosure on a mortgage or loan	7 (2%)	3.17 (.98)	0	ND	1 (< 1%)	4.0 (ND)	1 (< 1%)	3.0 (ND)
e. had credit rating difficulties	75 (20%)	3.26 (.70)	23 (10%)	2.84 (.69)	19 (9%)	3.38 (.89)	10 (5%)	3.25 (.71)
8. Crime and Legal Matters								
a. robbed	49 (13%)	3.22 (.84)	22 (9%)	3.28 (.75)	26 (12%)	2.82 (.67)	11 (6%)	2.64 (.51)
b. a victim of a violent act (rape, assault, etc.)	3 (1%)	4.0 (0.00)	4 (2%)	3.75 (.50)	4 (2%)	3.33 (1.16)	2 (1%)	3.0 (ND)
c. involved in a car accident	45 (12%)	2.74 (.91)	31 (13%)	2.89 (.97)	27 (12%)	2.90 (.79)	29 (15%)	2.77 (.87)
d. involved in a law suit	35 (9%)	3.05 (.83)	14 (6%)	2.73 (1.01)	16 (7%)	3.80 (.45)	15 (8%)	3.0 (1.00)
e. involved in a minor violation of the law (traffic tickets, disturbing the peace, etc.)	75 (20%)	2.15 (.69)	37 (16%)	2.40 (.91)	30 (14%)	2.54 (.78)	23 (12%)	2.21 (1.12)
f. involved in legal troubles resulting in your being arrested or held in jail	0	ND	2 (1%)	4.0 (ND)	1 (< 1%)	3.0 (ND)	0	ND
9. Parenting								
a. had a change in child care arrangements	88 (23%)	3.11 (.90)	34 (15%)	3.60 (.89)	23 (10%)	2.86 (.90)	17 (9%)	3.0 (.82)
b. had conflicts with husband or partner about parenting	119 (31%)	3.13 (.84)	51 (22%)	2.68 (.85)	37 (17%)	2.86 (.83)	26 (14%)	2.74 (.87)
c. had conflicts with child's grandparents (or other important person) about parenting	40 (11%)	2.87 (.78)	17 (7%)	2.46 (.82)	10 (5%)	3.29 (.76)	5 (3%)	4.0 (0.00)
d. taken on full responsibility for parenting as a single parent	37 (10%)	3.0 (.93)	10 (4%)	3.67 (.58)	8 (4%)	4.0 (ND)	9 (5%)	4.0 (0.00)
e. custody battles with former husband or partner	6 (2%)	3.60 (.89)	2 (1%)	3.0 (ND)	3 (1%)	3.0 (1.41)	1 (< 1%)	4.0 (ND)

Acknowledgements
We acknowledge all the women who participated in the SMWHS. Only the authors of this paper contributed to this manuscript.

Funding
Not applicable.

Authors' contributions
AJT conducted the literature review, analyzed the data and had primary responsibility for writing the manuscript. NFW contributed to the design and literature review, analyzed the data and edited the manuscript. ESM edited the manuscript. ESM and NFW were PIs of the Seattle Midlife Women's Health Study and collected all data. All authors read and approved the final manuscript.

Authors' information
Annette Joan Thomas, College of Nursing, Seattle University.
Ellen Sullivan Mitchell, Department of Family and Child Nursing, University of Washington School of Nursing.
Nancy Fugate Woods, Department of Biobehavioral Nursing and Health Informatics, University of Washington School of Nursing.

Competing interests
NFW is guest editor of this journal. Peer review and all decisions made regarding this manuscript were made by an associate editor at a different institution. AJT and ESM have no competing interests.

Author details
[1]College of Nursing, Seattle University, Seattle, USA. [2]Family and Child Nursing, University of Washington, Seattle, USA. [3]Biobehavioral Nursing and Health Informatics, University of Washington, Seattle, USA.

References
1. Woods NF, Mitchell ES, Percival DB, Smith-Dejulio K. Is the menopausal transition stressful? Observations of perceived stress from the Seattle midlife Women's health study. Menopause. 2009;16(1):90–7.
2. Freeman EW, Sammel MD, Lin H, Gracia CR. Symptoms in the menopausal transition: hormone and behavioral correlates. Am Coll Obst and Gyn. 2008; 111(1):127–36.
3. Mitchell ES, Woods NF. Symptom experiences of midlife women: observations from the Seattle midlife women's health study. Maturitas. 1996; 25:1–10.
4. Thomas AJ, Mitchell ES, Woods NF. The challenges of midlife women: themes from the Seattle midlife women's health study. Midlife Women's Health. 2018;4(8):1–10.
5. Mitchell ES, Woods NF. Anticipating menopause: observations from the Seattle midlife women's health study. Menopause. 1999;6(2):167–73.
6. Seib C, Whiteside E, Lee K, Humphreys J, et al. Stress, lifestyle and quality of life in midlife and older women: results from the stress and health of women study. Womens Health Issues. 2014;24(1):e43–52.
7. Horri N, Haghighi S, Hosseini SM, Zare M, Paravesh E, Amini M. Stressful life events, education, and metabolic syndrome in women: are they related? A study in first-degree relatives of type 2 diabetes. Metab Syndr Relat Disord. 2010;8(6):483–7.
8. Rosman L, Dunsiger S, Salmoirago-Blotcher E. Cumulative impact of stressful life events on the development of Takotsubo cardiomyopathy. Annals of Behav Med. 2017;51(6):925–30.
9. Hall MH, Casement MD, Troxel WM, et al. Chronic stress is prospectively associated with sleep in midlife women: the SWAN sleep study. Sleep. 2014; 10(38):1645–55.
10. Holmes TH, Rahe RH. The social readjustment rating scale. J Psychosom Res. 1967;11(2):213–8.
11. Norbeck JS. Modification of life event questionnaires with female respondents. Res Nurs Health. 1984;7(1):61–71.
12. Woods NF, Mitchell ES. The Seattle midlife women's health study: a longitudinal prospective study of women during the menopausal transition and early postmenopause. Women's Midlife Health. 2016;2:6.
13. Mitchell ES, Woods NF, Mariella A. Three stages of the menopausal transition: toward a more precise definition. Menopause. 2000;7:334–9.
14. Soules MR, Sherman S, Parrott E, et al. Executive summary: stages of reproductive aging workshop (STRAW). Feril Steril. 2001;76:874–8.
15. Harlow SD, Gass M, Hall JE, et al. Executive summary of the stages of reproductive aging workshop +10: addressing the unfinished agenda of staging reproductive aging. Menopause. 2012;19(4):387–95.
16. Harlow SD, Mitchell ES, Crawford S, et al. The reSTAGE collaboration: defining optimal bleeding criteria for onset of early menopausal transition. Fertil Steril. 2008;89:129–40.
17. Harlow SD, Cain K, Crawford S, et al. Evaluation of four proposed bleeding criteria for the onset of late menopausal transition. J Clin Endocrin Metab. 2006;91:3432–8.
18. Harlow SD, Crawford S, Dennerstein L, Bulger HG, Mitchell ES, Sowers MF, ReSTAGE Collaboration. Recommendations from a multi-study evaluation of proposed criteria for staging reproductive aging. Climacteric. 2007;10:112–9.
19. Woods-Giscombé CL, Lobel M, Zimmer C, et al. Whose stress is making me sick? Network-stress and emotional distress in African American women. Issues Mental Health Nursing. 2015;36(9):710–7.
20. Miller JB, Stiver IP. The healing connection: how women form connections in therapy and in life. Boston: Beacon Press; 1997. Chapter 3
21. McDonough P, Walter V, Strohschein L. Chronic stress and the social patterning of women's health in Canada. Soc Sci Med. 2002;54:767–82.
22. Newton NJ, Ryan LH, King RT, Smith J. Cohort differences in the marriage-health relationship for midlife women. Soc Sci Med. 2014;116:64–72.
23. Bromberger JT, Kravitz HM, Chang Y-F, et al. Major depression during and after the menopausal transition: study of women's health across the nation (SWAN). Psychol Med. 2011:1–10.
24. Bromberger JT, Matthews KA, Schott LL, et al. Depression symptoms during the menopausal transition: the study of women's health across the nation (SWAN). J Affect Disord. 2007;103:267–72.

19

Neighborhood disorder, exposure to violence, and perceived discrimination in relation to symptoms in midlife women

Linda M Gerber[1,2]* and Lynnette Leidy Sievert[3]

Abstract

Background: Some symptoms at midlife are associated with stress, such as hot flashes, trouble sleeping, headaches, or depressed mood. Hot flashes have been studied in relation to laboratory stressors, physiological biomarkers, and self-reported stress, but less is known about hot flashes in relation to the larger context of women's lives. This study examined the risk of symptoms in relation to neighborhood disorder, exposure to neighborhood violence, social cohesion and perceived discrimination. We hypothesized that women exposed to more negative neighborhood characteristics and discrimination would be more likely to report hot flashes and other midlife symptoms.

Methods: Participants were black and white women, aged 40 to 60, drawn from a cross-sectional investigation of race/ethnicity, socioeconomic status, and blood pressure in New York City (n = 139). Demographic information, medical history, menopausal status, and symptoms were measured by questionnaire. Likert scales were used to measure neighborhood characteristics, specifically, the Neighborhood Disorder Scale, the Exposure to Violence Scale, the Perceived Violence Subscale, the Neighborhood Social Cohesion and Trust Scale, and the Everyday Discrimination Scale. Ten symptoms were included in analyses: lack of energy, feeling blue/depressed, backaches, headaches, aches/stiffness in joints, shortness of breath, hot flashes, trouble sleeping, nervous tension, and pins/needles in hands/feet. Each scale with each symptom outcome was examined using logistic regression analyses adjusting for significant covariates.

Results: Black women reported higher scores on all negative neighborhood characteristics and discrimination, and a lower score on the positive Neighborhood Social Cohesion and Trust. Neighborhood Disorder was associated with feeling blue/depressed, aches/stiffness in joints, and hot flashes, and Perceived Violence was associated with aches/stiffness in joints, after controlling for model-specific covariates. There was a lower risk of backaches with increasing Neighborhood Social Cohesion and Trust score. The Everyday Discrimination Scale was associated with lack of energy. Lack of energy, feeling blue/depressed, aches/stiffness in joints, and hot flashes appeared to be most vulnerable to negative neighborhood context and discrimination.

Conclusions: This study adds to the literature linking neighborhood environments to health outcomes. The associations between negative neighborhood contexts and discrimination with diverse symptoms, and the association between social cohesion and back pain, point to the need to expand analyses of stress to multiple physiological systems.

Keywords: Menopause, Hot flashes, Aches, Stress, Neighborhood disorder, Violence, Discrimination

* Correspondence: lig2002@med.cornell.edu
[1]Department of Healthcare Policy & Research, Division of Biostatistics and Epidemiology, Weill Cornell Medical College, 402 E. 67th St., LA-231, New York, NY 10065, USA
[2]Department of Medicine, Division of Nephrology and Hypertension, Weill Cornell Medical College, New York City, NY, USA
Full list of author information is available at the end of the article

Background

Multiple symptoms have been associated with the menopausal transition. Some, such as hot flashes, are clearly associated with hormonal changes [1–4]. Other symptoms, such as joint pain and headaches, may be associated with hormonal changes, but the evidence is less straight forward [5, 6]. Social, rather than hormonal, changes may be responsible for depressed mood or trouble sleeping in some women [7, 8]. Although not well established, certain studies suggest that stress may be associated with hot flashes [3, 9, 10], trouble sleeping, headaches, and depressed mood [11–13].

"Stress" can have multiple meanings, and has been measured in multiple ways. In relation to hot flashes, stress has been measured both inside the laboratory [14–16] and outside of the laboratory in relation to perceived stress scores [3, 9, 10], cortisol levels [17–21], measures of blood pressure [22–25], and C-reactive protein [10, 26]. Missing from these analyses is a consideration of the larger context of women's lives, specifically at the level of problems in the neighborhood and the social challenge of perceived discrimination.

A broad range of research links neighborhood social and economic environments to the health of residents [27–29]. Neighborhoods with high levels of poverty, violence, and disorder have been associated with detrimental effects on individuals residing in these areas [27, 30, 31]. Stress is related to the chronic difficulties encountered within neighborhoods, and this neighborhood stress has been reported to increase vulnerability to immune disorders and cardiovascular disease [32, 33]. Exposure to events known to elicit stressful emotions such as fear, anger, or depression have been assessed by two subscales (Neighborhood Disorder and Exposure to Violence) of the City Stress Inventory [34]. Studies among caregivers of children with asthma have shown an increase in asthma morbidity and depression in association with increasing levels of perceived violence [35, 36].

Neighborhoods with low levels of social cohesion have been associated with increased rates of depression in the Multi-Ethnic Study of Atherosclerosis (MESA) Study [37], coronary calcification in the CARDIA study [38], and to increased risk of acute myocardial infarction mortality in Scania, Sweden [39]. Additionally, the Jackson Heart Study found that, in disadvantaged neighborhoods, low social cohesion was associated with higher levels of cumulative biological risk among African American men [27].

Racial disparities in health have been posited to be linked to exposures of discrimination [40]. Self-reported unfair treatment or perceived discrimination has been reported to contribute to broad-based morbidity [41, 42]. Brondolo et al. [43] have reported that racial discrimination may also influence cardiovascular disease risk. It has been suggested that among African Americans, the experience of everyday unfair treatment leads to a cumulative biological "wear and tear" (or allostatic load [44]) as measured across 22 biomarkers, representing seven system levels, of biological disintegration [45]. The results of that study, conducted among midlife African Americans, adds to the literature linking the stress of discrimination to effects on multiple downstream physiological systems [45]. There is also evidence from the Study of Women's Health Across the Nation (SWAN) linking higher levels of discrimination to higher levels of allostatic load [46]. In addition, in SWAN, the Everyday Discrimination Scale was administered at baseline and at each of the 13 follow-up periods. Chronic everyday discrimination was associated with more bodily pain, in fully adjusted models, among African-American, Chinese, and non-Hispanic white women [47]. Higher allostatic load levels, in addition to contributing to increased risk for many health outcomes [48], may also contribute to greater reporting of midlife symptoms among both black and white women during this period of increased vulnerability.

The purpose of the study presented here was to examine the risk of symptoms at midlife in relation to neighborhood disorder, exposure to neighborhood violence, and perceived discrimination among black and white women living in New York City. We focused on hot flashes and night sweats because of previous studies that suggest a relationship between stress and vasomotor symptoms [3, 9, 10]. An additional reason for this focus was the suggestion that hot flashes and night sweats may be markers of cardiovascular disease risk [49, 50]. In addition, we examined other possible symptoms at midlife that could be associated with increasingly negative neighborhood characteristics and levels of discrimination. We hypothesized that women who report higher levels of neighborhood disorder, violence, and increasing experience of personal discrimination would be more likely to report hot flashes and other symptoms at midlife, even after controlling for age, ethnicity, BMI, and menopausal status. To our knowledge, this is the first study of symptoms at midlife among black and white women in relation to neighborhood context, beyond discrimination.

Methods

The Neighborhood Study of Blood Pressure and Sleep, conducted from September 1999 through July 2003, was a cross-sectional investigation of race/ethnicity, socioeconomic status, and diurnal blood pressure (BP) patterns [18, 51]. Data for this study were drawn from this parent study. Because this study examined both neighborhood characteristics and symptom experience at midlife, these data offer a unique opportunity to test our hypothesis that hot flashes are more frequently reported among those residing in a stressful environment.

Participants were recruited through fliers and word of mouth from Weill Cornell Medical College, Mount Sinai School of Medicine, Harlem Hospital, and North General Hospital using a common protocol and consent form approved by the institutional review committee at each of the four institutions. At recruitment, women were 18 to 65 years old, white or black, had no previous cardiovascular disease, and no major medical problems other than hypertension ($n = 211$). Those who were eligible and chose to participate completed informed consent before initiating study procedures. The analyses here focus on women aged 40 to 60 ($n = 139$) at the time of interview in order to better assess symptoms at midlife; thus, this is a subset of a larger study.

Data collected

Participants completed a self-administered demographic and medical history questionnaire that included questions about education, smoking habits, and menstruation. Age and race/ethnicity were self-reported. Questions about menopausal status queried the last menstrual cycle, whether menstruation had occurred in the previous 12 months, menstrual regularity, and whether cycles had changed in length. Post-menopausal status was defined as having had at least 12 months of amenorrhea. Peri-menopausal status was defined by missed menstrual periods and significant changes in menstrual cycle regularity and length. Pre-menopausal status was defined as having regular menstruation. These categories were used in lieu of the STRAW+ 10 stages [52] because of the cross-sectional nature of the study and the small number of women in the peri-menopausal group. Because of the small number of women in the peri-menopause category, women were grouped into two groups: pre- vs. peri/postmenopause for analyses. Height and weight were measured twice by a technician. The average of the two measurements was used, and body mass index (BMI) was calculated as weight divided by the square of height (kg/m^2).

The following Likert scales were used to measure neighborhood characteristics: (1) The Neighborhood Disorder (ND) Scale [34] assessed perceptions of neighborhood disorder with 11 items that served as a subset of City Stress Inventory, scaled as 0–33 (e.g., I heard neighbors complaining about crime in our neighborhood; People in the neighborhood complained about being harassed by police). (2) The Exposure to Violence (EV) Scale, [34], is a 7 items subset of the City Stress Inventory, scaled as 0–21 (e.g., A family member was attacked or beaten; A friend was robbed or mugged). (3) The Perceived Violence (PV) Subscale is from the Project on Human Development

in Chicago Neighborhoods: Community Survey, 1994–1995 [53], scaled 5–20, (e.g., During the past 6 months, how often was there a fight in this neighborhood in which a weapon was used; How often were their sexual assaults/rape). (4) The Neighborhood Social Cohesion and Trust (NSCT) Scale is a subscale of the Collective Efficacy instrument used to assess social cohesion among neighbors with 5 items, scaled 0–15 (e.g., This is a close-knit neighborhood; People around here are willing to help their neighbors) [54]. (5) The Everyday Discrimination Scale (EDS), scaled 0–45 [55] is a scale of 9 items that assesses chronic and routine experiences of unfair treatment (e.g., You are treated with less courtesy than other people; people act as if they are afraid of you; you are called names or insulted.)

Symptoms associated with menopause were queried with a frequently used questionnaire that embeds menopausal symptoms into a list of everyday complaints [56, 57]. Each participant was asked whether or not she had been bothered by each of 23 symptoms during the past 2 weeks, e.g., hot flashes, trouble sleeping, or feeling blue or depressed. Answers were assessed as yes/no.

We selected symptoms for study by first excluding 8 symptoms that were placed in the list to make the instrument less obviously about menopausal symptoms (diarrhea, persistent cough, upset stomach, sore throat, loss of appetite, menstrual problems, fluid retention, urinary tract/bladder infections). We also excluded one symptom, vaginal dryness, which was not expected to vary with contextual stress.

Statistical analysis

Exploratory factor analyses were carried out with the 14 remaining symptoms to examine how symptoms grouped in the entire sample. Our assumption was that symptoms clustering with hot flashes were our best candidates for the study of midlife symptoms. Scree plots were examined to identify the point at which eigenvalues began to level off. It was decided that three was the most informative number of factors. Three factors were extracted using the method of unweighted least squares with varimax rotation. Unweighted least squares was applied to achieve more conservative results (i.e., fewer symptoms with factor scores > 0.300).

We repeated the factor analyses and each time excluded one symptom that did not cluster with hot flashes. In this way, difficulty concentrating, rapid heartbeat, dizzy spells, and cold sweats were excluded. With each change, the total variance explained increased. The final 10 symptoms were: lack of energy, feeling blue/depressed, backaches, headaches, aches/stiffness in joints, shortness of breath, hot flashes, trouble sleeping, nervous tension, and pins/needles in hands/feet. With fewer than 10 symptoms, the total variance explained started to decline.

Bivariate Spearman correlations were examined among the scores for neighborhood disorder, violence, and discrimination. Spearman correlations were applied because scores were not normally distributed. We examined race/ethnicity in relation to neighborhood characteristics, and each symptom in relation to neighborhood characteristics using Mann-Whitney U tests. Symptoms significantly associated with neighborhood characteristics at the level of $p < 0.20$ were chosen for logistic regression analyses.

In those occasional situations where a participant was missing a subset of the items used to compute a scale score, we used a regression-based approach to estimate the expected value of the scale based on the non-missing items, and replaced/imputed the missing value with its expected value if the R^2 for the regression $\geq 70\%$. By definition, the resulting equation is the optimal linear function of the available items for estimating the scale score based on data from those who answered all items.

We examined race/ethnicity, smoking, menopausal status, and education (≤ 12, 13–16, > 16 years) in relation to each symptom by chi-square analysis, and age and BMI in relation to each symptom by t-test and included race/ethnicity, smoking, education, and/or BMI as covariates in logistic regression models if the relationship between the variable and the symptom was $p < 0.20$ in unadjusted analyses. We did not include all possible covariates in our models in order to increase the power of each model.

Logistic regression analyses were carried out with the symptom (yes/no) as the dependent variable, with each neighborhood or discrimination scale as the primary independent variable controlling for any significant covariate(s). In addition, linear regression was used to examine derived factor scores as outcome variables with each neighborhood or discrimination scale as a predictor variable while controlling for covariates. All analyses were conducted with IBM SPSS Statistics for Windows, Version 24.0. Armonk, NY: IBM Corp.

Results

Table 1 shows the sample characteristics for the total sample ($n = 139$), and for the white (45%) and black (55%) women. Mean age was 49.1 years and did not vary by race/ethnicity. White women had higher levels of education, but did not significantly differ with regard to smoking, BMI, or menopausal status. All of the neighborhood and discrimination scales differed by race/ethnicity so that black women reported higher scores on negative neighborhood characteristics and discrimination, and a lower score on the positive neighborhood social cohesion and trust scale.

Table 1 Sample characteristics

	Total sample $N = 139$	White women $N = 62$	Black women $N = 77$	p-value
Mean age (s.d.)	49.1 (5.7)	49.7 (6.0)	48.7 (5.5)	0.31
% Level of education				
≤ 12	16.3%	6.7%	24.6%	< 0.001
13–16	58.9%	50.0%	66.7%	
17+	24.8%	43.3%	8.7%	
% Smoking	22.1%	15.0%	28.2%	0.07
Mean BMI (s.d.)	29.6 (6.4)	28.5 (6.1)	30.6 (6.5)	0.06
% Menopause status				
Pre-	48.0%	39.6%	55.6%	0.09
Peri-	6.9%	4.2%	9.3%	
Post-	45.1%	56.3%	35.2%	
Neighborhood Disorder				
Scale range 0–28				
Means (s.d.)	8.3 (7.4)	5.1 (5.6)	11.1 (7.6)	< 0.001
Medians	6.00	3.23	10.00	< 0.001
Exposure to Violence				
Scale range 0–15				
Means (s.d.)	1.9 (3.0)	0.8 (1.5)	2.9 (3.5)	< 0.001
Medians	1.00	0.00	2.00	< 0.001
Perceived Violence				
Subscale range 5–18				
Means (s.d.)	9.4 (3.6)	8.4 (3.1)	10.4 (3.8)	0.002
Medians	9.00	7.10	10.25	0.004
Neighborhood Social Cohesion and Trust				
Scale range 1–14				
Means (s.d.)	8.4 (2.5)	9.3 (1.9)	7.6 (2.7)	< 0.001
Medians	8.63	10.00	8.00	< 0.001
Everyday Discrimination				
Scale range 0–39				
Means (s.d.)	8.7 (8.2)	6.2 (5.9)	11.1 (9.4)	0.001
Medians	6.00	5.00	7.50	0.002

There were no significant differences between white and black women with regard to symptom report. Only nervous tension approached significance ($p = 0.05$) (Table 2).

Factor analysis

After selecting the 10 symptoms of interest, among all women, the first factor comprised psychosomatic symptoms. Hot flashes loaded onto the second factor along with three somatic symptoms (backaches, aches/stiffness in joints, and pins/needles in hands/feet). A third factor captured some remaining somatic symptoms, including headaches and shortness of breath. Although sample

Table 2 Frequency of symptoms by race/ethnicity

	Total sample (n), %	White women (n), %	Black women (n), %	p-value
Lack of energy	(66), 55.0%	(31), 57.4%	(35), 53.0%	0.632
Feeling blue/ depressed	(42), 34.7%	(18), 32.7%	(24), 36.4%	0.676
Backaches	(58), 47.9%	(23), 42.6%	(35), 52.2%	0.291
Headaches	(66), 53.7%	(27), 49.1%	(39), 57.4%	0.361
Aches/stiffness in joints	(71), 58.7%	**(27), 50.9%**	**(44), 64.7%**	0.127
Shortness of breath	(22), 18.2%	(8), 14.8%	(14), 20.9%	0.389
Hot flashes	(49), 39.8%	**(18), 33.3%**	**(31), 44.9%**	0.192
Trouble sleeping	(58), 47.5%	**(30), 55.6%**	**(28), 41.2%**	0.114
Nervous tension	(42), 34.4%	**(24), 43.6%**	**(18), 26.9%**	0.052
Pins and needles in hands/feet	(30), 24.4%	**(10), 18.2%**	**(20), 29.4%**	0.149

Differences with a p value < 0.20 bolded for inclusion as a covariate in logistic regressions

sizes were small, there were differences in factor loadings between white and black women. White women reflected the total sample findings. Among black women, hot flashes clustered with lack of energy, feeling blue/depressed, backaches, and nervous tension in addition to aches/stiffness in joints and pins/needles in hands/feet. Of the 10 symptoms in Table 3, headaches, shortness of breath, and trouble sleeping did not group into a factor with hot flashes (Table 3).

Spearman correlations
The neighborhood scales were correlated with each other in the expected directions. Neighborhood Disorder correlated positively with Exposure to Violence ($r = .649$, $p < 0.001$), Perceived Violence ($r = .679$, $p < 0.001$), and Everyday Discrimination Scale ($r = .495$, $p < 0.001$), and correlated negatively with Neighborhood Social Cohesion and Trust ($r = -.300$, $p = 0.001$). Exposure to

Violence correlated positively with Perceived Violence ($r = .489$, $p < 0.001$) and Everyday Discrimination Scale ($r = .422$, $p < 0.001$), and negatively with Neighborhood Social Cohesion and Trust ($r = -.232$, $p = 0.009$). Neighborhood Social Cohesion and Trust correlated negatively with Perceived Violence ($r = -.283$, $p = 0.002$) and Everyday Discrimination Scale ($r = -.318$, $p < 0.001$).

Bivariate results
The following associations were found between symptoms and women's characteristics (data not shown). With regard to age at interview, women reporting aches/stiffness in joints ($p < 0.001$), hot flashes ($p < 0.001$) and nervous tension ($p = 0.04$) were older than women not reporting those symptoms. Women reporting headaches were younger ($p = 0.006$) than women not reporting headaches. With regard to menopausal status, peri- and post-

Table 3 Factor analyses of symptoms included in study

	Total sample 1	2	3	White women 1	2	3	Black women 1	2	3
Lack of energy	.712	.252	.270	.739	.160	.326	.712	.367	−.012
Feeling blue/ depressed	.842	.084	−.144	.776	−.073	−.071	.533	.490	.366
Backaches	.344	.510	.352	.326	.741	−.212	.533	.544	−.182
Headaches	−.058	.040	.803	.104	.098	.609	.162	−.020	−.844
Aches/stiffness in joints	.119	.808	.221	.093	.828	.186	.761	.030	.016
Shortness of breath	.280	.190	.467	−.005	.111	.775	.072	.801	−.051
Hot flashes	.055	.720	−.283	−.152	.631	.221	.485	−.097	.557
Trouble sleeping	.653	.060	.211	.752	.194	−.046	.205	.720	.073
Nervous tension	.717	.250	.002	.597	.045	.456	.713	.283	.329
Pins and needles in hands/feet	.359	.493	.157	.315	.377	.248	.652	.209	−.108
Variance explained (rounded)	25%	18%	13%	23%	19%	15%	29%	20%	13%
Cumulative variance explained	56.31%			56.70%			61.78%		

menopausal women (combined) were more likely to report a lack of energy ($p = 0.007$), aches/stiffness in joints ($p = 0.004$), and hot flashes ($p < 0.001$). Finally, with regard to BMI, women with aches/stiffness in joints ($p = 0.06$), and backaches ($p = 0.07$) tended to have a higher BMI than women not reporting those symptoms. No symptom frequencies differed by smoking status or level of education (≤ 12, 13–16, > 16 years) at $p < 0.20$.

Looking across bivariate results for symptoms (yes/no) in relation to measures of neighborhood disorder, violence, cohesion, and discrimination, Table 4 shows that the measures of Neighborhood Disorder were associated with 7 symptoms at the $p < 0.2$ level. In all instances, women with the symptoms had higher median levels of neighborhood disorder. The two measures of neighborhood violence (Exposure to Violence and Perceived Violence) were associated with 4 and 3 symptoms, respectively, at the $p < 0.20$ level. The Neighborhood Social Cohesion and Trust was associated with 2 symptoms so that women with more social cohesion and trust in the neighborhood were less likely to report backaches ($p < 0.05$) and aches/stiffness in joints ($p < 0.20$). The Everyday Discrimination Scale was associated with 4 symptoms at the $p < 0.20$ level.

Logistic regression results

Neighborhood Disorder remained significantly associated with feeling blue/depressed, aches/stiffness in joints, and hot flashes (OR 1.084, 95% CI 1.007–1.165) after controlling for model-specific independent variables (Table 5). Exposure to Violence did not remain associated with any symptom (Table 6), but aches/stiffness in joints remained associated with Perceived Violence after controlling for age, race/ethnicity, BMI and menopausal status (Table 7). There was a lower risk of backaches as the neighborhood cohesion score increased (Table 8). Finally, discrimination (Everyday Discrimination Scale) remained associated with lack of energy after controlling for model-specific independent variables (Table 9).

Looking across Tables 5, 6, 7, 8 and 9, in addition to neighborhood context and discrimination, increasing age reduced the risk of headaches, but elevated the risks of aches/stiffness in joints. Peri/post-menopausal status was associated with an increased likelihood of lack of energy in two models (OR 7.324 and OR 8.071) and an increased likelihood of hot flashes in three models (OR 4.734, OR 3.611, and OR 4.265). BMI was not associated with any symptom in logistic regression models after controlling for age, race/ethnicity, menopausal status, and neighborhood characteristics.

Linear regression results

Both Neighborhood Disorder and Everyday Discrimination scores were significantly associated with derived Factor 1 scores (data not shown). Symptoms loading onto Factor 1 included "Feeling blue or depressed" and "Lack of energy." These results are consistent with our logistic regression results where the associations were significant between "Feeling blue or depressed" and Neighborhood Disorder ($p = 0.011$) and between "Lack of energy" and Everyday Discrimination ($p = 0.006$).

Discussion

The results of this study suggest that neighborhood context and discrimination may be associated with midlife symptoms in a cohort of black and white women residing in a large urban environment. To our knowledge, this is one of very few studies to extend the investigation of perceived social features of neighborhoods to symptoms among women at midlife. A major strength of this study is the many measures of neighborhood context collected in relation to the broad range of symptoms examined. A novel approach used factor analysis to focus our examination on ten symptoms, clustered on three factors. Of those ten symptoms, five were found to be significantly associated with neighborhood context or discrimination.

As is often the case with midlife symptoms [58–61], the ten symptoms of interest did not separate cleanly

Table 4 Median level of each scale by symptom occurrence (yes/no)

	Lack of energy		Feeling blue/ depressed		Backaches		Headaches		Aches/ stiffness in joints		Short of breath		Hot flashes		Trouble sleeping		Nervous tension		Pins and needles in hands/feet	
	No	Yes	No	Yes	No	Yes	No	Yes	No	Yes	No	Yes	No	Yes	No	Yes	No	Yes	No	Yes
ND	5.09	6.00$^{\&}$	5.00	9.00*	6.00	6.00	4.50	8.00$^{\#}$	4.00	8.00$^{\#}$	5.04	9.00$^{\#}$	5.04	9.00*	5.54	6.00	6.00	6.00	5.09	10.00*
EV	0.00	1.00$^{\&}$	0.00	1.00$^{\&}$	1.00	1.00	1.00	1.00	0.00	1.00	1.00	1.00	0.50	2.00$^{\&}$	1.00	1.00	1.00	1.00	0.00	2.00*
PV	9.00	9.89	9.00	10.13	9.12	9.59	9.00	10.00	7.58	10.40*	9.16	9.33	8.43	10.00$^{\#}$	10.18	9.08$^{\&}$	9.00	10.13	9.00	10.00
NSCT	8.00	8.51	8.00	9.00	9.00	8.00$^{\#}$	8.00	8.57	9.00	8.00$^{\&}$	8.57	8.00	8.30	8.00	8.79	8.00	8.00	8.51	8.00	8.03
EDS	5.00	7.00*	6.00	7.00	6.00	7.00	5.00	7.00$^{\&}$	6.00	7.00*	6.50	6.50	7.00	6.50	6.00	7.50	6.00	8.00	6.00	9.00$^{\#}$

$^{*}p < 0.05$; $^{\#}p \leq 0.1$; $^{\&}p < 0.20$ using Mann-Whitney U test

ND Neighborhood Disorder Scale, EV Exposure to Violence Scale, PV Perceived Violence Scale, NSCT Neighborhood Social Cohesion and Trust, EDS Everyday Discrimination Scale

Table 5 Logistic regression results for Neighborhood Disorder (ND)[a]

	Lack of energy	Feeling blue/ depressed	Headaches	Aches/ stiffness in joints	Short of breath	Hot flashes	Pins and needles in hands/feet
	AOR[f] (95% CI)	AOR (95% CI)	AOR (95% CI)	AOR (95% CI)	AOR (95% CI)	AOR (95% CI)	AOR (95% CI)
Age	.92 (.82–1.03)		.86 (.77–.96)[c]	1.13 (.99–1.28)		1.05 (.94–1.18)	1.04 (.97–1.13)
Black				2.62 (.89–7.73)		1.70 (.62–4.69)	1.41 (.54–3.68)
BMI	1.04 (.97–1.12)			1.04 (.955–1.126)	1.04 (.06–1.12)		
Peri/Post[b]	7.32 (1.80–29.76)[d]		1.88 (.55–6.38)	2.66 (.62–11.36)		4.73 (1.25–17.93)[e]	
ND	1.07 (.997–1.145)	1.07 (1.02–1.13)[f]	1.06 (.99–1.12)	1.11 (1.01–1.21)[g]	1.06 (.997–1.13)	1.08 (1.01–1.17)[h]	1.06 (.99–1.13)

[a]Symptoms selected for logistic regression were those associated with the neighborhood characteristic in Table 4
[b]Pre is the reference
[c]$p = .007$; [d]$p = .005$; [e]$p = .022$; [f]$p = 0.011$; [g]$p = 0.030$; [h]$p = 0.031$
[f]AOR adjusted odds ratio

into distinct groups through factor analyses. Also consistent with other studies [58, 61], there is population variation in how symptoms cluster. In the study presented here, depressed mood and hot flashes grouped together among the Black sample, but not the White sample or in the sample as a whole.

Lack of energy, feeling blue/depressed, aches/stiffness in joints, and hot flashes were the symptoms most vulnerable to the effect of negative neighborhood context. Each of these four symptoms remained significantly associated with different neighborhood characteristics after adjusting for model-specific covariates. All but lack of energy were associated with Neighborhood Disorder.

Why these symptoms would be most affected by neighborhood context is not immediately clear. Looking at the factor analyses, aches/stiffness in joints consistently clustered together with hot flashes, but feeling blue/depressed only clustered with hot flashes among Black women. Backaches and pins/needles also clustered with hot flashes, but backaches were only significantly associated with the Neighborhood Social Cohesion and Trust, and pins/needles were not associated with any measure of neighborhood context or discrimination. The factor analyses did not help us predict how symptoms would be associated with neighborhood stress.

Neighborhood Disorder remained significantly associated with feeling blue/depressed, aches/stiffness in joints, and hot flashes after controlling for model-specific independent variables. This suggests that stress related to neighborhood disorder may be expressed as emotional, somatic, and vasomotor experience. Somatization of emotional symptoms may at times serve as psychosomatic "idioms of distress," calling attention to difficulties that are hard to verbally express [62–64].

Aches/stiffness in joints remained associated with Perceived Violence, but not Exposure to Violence, after controlling for age, race/ethnicity, BMI and menopausal status. Because of differences in the scales, as well as the relatively modest correlation between them ($r = .489$), it is not surprising that they are not similarly associated with midlife symptoms.

Only backaches were associated with the neighborhood cohesion score, decreasing the risk of backaches as the score increased (Table 8). Women were 15% less likely to report having had backaches for each unit increase (1 point on a 0–15 point scale) on the Neighborhood Social Cohesion and Trust scale. Backaches may also be indicative of depression and somatization [65, 66]. The Multi-Ethnic Study of Atherosclerosis (MESA) found that neighborhoods with low levels of social

Table 6 Logistic regression results for Exposure to Violence (EV)[a]

	Lack of Energy	Feeling blue/depressed	Hot flashes	Pins and needles in hands/feet
	AOR[c] (95% CI)	AOR (95% CI)	AOR (95% CI)	AOR (95% CI)
Age	.93 (.83–1.04)		1.07 (.96–1.20)	1.05 (.97–1.13)
Black			2.02 (.74–5.47)	1.47 (.57–3.77)
BMI	1.05 (.97–1.13)			
Peri/Post[a]	5.82 (1.52–22.38)[d]		3.61 (1.01–12.92)[e]	
EV	1.13 (.96–1.33)	1.06 (.94–1.20)	1.11 (.95–1.304)	1.13 (.99–1.30)

[a]Symptoms selected for logistic regression were those associated with the neighborhood characteristic in Table 4
[b]Pre is the reference
[c]AOR adjusted odds ratio
[d]$p = 0.010$; [e]$p = 0.048$

Table 7 Logistic regression results for Perceived Violence (PV)[a]

	Aches/ stiffness in joints AOR[e] (95% CI)	Hot flashes AOR (95% CI)	Trouble sleeping AOR (95% CI)
Age	1.13 (.99–1.29)	1.05 (.93–1.18)	
Black	2.55 (.85–7.63)	2.54 (.90–7.20)	.69 (.31–1.54)
BMI	.998 (.91–1.09)		
Peri/Post[b]	1.57 (.35–7.05)	4.27 (1.09–16.68)[c]	
PV	1.17 (1.01–1.36)[d]	1.10 (.96–1.25)	.95 (.85–1.06)

[a]Symptoms selected for logistic regression were those associated with the neighborhood characteristic in Table 4
[b]Pre is the reference
[c]p = 0.037; [d]p = 0.035
[e]AOR adjusted odds ratio

cohesion had increased rates of depression [37], but that was not the case here. It should be noted that the Neighborhood Social Cohesion and Trust scale in the MESA study was evaluated as tertiles, and a different measure of depressed mood (the Centers of Epidemiologic Studies Depression scale) was used.

Finally, the Everyday Discrimination Scale remained associated with lack of energy after controlling for model-specific independent variables (Table 9). A number of studies have documented associations between discrimination and physical symptoms The SWAN study found everyday discrimination was significantly associated with bodily pain in all ethnic groups [47]. In contrast, data from the Midlife Development in the United States study (MIDUS) did not show a significant association in whites, but demonstrated a significant positive relationship between perceived discrimination and frequency of back pain among African Americans, with a stronger association observed among African-American women [67].

In examining the relation between neighborhood social environments and discrimination with midlife symptoms, there were also contributions of age, race/ethnicity, and menopausal status. Older women had a reduced risk of headaches compared to younger women, in contrast to

Table 8 Logistic regression results for the Neighborhood Social Cohesion and Trust (NSCT) Scale[a]

	Backaches AOR[*] (95% CI)	Aches/ stiffness in joints AOR (95% CI)
Age	.	1.14 (1.01–1.29)[c]
Black		3.40 (1.16–9.97)[d]
BMI	1.05 (.98–1.12)	1.03 (.95–1.12)
Peri/Post[b]		2.03 (.49–8.46)
NSCT	.85 (.72–.99)[e]	.94 (.78–1.13)

[*]AOR adjusted odds ratio
[a]Symptoms selected for logistic regression were those associated with the neighborhood characteristic in Table 4
[b]Pre is the reference
[c]p = 0.042; [d]p = 0.026; [e]p = 0.035

studies of tension-related headaches [68]. Older women had an elevated risk of aches/stiffness in joints, as would be expected [69]. Although higher rates of reported pain among African-Americans was noted in Dugan et al. [47], the differences of 65% among black women vs 50% among white women in the frequency of aches/stiffness of joints observed in this study did not reach statistical significance, perhaps due to small numbers. Nervous tension was reported less frequently among black than white women (27% vs 44%, respectively), approaching statistical significance (p = 0.052). It is interesting to note, however, in models where neighborhood context or discrimination were significantly associated with a midlife symptom, race/ethnicity did not significantly add risk.

Peri/post-menopausal status was associated with an increased likelihood of lack of energy and, in three models, an increased likelihood of hot flashes. Lack of energy is frequently one of the most commonly reported symptoms among women at menopause [56, 70, 71], and it is well established that the loss of estrogen during the late menopausal transition is associated with hot flashes [1].

This study has several limitations. There is limited assessment of symptoms (i.e., presence in past 2 weeks, without assessment of frequency or bothersomeness.) Given the cross-sectional design of this study, we are unable to determine the temporal sequence of the reported relationships. This study posited that the effects of neighborhood context would be related to symptoms at midlife; however, a depressed person might perceive her neighborhood more negatively than a person without depressive symptoms [72]. Longitudinal studies are needed to address the direction of any causal association.

There is a potential for spurious associations given the multiplicity of outcomes. We were careful, however, to limit just those covariates into multivariable models that were significant or marginally significant in bivariate analyses. An additional limitation is the potential lack of power to detect significant findings due to the small sample size. Among the strengths of this study is the fact that participants were drawn

Table 9 Logistic regression results for Everyday Discrimination Scale (EDS)[a]

	Lack of energy	Headaches	Aches/ stiffness in joints	Pins and needles in hands/feet
	AOR[*] (95% CI)	AOR (95% CI)	AOR (95% CI)	AOR (95% CI)
Age	.92 (.82–1.04)	.87 (.78–.97)[c]	1.14 (.998–1.29)	1.05 (.97–1.13)
Black			2.75 (.94–8.07)	1.80 (.71–4.55)
BMI			1.03 (.95–1.12)	
Peri/Post[b]	8.07 (1.93–33.81)[d]	1.63 (.48–5.54)	2.26 (.51–9.98)	
EDS	1.10 (1.03–1.18)[e]	1.05 (.99–1.11)	1.08 (.996–1.17)	1.05 (.997–1.11)

[*]AOR adjusted odds ratio
[a]Symptoms selected for logistic regression were those associated with the neighborhood characteristic in Table 4
[b]Pre is the reference
[c]$p = 0.010$; [d]$p = 0.004$; [e]$p = 0.006$

from four distinct sites from a large and diverse city. Additionally, standardized data collection protocols were used across sites to assess multiple measures of neighborhood characteristics.

Conclusions

This study adds to the literature linking neighborhood environments to health outcomes. We have extended this literature to a number of women's midlife symptoms that have not been previously examined. In our sample comprised of both black and white women, we found that negative neighborhood context increased the risk of self-reported depression, aches/stiffness in joints, and hot flashes while greater social cohesion lowered the risk of backaches. The association between discrimination and lack of energy is intriguing, and points to the need to further examine links between exposure to everyday discrimination, and other measures of neighborhood context, and multiple physiological systems.

Acknowledgments
The authors thank the other investigators, and particularly Joseph E. Schwartz, PhD, for his valuable contributions. We also thank the participants of the Neighborhood Study of Blood Pressure and Sleep for their cooperation.

Funding
The study was supported by grants NIH P01HL175 10, R21HL76057, and M01RR00047.

Authors' contributions
LMG designed this study and supervised data collection; LMG and LLS carried out all analyses, drafted the manuscript, and approved the final manuscript.

Competing interests
The authors declare that they have no competing interests.

Author details
[1]Department of Healthcare Policy & Research, Division of Biostatistics and Epidemiology, Weill Cornell Medical College, 402 E. 67th St., LA-231, New York, NY 10065, USA. [2]Department of Medicine, Division of Nephrology and Hypertension, Weill Cornell Medical College, New York City, NY, USA. [3]Department of Anthropology, UMass Amherst, Amherst, MA, USA.

References
1. Freedman RR. Pathophysiology and treatment of menopausal hot flashes. Semin Reprod Med. 2005;23:117–25.
2. Freeman EW, Sammel MD, Lin H. Temporal associations of hot flashes and depression in the transition to menopause. Menopause. 2009;16:728–34.
3. Gold EB, Block G, Crawford S, Lachance L, FitzGerald G, Miracle H, Sherman S. Lifestyle and demographic factors in relation to vasomotor symptoms: baseline results from the Study of Women's Health Across the Nation. Am J Epidemiol. 2004;159(12):1189–99.
4. Randolph JF, Sowers M, Bondarenko I, Gold EB, Greendale GA, Bromberger JT, Brockwell SE, Matthews KA. The relationship of longitudinal change in reproductive hormones and vasomotor symptoms during the menopausal transition. J Clin Endocrinol Metab. 2005;90:6106–12.
5. Sacco S, Ricci S, Degan D. Carolei. Migraine in women: the role of hormones and their impact on vascular diseases. J Headache Pain. 2012; 13(3):177–89.
6. Szoeke CE, Cicuttini F, Guthrie J, Dennerstein L. Self-reported arthritis and the menopause. Climacteric. 2005;8(1):49–55.
7. Bromberger JT, Kravitz HM. Mood and menopause: findings from the Study of Women's Health Across the Nation (SWAN) over ten years. Obstet Gynecol Clin N Am. 2011;38(3):609–25.
8. Tom SE, Kuh D, Guralnik JM, Mishra C. Self reported sleep difficulty during the menopausal transition: results from a prospective cohort study. Menopause. 2010;17(6):1128–35.
9. Freeman EW, Sammel MD, Lin H, Liu Z, Gracia CR. Duration of menopausal hot flushes and associated risk factors. Obstet Gynecol. 2011;117(5):1095–104.
10. Sievert LL. Huicochea-Gómez L, Cahuich-Campos D, Koomoa D-L, Brown DE. Stress and the menopausal transition in Campeche. Mexico Women's Midlife Health. 2018. http://doi.org/10.1186/s40695-018-0038-x.
11. Han KS, Kim L, Shim I. Stress and sleep disorder. Exp Neurobiol. 2012;21(4): 141–50.
12. Martin PR, Lae L, Reece J. Stress as a trigger for headaches: relationship between exposure and sensitivity. Anxiety Stress & Coping. 2007;20(4): 393–407.

13. Tafet GE, Nemeroff CB. The links between stress and depression: psychoneuroendocrinological, genetic, and environmental interactions. J Neuropsychiatry Clin Neurosci. 2016;28(2):77–88.

14. Cignarelli M, Cicinelli E, Corso M, et al. Biophysical and endocrinemetabolic changes during menopausal hot flashes: increase in plasma free fatty acid and norepinephrine levels. Gynecol Obstet Investig. 1989;27:34–7.

15. Meldrum DR, Defazio JD, Erlik Y, et al. Pituitary hormones during the menopausal hot flash. Obstet Gynecol. 1984;64:752–6.

16. Swartzman LC. Impact of stress on objectively recorded menopausal hot flushes and on flush report bias. Health Psychol. 1990;9(5):529–45.

17. Cagnacci A, Cannoletta M, Caretto S, Zanin R, Xholli A, Volpe A. Increased cortisol level: a posible link between climacteric symptoms and cardiovascular risk factors. Menopause. 2011;18(3):273–8.

18. Gerber LM, Sievert LL, Schwartz JE. Hot flashes and midlife symptoms in relation to levels of salivary cortisol. Maturitas. 2017;96:26–32.

19. Gibson CJ, Thurston RC, Matthews KA. Cortisol dysregulation is associated with daily diary-reported hot flashes among midlife women. Clin Endocrinol. 2016;85:645–51.

20. Reed SD, Newton KM, Larson JC, Booth-LaForce C, Woods NF, Landis CA, Tolentino E, Carpenter JS, Freeman EW, Joffe H, Anawalt BD, Guthrie KA. Daily salivary cortisol patterns in midlife women with hot flashes. Clin Endocrinol. 2016;84(5):672–9.

21. Woods NF, Carr MC, Tao EY, Taylor HJ, Mitchell ES. Increased urinary cortisol levels during the menopause transition. Menopause. 2006;13(2):212–21.

22. Brown DE, Sievert LL, Morrison LA, Rahberg N, Reza A. Relationship between hot flashes and ambulatory blood pressure: the Hilo Women's health study. Psychosom Med. 2011;73(2):166–72.

23. Gerber LM, Sievert LL, Warren K, Pickering TG, Schwartz JE. Hot flashes are associated with increased ambulatory systolic blood pressure. Menopause. 2007;14(2):308–15.

24. Jackson EA, El Khoudary SR, Crawford SL, Matthews K, Joffe H, Chae C, Thurston RC. Hot flash frequency and blood pressure: data from the Study of Women's Health Across the Nation. J Women's Health. 2016;25(12):1204–9.

25. James GD, Sievert LL, Flanagan E. Ambulatory blood pressure and heart rate in relation to hot flash experience among women of menopausal age. Ann Hum Biol. 2004;31(1):49–58.

26. Thurston RC, El Koudary SR, Sutton-Tyrrell K, Crandall CJ, Gold E, Sternfeld B, Selzer F, Matthews KA. Are vasomotor symptoms associated with alterations in hemostatic and inflammatory markers? Findings from the Study of Women's Health Across the Nation. Menopause. 2011;18(10):1044–51.

27. Barber S, Hickson DA, Kawachi I, Subramanian SV, Earls F. Double-jeopardy: the joint impact of neighborhood disadvantage and low social cohesion on cumulative risk of disease among African American men and women in the Jackson Heart Study. Soc Sci Med. 2016;153:107–15.

28. Diez Roux AV, Mair C. Neighborhoods and health. Ann N Y Acad Sci. 2010; 1186(1):125–45.

29. Diez-Roux AV, Merkin SS, Arnett D, Chambless L, Massing M, Nieto FJ, Watson RL. Neighborhood of residence and incidence of coronary heart disease. N Engl J Med. 2001;345(2):99–106. https://doi.org/10.1056/NEJM200107123450205.

30. Sternthal MJ, Jun H-J, Earls F, Wright RJ. Community violence and urban childhood asthma: a multilevel analysis. Eur Respir J. 2010;36(6):1400–9.

31. Ewart CK, Elder GJ, Smyth JM. How neighborhood disorder increases blood pressure in youth: agonistic striving and subordination. J Behav Med. 2014; 37(1):113–26.

32. Suchday S, Kapur S, Ewart CK, Friedberg JP. Urban stress and health in developing countries: development and validation of a neighborhood stress index for India. Behav Med. 2006;32(3):77–86.

33. Gallo LC, Fortmann AL, de los Monteros KE, Mills PJ, Barrett-Connor E, Roesch SC, Matthews KA. Individual and neighborhood socioeconomic status and inflammation in Mexican-American women: what is the role of obesity? Psychosom Med. 2012;74(5):535–42.

34. Ewart CK, Suchday S. Discovering how urban poverty and violence affect health: development and validation of a Neighborhood Stress Index. Health Psychol. 2002;21(3):254–62.

35. Wright RJ, Mitchell H, Visness CM, Cohen S, Stout J, Evans R, Gold DR. Community violence and asthma morbidity: the Inner-City Asthma Study. Am J Public Health. 2004;94(4):625–32.

36. Tonorezos ES, Breysse PN, Matsui EC, McCormack MC, Curtin-Brosnan J, Williams D, et al. Does neighborhood violence lead to depression among caregivers of children with asthma? Soc Sci Med. 2008;67(1):31–7.

37. Echeverría S, Diez-Roux AV, Shea S, Borrell LN, Jackson S. Associations of neighborhood problems and neighborhood social cohesion with mental health and health behaviors: the multi-ethnic study of atherosclerosis. Health & Place. 2008;14(4):853–65.

38. Kim D, Diez Roux AV, Kiefe CI, Kawachi I, Liu K. Do neighborhood socioeconomic deprivation and low social cohesion predict coronary calcification?: the CARDIA study. Am J Epidemiol. 2010;172(3):288–98.

39. Chaix B, Lindström M, Rosvall M, et al. Neighbourhood social interactions and risk of acute myocardial infarction. J Epidemiol Comm Health. 2008;62: 62–8.

40. Colen CG, Ramey DM, Cooksey EC, Williams DR. Racial disparities in health among nonpoor African Americans and Hispanics: the role of acute and chronic discrimination. Soc Sci Med. 2018;199:167–80.

41. Krieger N. Embodying inequality: a review of concepts, measures, and methods for studying health consequences of discrimination. International J Health Services. 1999;29:295–352.

42. Williams DR, Mohammed SA. Discrimination and racial disparities in health: evidence and needed research. J Behavioral Med. 2009;32(1):20–47.

43. Brondolo E, Libby DJ, Denton E, Thompson S, Beatty DL, Schwartz J, et al. Racism and ambulatory blood pressure in a community sample. Psychosom Med. 2008;70(1):49–56.

44. McEwen BS, Seeman T. Protective and damaging effects of mediators of stress: elaborating and testing the concepts of allostasis and allostatic load. Ann N Y Acad Sci. 1999;896:30–47.

45. Ong AD, Williams DR, Nwizu U, Gruenewald TL. Everyday unfair treatment and multisystem biological dysregulation in African American adults. Cult Divers Ethn Minor Psychol. 2017;23(1):27–53.

46. Upchurch DM, Stein J, Greendale GA, Chyu L, Tseng CH, Huang MH, Seeman T. A longitudinal investigation of race, socioeconomic status, and psychological mediators of allostatic load in midlife women: findings from the study of women's health across the nation. Psychosom Med. 2015;77:402–12.

47. Dugan SA, Lewis TT, Everson-Rose SA, Jacobs EA, Harlow SD, Janssen I. Chronic discrimination and bodily pain in a multiethnic cohort of midlife women in the Study of Women's Health Across the Nation. Pain. 2017; 158(9):1656–65.

48. Seeman TE, Crimmins E, Huang MH, Singer B, Bucur A, Gruenewald T, Reuben DB. Cumulative biological risk and socio-economic differences in mortality: MacArthur studies of successful aging. Soc Sci Med. 2004; 58:1985–97.

49. Gast GC, Grobbee DE, Pop VJ, Keyzer JJ, Wijnands-van Gent CJ, Samsioe GN, Nilsson PM, van der Schouw YT. Menopausal complaints are associated with cardiovascular risk factors. Hypertension. 2008;51:1492–8.

50. Thurston RC, Chang Y, Barinas-Mitchell E, Jennings JR, Landsittel DP, Santoro N, von Känel R, Matthews KA. Menopausal hot flashes and carotid intima media thickness among midlife women. Stroke. 2016;47(12):2910–5.

51. Spruill TM, Gerber LM, Schwartz JE, Pickering TG, Ogedegbe G. Race differences in the physical and psychological impact of hypertension labeling. Am J Hypertens. 2012;25(4):458–63.

52. Harlow SD, Gass M, Hall JE, Lobo R, Maki P, Rebar RW, Sherman S, Sluss PM, de Villiers TJ. STRAW+10 collaborative group. Executive summary of the stages of reproductive aging workshop + 10: addressing the unfinished agenda of staging reproductive aging. Menopause. 2012;19(4):387–95.

53. Earls FJ, Brooks-Gunn J, Raudenbush SW, Sampson RJ. Project on human development in Chicago neighborhoods (PHDCN): master file, wave 1, 1994–1997 [Computer file]. ICPSR13580-v3. Boston, MA: Harvard Medical School [producer], 2002d. Ann Arbor, MI: Interuniversity Consortium for Political and Social Research [distributor], 2005:12–06.

54. Sampson RJ, Raudenbush SW, Earls F. Neighborhoods and violent crime: a multilevel study of collective efficacy. Science. 1997;277:918–24.

55. Williams DR, Yu Y, Jackson JS, Anderson NB. Racial differences in physical and mental health socio-economic status, stress and discrimination. J Health Psychol. 1997;2(3):335–51.

56. Avis NE, Kaufert PA, Lock M, McKinlay SM, Vass K. The evolution of menopausal symptoms. Baillieres Clin Endocrinol Metab. 1993;7:17–32.

57. Obermeyer CM, Reher D, Saliba M. Symptoms, menopausal status, and country differences: a comparative analysis from the DAMeS project. Menopause. 2007;14(4):788–97.

58. Lerner-Geva L, Boyko V, Blumstein T, Benyamini Y. The impact of education, cultural background, and lifestyle on symptoms of the menopausal

transition: the Women's health at midlife study. J Women's Health. 2010;19: 975–85.

59. Melby MK. Factor analysis of climacteric symptoms in Japan. Maturitas. 2005; 52:205–22.

60. Sievert LL, Obermeyer CM. Symptom clusters at midlife: a four-country comparison of checklist and qualitative responses. Menopause. 2012;19(2): 133–44.

61. Sievert LL, Obermeyer CM, Saliba M. Symptom groupings at midlife: cross-cultural variation and association with job, home, and life change. Menopause. 2007;14(4):798–807.

62. Gureje O, Simon GE, Ustun TB, Goldberg DP. Somatization in crosscultural perspective: a World Health Organization study in primary care. Am J Psychiatry. 1997;154:989–95.

63. Keyes CL, Ryff CD. Somatization and mental health: a comparative study of the idiom of distress hypothesis. Soc Sci Med. 2003;57:1833–45.

64. Kleinman A, Kleinman J. Somatization: the interconnections in Chinese society among culture, depressive experiences, and the meanings of pain. In: Kleinman A, Good B, editors. Culture and depression. Berkeley, CA: University of California Press; 1985. p. 429–90.

65. Licciardone JC, Gatchel RJ, Kearns CM, Minotti DE. Depression, somatization, and somatic dysfunction in patients with nonspecific chronic low back pain: results from the OSTEOPATHIC trial. J Am Osteopath Assoc. 2012;112(12): 783–91.

66. Pincus T, Burton AK, Vogel S, Field AP. A systematic review of psychological factors as predicators of chronicity/disability in prospective cohorts of low back pain. Spine. 2002;27(5):E109–20.

67. Edwards RR. The association of perceived discrimination with low back pain. J Behav Med. 2008;31:379–89.

68. Neri I, Granella F, Nappi R, Manzoni G, Facchinetti F, Genazzani A. Characteristics of headache at menopause: a clinico-epidemiologic study. Maturitas. 1993;17(1):31–7.

69. Gao HL, Lin SQ, Chen Y, Wu ZL. The effect of age and menopausal status on musculoskeletal symptoms in Chinese women aged 35-64 years. Climacteric. 2013;16(6):639–45.

70. Dennerstein L, Smith AMA, Morse C, Burger H, Green A, Hopper J, Ryan M. Menopausal symptoms in Australian women. Med J Aust. 1993;159:232–6.

71. Sievert LL, Anderson D, Melby MK, Obermeyer CM. Methods used in cross-cultural comparisons of somatic symptoms and their determinants. Maturitas. 2011;70:127–34.

72. Mair C, Diez Roux AV, Shen M, Shea S, Seeman T, Echeverria S, O'Meara ES. Cross-sectional and longitudinal associations of neighborhood cohesion and stressors with depressive symptoms in the multiethnic study of atherosclerosis (MESA). Ann Epidemiol. 2009;19(1):49–57.

Permissions

List of Contributors

Karen Oppermann
School of Medicine, Passo Fundo University, Passo Fundo, RS, Brazil
Hospital São Vicente de Paulo, Passo Fundo, RS, Brazil

Verônica Colpani and Poli Mara Spritzer
Gynecological Endocrinology Unit, Division of Endocrinology, Hospital de Clinicas de Porto Alegre, Porto Alegre, RS, Brazil

Sandra C. Fuchs
Department of Social Medicine, School of Medicine, Federal University of Rio Grande do Sul, Porto Alegre, RS, Brazil

Poli Mara Spritzer
Department of Physiology, Federal University of Rio Grande do Sul, Porto Alegre, RS, Brazil

Mags E. Beksinska and Jenni A. Smit
MatCH Research Unit [Maternal, Adolescent and Child Health Research Unit], Department of Obstetrics and Gynaecology, Faculty of Health Sciences, University of the Witwatersrand, 40 Dr AB Xuma Street,11th floor, Suite 1108-9,Commercial City, Durban 4001, South Africa

Immo Kleinschmidt
London School of Hygiene and Tropical Medicine, Keppel Street, London WC1E, England

Ayelet Ziv-Gal
School of Health Sciences, Massey University, Palmerston North, New Zealand

Rebecca L. Smith
Department of Pathobiology, University of Illinois, Urbana, Illinois, USA

Lisa Gallicchio
Epidemiology and Genomics Research Program, Division of Cancer Control and Population Sciences, National Cancer Institute, Bethesda, Maryland, USA

Susan R. Miller and Howard A. Zacur
Johns Hopkins University School of Medicine, Baltimore, Maryland, USA

Jodi A. Flaws
Department of Comparative Biosciences, University of Illinois, 2001 S. Lincoln Avenue, Urbana, Illinois 61802, USA

Ellen Sullivan Mitchell
Family and Child Nursing, University of Washington, Seattle, USA

Nancy Fugate Woods
Biobehavioral Nursing and Health Informatics, University of Washington, Seattle, USA

Elizabeth Hedgeman, Carrie A. Karvonen-Gutierrez and Siobán D. Harlow
Department of Epidemiology, School of Public Health, University of Michigan, 6610B SPH I, 1415 Washington Heights, Ann Arbor, MI 48109-2029, USA

Rebecca E. Hasson
School of Kinesiology, School of Public Health, University of Michigan, Ann Arbor, USA

William H. Herman
Department of Internal Medicine, School of Public Health, University of Michigan, Ann Arbor, USA

Susanna D. Mitro and Siobán D. Harlow
Department of Epidemiology, School of Public Health, 1415 Washington Heights, Ann Arbor, MI 48109, USA

John F. Randolph and Barbara D. Reed
School of Medicine, University of Michigan Ann Arbor, Ann Arbor, MI, USA

Claire Hardy, Eleanor Thorne and Myra S. Hunter
Department Psychology (at Guy's), Institute of Psychiatry, Psychology and Neuroscience, Kings College London, 5th Floor Bermondsey Wing, Guy's Campus, London SE1 9RT, UK

Amanda Griffiths
Division of Psychiatry & Applied Psychology, School of Medicine, University of Nottingham, Nottingham, UK

Gita D. Mishra, Hsin-Fang Chung and Yalamzewod Assefa Gelaw
School of Public Health, The University of Queensland, Herston Road, Herston, Brisbane, QLD 4006, Australia

Deborah Loxton
Research Centre for Generational Health and Ageing, The University of Newcastle, Callaghan, NSW, Australia

Zarah Batulan, Nadia Maarouf and Vipul Shrivastava
Department of Cardiac Sciences, Libin Cardiovascular Institute of Alberta, University of Calgary, Health Research Innovation Centre, GB42, 3280 Hospital Dr NW, Calgary, AB T2N 4Z6, Canada

Edward O'Brien
Department of Cardiac Sciences, Libin Cardiovascular Institute of Alberta, Health Research Innovation Centre, Room GAA16, 3280 Hospital Drive NW, Calgary, AB T2N 4Z6, Canada

Versie Johnson-Mallard
Department of Family, Community, and Health System Science, Robert Wood Johnson Nurse Faculty Scholar Alum, University of Florida, College of Nursing, Gainesville, FL, USA

Elizabeth A. Kostas-Polston
Daniel K. Inouye Graduate School of Nursing, Uniformed Services University of the Health Sciences, Bethesda, MD, USA

Nancy Fugate Woods
Biobehavioral Nursing and Health Informatics, Interim Associate Dean for Diversity, Equity, and Inclusion, University of Washington School of Nursing, Seattle, WA, USA

Katherine E. Simmonds
MGH Institute of Health Professions, Boston, MA, USA

Ivy M. Alexander
Director of Advance Practice Programs, Storrs, CT, USA

Diana Taylor
UCSF School of Nursing, Research Faculty, Advancing New Standards in Reproductive HealthProgram (ANSIRH), UCSF Bixby Center for Global Reproductive Health, University of California, San Francisco, CA, USA

Ellen W. Freeman
Department of Obstetrics/Gynecology and Department of Psychiatry, 3701 Market Street, Suite 820 (Mudd Suite), Philadelphia, PA 19104, USA

Mary D. Sammel
Center for Clinical Epidemiology and Biostatistics, Perelman School of Medicine, University of Pennsylvania, U.S, Philadelphia, USA

Lynnette Leidy Sievert
Department of Anthropology, Machmer Hall, 240 Hicks Way, UMass Amherst, Amherst, MA 01003-9278, USA

Laura Huicochea-Gómez and Diana Cahuich-Campos
Departamento de Sociedad y Cultura, El Colegio de la Frontera, ECOSUR, Campeche, México

Dana-Lynn Ko'omoa-Lange
Department of Pharmaceutical Science, University of Hawai'i at Hilo, Hilo, HI, USA

Daniel E. Brown
Department of Anthropology, University of Hawai'i at Hilo, Hilo, HI, USA

Catherine Kim
Departments of Medicine and Obstetrics & Gynecology, University of Michigan, 2800 Plymouth Road, Building 16, Room 430W, Ann Arbor, MI 48109, USA

Siobàn D. Harlow, Huiyong Zheng and Daniel S. McConnell
Department of Epidemiology, University of Michigan, Ann Arbor, MI, USA

John F. Randolph Jr
Department of Obstetrics & Gynecology, University of Michigan, Ann Arbor, MI, USA

Nancy Fugate Woods
Department of Biobehavioral Nursing, University of Washington, Seattle, WA 98195, USA

Ellen Sullivan Mitchell
Department of Family and Child Nursing, University of Washington, Seattle, WA98195 USA

Maria E. Bleil
Department of Family and Child Nursing, University of Washington, Seattle, WA 98195, USA

Paul English and Jhaqueline Valle
California Department of Public Health, California Environmental Health Tracking Program, Richmond, CA 94804, USA

Nancy F. Woods
Department of Biobehavioral Nursing and Health Informatics, University of Washington, Seattle, WA 98195, USA

Kyle D. Crowder
Department of Sociology, University of Washington, Seattle, WA 98195, USA

Steven E. Gregorich
Department of Medicine, University of California San Francisco, San Francisco, CA 94143, USA

Marcelle I. Cedars
Department of Obstetrics, Gynecology, & Reproductive Sciences, University of California San Francisco, San Francisco, CA 94143, USA

Catherine Kim
Departments of Medicine, Obstetrics & Gynecology, and Epidemiology, University of Michigan, 2800 Plymouth Road, Building 16, Room 430W, Ann Arbor, MI 48109-2800, USA

Yuanyuan Pan and Barbara H. Braffett
The Biostatistics Center, George Washington University, Rockville, MD, USA

Valerie L. Arends and Michael W. Steffes
Department of Laboratory Medicine and Pathology, University of Minnesota, Minneapolis, MN, USA

Hunter Wessells
Department of Urology, University of Washington, Seattle, WA, USA

Aruna V. Sarma
Department of Urology, University of Michigan, Ann Arbor, MI, USA

Annette Joan Thomas
College of Nursing, Seattle University, Seattle, Washington, USA

Ellen Sullivan Mitchell
Family and Child Nursing, University of Washington, Seattle, Washington, USA

Nancy Fugate Woods
Biobehavioral Nursing and Health Informatics, University of Washington, Seattle, Wahsington, USA

Annette Joan Thomas
College of Nursing, Seattle University, Seattle, USA

Ellen Sullivan Mitchell
Family and Child Nursing, University of Washington, Seattle, USA

Nancy Fugate Woods
Biobehavioral Nursing and Health Informatics, University of Washington, Seattle, USA

Linda M. Gerber
Department of Healthcare Policy & Research, Division of Biostatistics and Epidemiology, Weill Cornell Medical College, 402 E. 67th St., LA-231, New York, NY 10065, USA
Department of Medicine, Division of Nephrology and Hypertension, Weill Cornell Medical College, New York City, NY, USA

Lynnette Leidy Sievert
Department of Anthropology, UMass Amherst, Amherst, MA, USA

Index

www.ingramcontent.com/pod-product-compliance
Lightning Source LLC
Chambersburg PA
CBHW082035190326
41458CB00010B/3376